Fitness and Health ProMOTION

Author/Editor
Tom R. Thomas

Chapter Contributors
Debra A. Bemben
Richard A. Fee
Steve D. Houseworth
Jerry L. Mayhew
Parris R. Watts
Carole J. Zebas

eddie bowers publishing inc.
2600 Jackson Street
Dubuque, IA 52001

eddie bowers publishing, inc.
2600 Jackson Street
Dubuque, Iowa 52001

ISBN 0-945483-26-0

Printed in the United States of America.

9 8 7 6 5 4 3 2 1

PREFACE

Interest in physical fitness and personal health has exploded into pursuit of **total health and wellness**. This book is an attempt to bring topics of fitness and wellness together for those people seeking to maximize the benefits of a healthy life-style. The text is divided into five parts. In the initial chapters, the discussion focuses on life-styles, associated diseases, and changing behaviors. In the second part, the emphasis is on exercise and physical activities which can be incorporated into an active life-style. The third section contains special topics related to wellness pursuits, including weight control and female health. The fourth section relates to the psychological aspects of wellness, and in the final section, sports injuries and wellness evaluation/inventories are the key topics.

This text represents the work of a host of individuals. The chapter authors were selected because of their expertise in a specific area of fitness and health promotion. They are all excellent professionals, and I have thoroughly enjoyed this association. The reviewers were very helpful in refining the product and their efforts are appreciated. In addition, special thanks go to Eddie Bowers for his creativity and perseverance, Carla Pfab for her dedication to the project, Jane Williams for her help on the manuscript, and Carole Zebas for taking many of the photographs and for being a good sounding board for the text ideas. Universal Gym Equipment, Inc., provided many of the photographs, including those used on the back cover, and their assistance and professional courtesy are greatly appreciated.

Tom R. Thomas

CONTENTS

Chapter 1
Fitness and Wellness Concepts 2
(Parris Watts)
Learning Objectives 2
Important Terms 2
Introdution 3
What is Wellness 3
Dimensions of Health and the Total Person 4
Determinants of Health 5
Assumption of Responsibility for Personal Health 6
Meaning and Application of the Human Wholeness Concept 7
How to Achieve Wellness 7
Wellness - a Passing Fancy 10
Brief History of the Wellness Movement 10
Wellness for the Future 11
Wellness Research and Its Implications 12
Suggested Readings 15

Chapter 2
The Life-Style Diseases 16
(Judith Hurley, Richard Schlaadt)
Learning Objectives 16
Important Terms 16
Introduction 17
Cardiovascular Disease 17
- Smoking 18
- Cholesterol 19
- Exercise 19

Cancer 21
- Tobacco 21
- Diet and Exercise 22
- Sun Worshiping 22

Cerebrovascular Disease 22
- Hypertension 23

Osteoporosis 24
Overweight 26
Stress 26
Injuries 26
Choice is Yours 27
Suggested Readings 27

Chapter 3
Changing Personal Life-Style Behaviors 28
(Parris Watts)
Learning Objectives 28
Important Terms 28
Introduction 29
Barriers to Changing Life-Style Behaviors 30
Precursors to Health Behavior Change 31
Health Behavior Change: Models and Theory 33
Health Behavior Change: Goals and Objectives 35
Health Behavior Change: Strategies 37
- Stimulating Motivation 37
- Formulating Objectives 38
- Implementing an Action Plan 38
- Keeping Records 40
- Maintaining New Health Behaviors 41
- Assessing Personal Wellness 41
- Formulating a Personal Wellness Life-Style Plan 41

Maintenance of Health Behavior Change 42
Suggested Readings 45

Chapter 4
Specificity of Exercise Training 46
(Tom Thomas)
Learning Objectives 46
Important Terms 46
Specificity of Exercise Training 47
- Anaerobics 47
- Aerobics 49
- Carbohydrate and Fat as Energy Sources 49

Physiological Effects of Exercise 52
Exercise and Cardiovascular Fitness 56
Cardiovascular Detraining 57
Suggested Readings 59

Chapter 5
Starting and Maintaining Activity 60
(Tom Thomas)
Learning Objectives 60
Important Terms 60
Introduction 61
Principles of Comfortable Exercise 61
    Getting Started 61
    Timing 62
    Clothing 62
    Warm-Up 62
    Cool-Down 62
    Breathing 63
Determining Exercise Intensity 63
    Target Heart Rate 63
    Metabolic Equivalents 64
    Rating of Perceived Exertion (RPE) 65
    Talk Test 66
    Lactate Threshold 66
Determining Exercise Duration 66
Staying Power 67
Potentially Dangerous Activities 67
    Hot Weather Exercise 67
    Cold Weather Exercise 69
    Problem Practices 70
Suggested Readings 71

Chapter 6
Exercises for Fitness and Health 72
(Tom Thomas)
Learning Objectives 72
Important Terms 72
General Considerations 73
Jogging/Running 73
Aerobic Dance 74
    Precautions and Benefits 74
    Selecting Classes 75
    Low Impact 76
Walking 77
Stair Climbing/Stepping 78
Cross-Country Skiing 79
Rebounding 80
Cycling 80
Rowing 82
Swimming 83
Circuit Resistance Training 84
Healthy Activities 85
Suggested Readings 87

Chapter 7
Flexibility and Stretching 88
(Carole Zebas)
Learning Objectives 88
Important Terms 88
Introduction 89
Defining the Terminology 89
Benefits of Flexibility Training 90
Physiological and Biomechanical Changes 90
    Physiology of Muscle Temperature Elevation 90
    Biomechanics of Muscle Elasticity 91
Types of Stretching Exercises 91
    Ballistic Stretching Exercises 91
    Static Stretching Exercises 92
    Passive Stretching Exercises 93
    Proprioceptive Neuromuscular Facilitation Exercises 93
When to Stretch 95
Designing A Flexibility Program 95
Sample Stretching Exercises 96
Suggested Readings 103

Chapter 8
Muscular Fitness 104
(Tom Thomas)
Learning Objectives 104
Important Terms 104
Introduction 105
Types of Muscular Contraction 105
Methods of Providing Resistance 107
    Static Resistance 107
    Isotonic Resistance 108
    Variable Resistance 109
    Isokinetic Resistance 111
    Body Weight Resistance Exercises 112
Resistance Training Programs 112
    Workout Terms 112
    Strength Training 113
    Muscular Endurance 117
    Muscular Balance 117
    Muscular Tone 118
    Cardiovascular Fitness 119
Suggested Readings 123

Chapter 9
Weight Management Strategies 124
(Jerry Mayhew)
Learning Objectives 124
Important Terms 124
Body Composition 125
- Reference Standards 126
- Measurement Techniques 127

Nutrients Related to Exercise 130
- Carbohydrates 131
- Fats 132
- Proteins 134
- Vitamins 135
- Minerals 137
- Water 137

Dieting to Change Body Composition 138
- Losing Weight 138
- Body Composition Changes with Dieting 139

Exercise in Weight Management 142
- Aerobic versus Anaerobic 143
- Using Fat Stores 143

Combination Programs for Controlling Weight 143
Suggested Readings 145

Chapter 10
Female Health and Fitness 146
(Debra Bemben)
Learning Objectives 146
Important Terms 146
Introduction 147
Training Responses 147
- Weight Training 147
- Endurance Training 148

Exercise and the Menstrual Cycle 148
- Effects on Exercise Performance 148
- Effects on Reproductive Function 149
- Oral Contraceptive Use 150

Pregnancy 150
- Maternal Responses 151
- Outcomes 151
- Fetal Responses 151
- Recommendations 152

Menopause 153
- Cardiovascular Function 153
- Osteoporosis 153

Nutrition and the Exercising Female 155
- Iron Deficiency 155
- Calcium Intake 156
- Eating Disorders 157

Summary 158
Suggested Readings 159

Chapter 11
Stress Management 160
(Richard Fee)
Learning Objectives 160
Important Terms 160
Introduction 161
- Body's Response 161
- Immune System 163
- Cardiovascular System 165
- Gastrointestinal System 166
- Muscles 167
- Epidermal System 167

Sources of Stress 168
- Psychological 168
- Social 171
- Environmental 172

Techniques for Reducing Stress 174
- Relaxation 174
- Cognitive Methods 177
- Journaling 179
- Humor 180
- Exercise 180
- Music 182

Summary 182
Suggested Readings 183

Chapter 12
Exercise Motivation and Adherence 184
(Steve Houseworth)
Learning Objectives 184
Important Terms 184
Importance of Motivation to Exercise 185
- Nature of Motivation 185
- Relationship of Exercise Motivation to Exercise/Health Behavior 185

Why People Initiate Exercise 186
- Functional Reasons 186
- Role of Expectancy 187

Maintaining Exercise Programs 187
- Expectancies versus Outcomes 187
- Barriers to Maintaining Exercise Programs 188

Exercise Addiction 191
- Causes 191
- Working with Exercise Addiction 194

Suggested Readings 195

Chapter 13
Preventing Fitness-Related Injuries 196 (Carole Zebas)
Learning Objectives 196
Important Terms 196
Introduction 197
Acute vs. Overuse Injuries 197
- Acute Injuries 197
- Overuse Injuries 199

Mechanisms of Injury 202
Common Fitness Related Injuries 204
- Knee Pain 204
- Achilles Tendinitis 204
- Iliotibial Band Syndrome 205
- Low Back Pain 206
- Plantar Fasciitis 206
- Shin Splints 206

Miscellaneous Fitness Related Injuries 207
- Blisters 207
- Muscle Cramps 207
- Muscle Soreness 207
- Stitch-in-the-Side 208
- Nerve Related Injuries 208

Heat Related Injuries 208
- Heat Exhaustion 210
- Heat Stroke 210

Cold Related Injuries 210
- Hypothermia 211
- Frostbite 211

Prevention of Musculoskeletal Injuries 212
Suggested Readings 213

Chapter 14
Inventories for Fitness and Health Promotion 214
1) Hamstring Flexibility 215
2) Iliopsoas Flexibility 217
3) Adductor Flexibility 219
4) Shoulder Flexibility 221
5) Shoulder and Upper Arm Flexibility 223
6) Upperback Flexibility 225
7) Abdominal Flexibility 227
8) Sit & Reach 229
9) Posture Assessment 231
10) Health Risk Appraisal 233
11) Stress Inventory 237
12) Nutrition Survey 239
13) Exercise Survey 241
14) Relaxation Survey 243
15) Stress Symptom Checklist 245
16) Guidelines for Effective Stress Management 247
17) Type A/B Behavior Evaluation 249
18) Hostility Evaluation 251
19) Body Fat Assessment 253
20) Waist/Hip Ratio (WHR) 257
21) Ideal Body Weight 259
22) Caloric Balance 261
23) Diet Analysis Software 265
24) One Mile Walk Test 267
25) Adult Fit N Dex 269
26) Personal Wellness Life-Style Plan 271
27) Strength Assessment 273
28) Exercise Log 277
29) Resistance Training Workout Records 279
30) Fat, Fiber, and Sodium Log 281

Appendix A
Approximate Caloric Expenditure per Minute for Various Physical Activities 282

Appendix B
Nutritive Value of Foods (USDA) **288**

Glossary 353

Index 363

Fitness
and
Health
Pro*MOTION*

CHAPTER

1

FITNESS AND WELLNESS CONCEPTS

Parris Watts

Learning Objectives

- Understand wellness as it relates to the concept of "health for human wholeness."
- Understand the four primary determinants of health/wellness and how they impact the six dimensions of the whole human being.
- Understand wellness as not just another passing fancy but as a movement that is here to stay.
- Discuss the three major steps on the pathway to human wholeness and realize that they are extremely important in achieving the highest attainable level of wellness.
- Understand the important wellness research studies which have been conducted to date that have definite implications for the future of wellness.

Important Terms

determinents of health
dimensions of health
dimensions of physical fitness
healthful living
human wholeness
life-style diseases
personal health responsibility (PHR)
self-image
wellness
wellness life-style behaviors

INTRODUCTION

Several years ago in the introductory health education course a student from Egypt shared an ancient proverb from his country. The proverb stated that "health is a crown on a rich person's head, taken for granted until he or she becomes a pauper." Embodied within these words of great wisdom are the concepts of fitness and wellness upon which this book is based and to which this chapter is devoted.

Four Dimensions of Physical Fitness

1. cardiorespiratory endurance (aerobic capacity)
2. muscular strength and endurance
3. flexibility
4. body composition

All of the **dimensions of physical fitness** are discussed in detail in the following chapters of this book. Many questions and even some controversies abound with regard to physical fitness issues. Because the majority of the additional chapters in this book, written by exercise science experts, will discuss fitness principles in considerable depth, the emphasis of this chapter will be placed on the concept of "overall wellness" (Inventory #10 on page 233).

In no way does this approach demean the value of physical fitness which is an extremely important contributor to wellness. It is evident that physical fitness is an invaluable precursor to the attainment of personal wellness and to the establishment and/or maintenance of a wellness lifestyle. The reader should keep these facts in mind while perusing this chapter.

Overall Wellness
↑
↓
Physical Fitness

WHAT IS WELLNESS

Wellness is a quality of life involving the dynamic interaction, interdependency, and intersupportiveness of the physical, intellectual, emotional, social, spiritual, and vocational dimensions of the whole human being. Based on this definition of wellness a conceptual model has been developed. See Figure 1.1 for an illustration of that definitional prototype, known as the Health for Human Wholeness Model.

An interpretation of the meaning and applicability of the Health for Human Wholeness Model should first be concerned with the six interlocking circles within the illustration. There is no significance attached to their relative positions, but it is important

Health for Human Wholeness Model

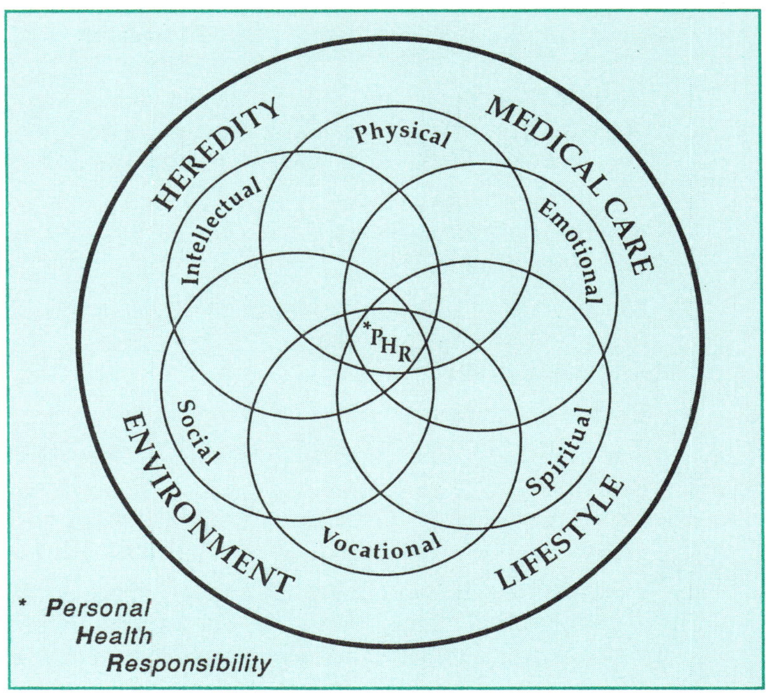

Figure 1.1. A conceptual model of total wellness.

Optimum Health

to note that the circles are equal in size. This is intended to depict the need for the whole individual to emphasize the establishment and/or maintenance of all aspects of his/her total being as equally as possible. Certainly the advantages of promoting a balanced approach to establishing and maintaining an optimum health state of the body, mind, and spirit are obvious. There is much more to wellness than just learning about how to live healthfully, eating nutritionally, becoming aware of managing stress, developing a positive **self-image**, or for that matter, being physically fit.

What is Wellness

In spite of the inherent value in each of the wellness life-style behaviors delineated above, none of them by itself constitutes wellness. The same is true of the physical, intellectual, emotional and other dimensions of health. Positive life-style behaviors contribute to wellness and the dimensions of health impact it. Nevertheless, the attainment of wellness is greater than the sum of its "contributors" or "impactors." Health for Human Wholeness, the ultimate form of overall wellness, is the product of the synergistic action of all factors which combine to create a means through which optimum wellness can be achieved.

DIMENSIONS OF HEALTH AND THE TOTAL PERSON

For clarification purposes, the following descriptions of the six **dimensions of health** are offered. Although the reader could undoubtedly describe each, descriptions have been included to assist in forming a consistent frame of reference. The following delineation is provided with that goal in mind.

Six Dimensions of Health

1. **Physical**—Related to levels of conditioning within the cardiovascular, respiratory, muscular, and other body systems. Generally considered in terms of physical fitness but also involves nutritional and numerous disease prevention elements.
2. **Intellectual**—Associated with the mind's ability to comprehend the nature of one's self and his/her environment, to make decisions, and to solve problems. Often thought of as intellectual capacity.
3. **Emotional**—Pertaining to feelings of love and worth which render the individual better able to cope with the stresses and strains of daily life. Customarily viewed in the context of emotional stability.
4. **Social**—Concerned with the ability to relate to people of all ages and walks of life in a meaningful and acceptable manner. Frequently referred to as social balance.
5. **Spiritual**—Linked to the presence of a spirit within humankind and an awareness of a higher purpose in life with aspirations toward it for oneself and for society. Commonly regarded in the realm of spiritual "attunement."
6. **Vocational**—Emphasizing the rather recently acknowledged importance of the workplace in relationship to the felt value, personal satisfaction, and overall wellness of employees. Most likely to be perceived as vocational fulfillment.

Another important feature portrayed within the Health for Human Wholeness Model is the relationship between the six components of the total person. The overlapping, interlocking arrangement of the circles is representative of the interdependency and intersupportiveness of the respective aspects of the whole individual. The relationship of the various components is dependent upon the continued growth and development of each. Likewise, the support necessary for each of the components to grow and develop, and in the process become dimensions of personal health, has its source in the close relationship that exists among those components.

Interlocking Components

DETERMINANTS OF HEALTH

The model also includes what appropriately could be called **determinants of health**. Heredity, medical care, environment, and life-style all can potentially impact the wellness status of an individual. Furthermore, the determinants of health can have either positive or negative influences on each dimension of the whole person. Those effects can be felt either directly or indirectly, because of the already discussed interaction, interdependency, and intersupportiveness which exists among these dimensions. The reader should visualize the Health for Human Wholeness Model in 3-D to encourage simultaneous conceptualization of all four of the health determinants having an impact on all six dimensions of health.

What Determines Health

Health Interactions and Impact

Heredity
Medical Care
Environment
Life-Style

Physical
Intellectual
Emotional
Vocational
Spiritual
Social

PHR*
Impact

* Personal Health Responsibility

The influences of the health determinants on each of the dimensions of health has significance. For example, it is impossible to isolate the effects of hereditary factors or medical care services in terms of the physical dimension alone. Moreover, it is not possible to separate the emotional response to a given environmental stressor from what will be evoked physically, intellectually, socially, spiritually, or vocationally as the whole person responds to that stressor.

The Positives and Negatives

Yet perhaps the most important point to be made regarding the determinants of health is their relative impact on the wellness state of any individual, currently or in the future. As improbable as it may seem, the effects of heredity, medical care, and environment combined do not have as much of an impact on the wellness state of Americans as does life-style

Personal Control

alone. That fact has both a positive and a negative side. On the down side are powerful effects of smoking, high fat, high calorie and high sodium consumption, sedentary living habits, maladaptive stress responses, and other abusive behaviors. Conversely, there is a tremendous potential for an improved state of wellness as a result of positive health related decisions and behaviors. Because of the internal focus of control inherent within the life-style determinant of health, the exciting message which needs to be delivered to human beings everywhere is that they have personal control over their own wellness destiny. If they make informed choices and follow healthful living principles, individuals can make a quantum leap toward the highest attainable level of wellness. Later in this chapter practical and realistic steps which can be taken on the pathway leading to health for human wholeness will be presented.

ASSUMPTION OF RESPONSIBILITY FOR PERSONAL HEALTH

PHR

Within the core of the Health for Human Wholeness Model are found the letters **PHR**, which stand for **Personal Health Responsibility.** The necessity to accept responsibility for one's personal health is possibly the most notable feature of the model. The position of PHR in the middle of the prototype, where all six dimensions of the whole being overlap, symbolizes the need for the individual to assume responsibility for his/her health in each aspect of their total personhood.

Personal Health Responsibility (PHR)

1. **Physically**—individuals cannot attain/maintain overall wellness unless they exercise regularly, eat wisely, get adequate amounts of sleep, avoid abusive behaviors, etc.
2. **Intellectually**—they must continue to learn and expand their mental horizons.
3. **Emotionally**—the development of a positive self-image is a precursor to health for human wholeness.
4. **Socially**—experiences which are satisfying and meet the human need for interpersonal relationships are necessary for optimum wellness.
5. **Spiritually**—failure to acknowledge the spiritual dimension of life and the inability to find a meaningful way to fill the void created if it is left unaddressed, may cause humans to settle for less than the highest achievable level of personal wholeness.
6. **Vocationally**—choices and health related decisions made daily in the workplace can have an incredible impact on one's health status, both in the present and in the future.

Assumption of personal health responsibility challenges the individual to acquire new health knowledge, to carefully evaluate current health related attitudes and to perhaps modify certain health practices and behaviors. Acceptance of the challenge to assume such responsibility for one's health brings to mind the words of an eighteenth century English philosopher, Charles Dubois. Dubois once stated that "the most important thing in life is to be able, at any moment, to sacrifice what we are for what we should become." Within the context of this discussion, it seems appropriate to amplify that statement even further. Perhaps it could be said that the most precious of all the principles of wellness is to be able and willing, at any given point in one's life, to sacrifice what we want and believe, for what we could and should become. Therein lies the true acid test and the real bottom line on the contract for a healthier life.

Accept the Challenge

MEANING AND APPLICATION OF THE HUMAN WHOLENESS CONCEPT

In approaching the conclusion of the interpretation of the Health for Human Wholeness Model, the term **human wholeness** still needs to be defined. Human wholeness is simply a matter of becoming the best a person can become physically, intellectually, emotionally, socially, spiritually, and vocationally, in light of and in spite of their limitations. Human wholeness is not a product, but instead it is a process. As a process, it is a dynamic outgrowth of what an individual thinks, feels, and does with respect to all six dimensions of their total self and their health. Human wholeness offers both an invitation and a challenge to be the best that one can be, in place of concentrating on the attainment of a "perfection level" which never can be reached. The reference in the definition to "limitations" is intended to raise the reader's consciousness regarding the need to honestly identify and accept those limitations, and more importantly, to compensate for them in positive ways.

Dynamic Process

Because of the emphasis on "building" from where a person currently is, the human wholeness idea has unlimited applicability. For example, a paraplegic, a person recovering from an emotional illness, or individuals perceiving themselves as having little spiritual depth, all have as much of an opportunity to become whole human beings as would seemingly "well together" people. Therein lies one of the most appealing qualities of the Health for Human Wholeness Model. Within its parameters is found the potential to create hope in the mind of any person who will take the time and expend the energy to consider what the concept has to offer.

Create Hope

HOW TO ACHIEVE WELLNESS

As indicated earlier in this chapter, a series of steps can be taken by an individual which will ultimately lead them to the highest achievable level of wellness.

Practical and Realistic Steps on the Pathway to Human Wholeness

1. Wellness oriented people must want to be healthy.
2. Individuals striving for overall wellness must believe they can be healthy.
3. Persons committed to living the wellness life-style must be able and willing to make behavioral choices, changes, and even sacrifices necessary to be healthy.

Following is a list of the most important **wellness life-style behaviors** which can be adopted. The list is based on research studies which have been conducted throughout the world. These studies have identified a close relationship between the listed behaviors and the health status of the research subjects involved.

Wellness Life-Style Behaviors

1. Do not smoke or use smokeless tobacco.
2. Do not misuse or abuse alcohol and other drugs (including caffeine and over-the-counter drugs).
3. Exercise (aerobically) a minimum of three times per week.
4. Eat at least three times every day (including breakfast) and know your food (Figure 1.2).
   a. Eat a variety of foods.
   b. Maintain a healthy body fat percentage.
   c. Choose a diet low in fat, saturated fat and cholesterol.
   d. Choose a diet with plenty of vegetables, fruits and grain products.
   e. Use sugars only in moderation.
   f. Use salt and sodium only in moderation.
5. Sleep seven to eight hours in each 24 hour period.
6. Always wear seatbelts.
7. Learn and apply effective stress awareness and stress management skills (Figure 1.3).

The steps on the pathway to human wholeness as shown on page 8 are essentially common sense principles for **healthful living**. Their practicality makes them both appealing and effective. Yet the most important point related to these steps is that those who stay on the path, realistically can reach their destination. They do not have to run a marathon on their hands, climb Mount Everest without any equipment, or swim the English Channel with arms tied behind their backs to traverse the pathway to human

Grocery Store Tour with a Nutritionist

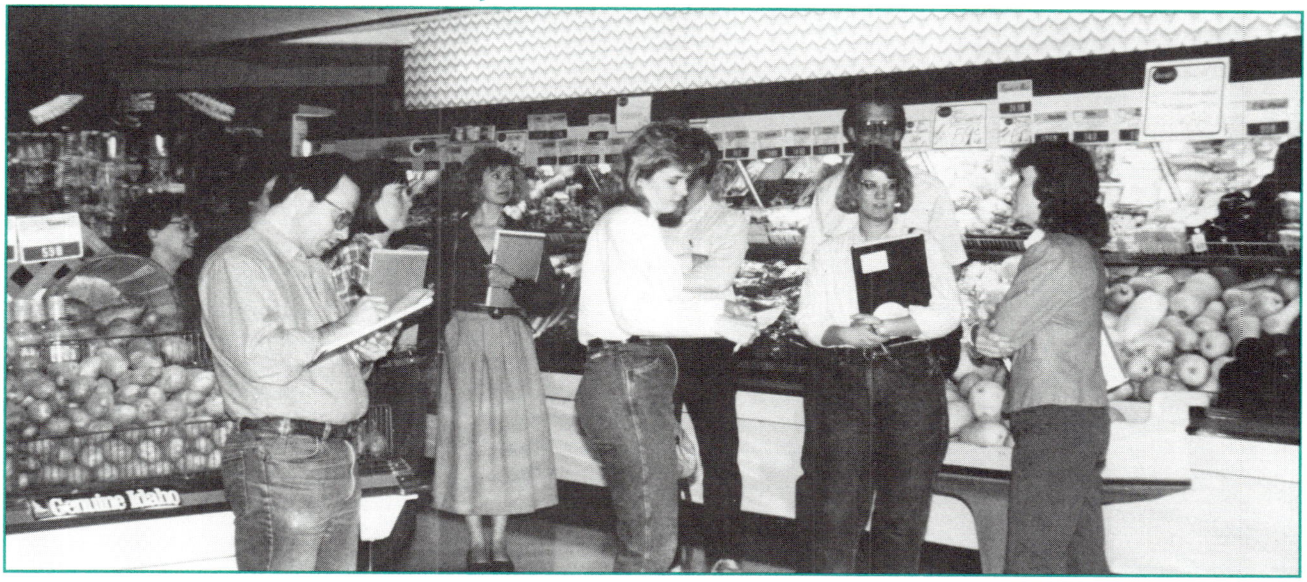

Figure 1.2. This education experience focusing on proper food selections can be an important step in changing diet.

wholeness. Ordinary people who want to be healthy, who believe they can be healthy, and who are willing to make some important life-style choices, changes, or even a few sacrifices, can walk in the footsteps of countless others who have already demonstrated that the ultimate level of wellness can be reached.

Path to Wellness

Not long ago a person who was obviously skeptical of "this wellness business" as he termed it, asked about the type of people who come to wellness life-style seminars. A response could be that most frequently the individuals who attend are the smart ones! The same is true of the persons who follow the steps on the pathway to human wholeness.

Relaxation Seminar

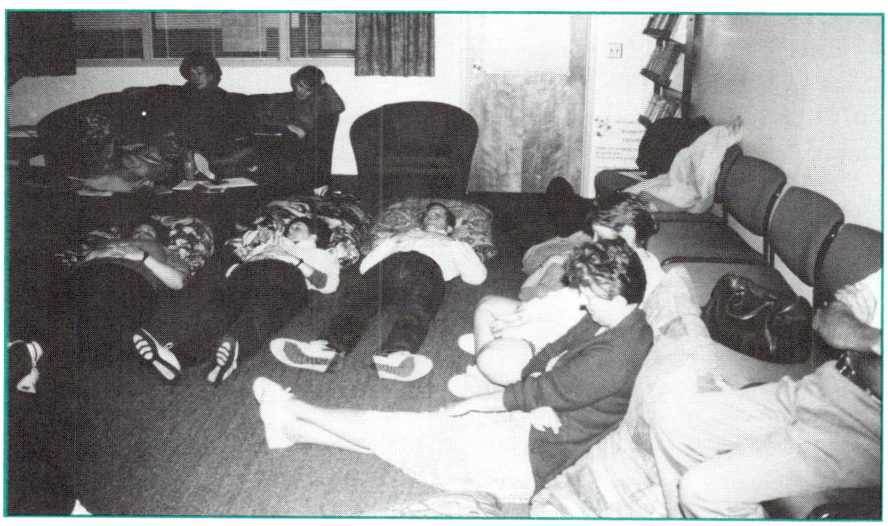

Figure 1.3. Relaxation skills can counter the effects of daily stress.

WELLNESS - A PASSING FANCY

Here to Stay

There are certain professionals in the various health related fields who would argue vehemently that wellness does not possess the necessary qualities to be sustained over time. It has already been clearly established in this chapter that wellness is much more than "the absence of disease or infirmity." As stated previously in its definition, wellness is a quality of life. Like a beautiful masterpiece of art, quality of life is difficult to describe. Nevertheless, people recognize real art when they see it and know true quality of life when they experience it. All over the United States and throughout other parts of the world, individuals who have adopted a wellness life-style are enjoying a higher quality of life than they have ever known before. Some will continue to consider wellness as a passing fancy, expecting it to fade away with time. Others are convinced that wellness is a movement which is here to stay.

BRIEF HISTORY OF THE WELLNESS MOVEMENT

Historical Foundation

An appreciation of the contemporary wellness movement is further enriched by acknowledging the historical foundation upon which it has been built. The beginning of the wellness movement can be traced to Halbert Dunn, a retired public health service physician. Dr. Dunn began lecturing about practical and timely health issues during the 1950's in the Washington, D.C. area. Within that same decade he wrote articles discussing what he chose to call "high level wellness." In 1961, a series of 29 of his lectures were published in a book with that title. Dunn's lectures and writings emphasized what he believed to be a very close relationship between the body, mind and spirit. He stressed that humans have a need for personal fulfillment and valued purposes. Dunn also believed that health should be extended beyond the traditional medical model where non-illness was the final goal to be attained.

Body Mind and Spirit

From the mid 1970's to the present, the wellness movement has advanced by leaps and bounds. Carefully nutured by such individuals as John Travis, Donald Ardell, and William Hettler, wellness has sprouted from the seeds planted by Halbert Dunn and has grown to become a thriving plant which is just beginning to blossom. John Travis was the first physician in the United States to provide wellness services and educational experiences to other health professions. He eventually extended his outreach efforts to the general public. Donald Ardell was a Travis contemporary and with his 1977 book, *High Level Wellness: An Alternative to Doctors, Drugs, and Disease*, he became a highly sought after seminar presenter, workshop facilitator and corporate consultant. William Hettler, another physician who is the director of the Student Health Service at the University of Wisconsin at Stevens Point, was the first person to establish a comprehensive wellness program in a university setting. Hettler's efforts culminated in the development of the initial student led wellness model which has been replicated in various forms in hundreds of colleges and universities throughout North America.

More recently, health professionals like Neil Schmottlach and David Gobble at Ball State University and James Rogers, George Oberle and Mac McCrary at Oklahoma State University have created other outstanding university based wellness programs for faculty, staff and students. Unique to Ball State and Oklahoma State is the delivery of wellness programming as a part of a graduate degree curriculum which prepares students for a wide variety of positions in the wellness field. Oklahoma State University also has what is perhaps the most innovative and technologically advanced wellness facility currently operational in the United States.

Wellness Explosion

Throughout the decade of the 1980's, an explosion of wellness program development in business and industry occurred. Although the primary motivation to establish such programs was to contain rapidly escalating corporate medical care costs, there were also other motives. Reduction of employee absenteeism and turnover, enhancement of the companies' public image and improvement in worker productivity and morale were all reasons for corporations to jump onto the wellness bandwagon. Among the most noteworthy corporations currently involved in promoting wellness for their employees known to this author are AT & T, Coors, General Foods, IBM, Johnson and Johnson, Kimberly Clark, Metropolitan Life, Moog Automotive, Pepisco, PET, Sentry Insurance, Tenneco, and Xerox.

WELLNESS FOR THE FUTURE

There is certainly no question in the mind of enlightened health professionals that the wellness movement is here to stay. It is far more than just another fad or passing fancy. There are simply too many reasons justifying the need for and extolling the virtues of wellness programs for them to slip into oblivion. Donald Ardell in his book, *The History and Future of Wellness* listed the following four factors as those which will cause wellness to continue to be a prominent concept during the remainder of the 1990's and beyond.

Factors Promoting the Wellness Concept

1. **High medical care costs.** Throughout the decade of the 80's expenditures for medical care increased astronomically while inflation in other segments of the economy was effectively being contained. Such a pattern continues to place additional pressure on an already ailing economy, and personal wellness efforts offer one of the few palatable ways to reverse that trend.
2. **Dissatisfaction with the current status of the medical care system.** It is not news to anyone that the American public is displeased with the quality of medical care received for what it costs. Many persons are asking and even demanding that this situation be improved. Adoption of wellness lifestyles by more people could help ease the strain on the currently overworked system. As members of the baby boom era continue to age, the necessity for greater emphasis and assumption of personal health responsibility will be further amplified.
3. **Expanded public awareness and interest in self-care and wellness.** This has been observed by in an ever increasing form. Wellness seminars conducted throughout the nation have been well attended and interest in personal health expressed by participants has been exceptional.
4. **The leadership assumed by business, industry, and hospitals.** This has been somewhat of a surprise, albeit a pleasant one. However, a concern about the effects that economic downturns will have on wellness programs in these settings have surfaced recently. Hopefully not all decisions related to such programming will be tied only to the bottom line.

WELLNESS RESEARCH AND ITS IMPLICATIONS

Life-Style Diseases

Since the turn of the 20th century, a number of major improvements in the health of Americans have occurred. The most evident improvements include more hygienic environmental health practices, the development of vaccines and antibiotics, and the discovery of the relationship between better nutrition and disease reduction. Many of these and other health advances in the United States, which are often simply taken for granted, were the results of research studies. Wellness, as the next important health related revolution which is perhaps already in progess, will require research findings to guide its future development.

It is common knowledge that the major health problems in contemporary America are clearly the result of the way its people live. Frequently referred to as **life-style diseases**, at least eight of the ten leading causes of death in the United States today are generally preventable. In fact the first five accounted for more than three fourths of all deaths in America during the past year. Information available from the National Center for Health Statistics verifies that those "fatal five"—heart diseases, cancer, cerebrovascular diseases, accidents, and chronic obstructive lung diseases—combine to create a monumental challenge to the citizens of the nation and the health professionals who serve them.

Are You the Prey

Within recent decades the shifting patterns of death and disease from acute, infectious conditions to chronic diseases have been duly noted. Research indicates that rather than being victims of devastating communicable diseases like former generations, today's Americans have fallen prey to sedentary work, spectator sports, high fat, high sugar, high sodium and low fiber diets, stress, smoking and the misuse and abuse of alcohol and other drugs. Numerous research studies have demonstrated that if behaviors associated with physical activity, diet and nutrition, stress management and seat belt usage were improved and if health impairing habits such as smoking and alcohol/drug misuse and abuse were eliminated, many pressing health problems could be reduced substantially. Surprisingly, some very small life-style changes can have a huge impact on health (Figure 1.3).

Beginning in the mid 1960's and particularly during the 1970's and 1980's there has been an escalation in the number of wellness related research studies conducted. As a result, more and better wellness data is now available.

Better Information

In 1964 the Surgeon General's Advisory Committee on Smoking and Health concluded in its now famous report, that "cigarette smoking is a health hazard of sufficient importance in the United States to warrant remedial action." Twenty years and more than 30,000 research studies later, the 1984 Surgeon General's report entitled *The Health Consequences of Smoking* concluded that "cigarette smoking is the major cause of chronic obstructive lung disease in both men and women." This research provided the basis upon which former Surgeon General C. Everett Koop later declared that "cigarette smoking is the single, most preventable cause of premature death and disability in the United States today."

In 1972 Nedro Belloc's and Lester Breslow's blockbuster article entitled "Relationship of Physical Health Status and Health Practice" was printed in *Preventive Medicine*. The Belloc and Breslow research done at UCLA, was the first published longitudinal study which correlated the health habits of a relatively large sample of subjects with verifiable health status measures. Incidentally, many of the steps on the pathway toward human wholeness presented earlier in this chapter were based on the research findings of Belloc and Breslow.

Another important wellness research study was conducted by Paffenbarger and Hale. Their article entitled "Work Activity and Coronary Heart Disease," was published during 1976 in the *New England Journal of Medicine*. The Paffenbarger and Hale research, which studied the exercise habits of longshoremen and alumni of Harvard University, demonstrated the value of wellness lifestyling, with an emphasis on sustained exercise patterns.

Surgeon General's Report

1978 and 1979 were significant years in terms of wellness research publications. During those two years a series articles on the three decade longitudinal study done in Framingham, Massachusetts and *Healthy People: The Surgeon General's Report on Health Promotion and Disease Prevention* were published. The Framingham studies focused on risk factors associated with coronary heart disease and became the basis upon which health risk appraisals were developed. The "Healthy People Report" contained the Surgeon General's goals for the reduction of mortality and morbidity rates to be achieved by 1990. The 1979 report also established priority areas in which resources were concentrated to attain the stated goals. Ten years later the entire process was repeated and refined to produce "Healthy People 2000." Employing the specific death and disease percentages reached by 1990 as baseline data, new goals have been set for Americans to achieve by the turn of the century.

Still another important Surgeon General's Report was released in 1988. The report on "Nutrition and Health" indicated that the majority of the nutritional problems in the United States today are linked not to nutritional deficiencies but instead to nutritional excesses and imbalances. The 1988 report provided recommendations that were essentially compatible with those which had been made by the Senate Select Committee on Nutrition and Human Needs in 1977.

The Multiple Risk Factor Intervention Trial (MRFIT) was a comprehensive investigation which spanned the decade of the 1980's and has made a valuable contribution to the wellness literature. Although many aspects of the project could be highlighted, the most outstanding result is that it took 10.5 years after the intervention trial began to demonstrate a statistically significant difference between the control and treatment groups relative to a number of the risk factors studied. That finding alone emphasizes the fact that wellness interventions are neither a quick fix nor a

Lawn and Garden Work

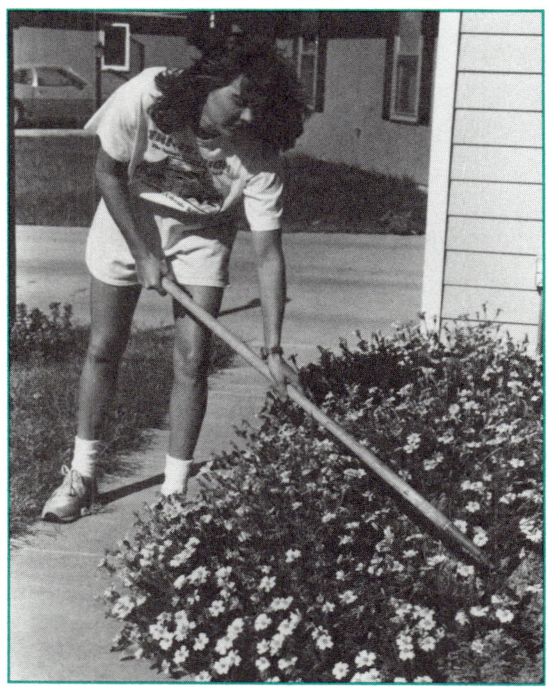

Low-intensity relaxing activity can be an important part of a healthy life-style.

universal panacea to cure all which currently ails the health care system in the United States. On the other hand, it is apparent that wellness must become a part of the solution to America's contemporary health problems.

The implications of the research reported herein and in other studies which have been or are yet to be conducted, are no doubt obvious to the reader. As lifelong advocates for their own health and for the wellness of others who will be served by them, the readers of this chapter already know that they must continue to be informed of new wellness research findings.

Keep Thinking and Reading

There are no silver wellness bullets to be shot, no mysterious wellness potions to be imbibed and no magic wellness wands to wave to assure that individuals and society will reach the goal of health for human wholeness. One by one the research studies must be conducted and their findings applied in personal wellness programs. Individually people will have to want to be healthy and believe that they can be. Within the heart and mind of each person must be assumed the responsibility to promote and protect one's own health. All by themself, a person must take that initial step on the pathway to human wholeness will have to be taken—and the next, and the next . . .

The future of wellness as a personal life-style and as a movement rests within the internal locus of control of each person who has read the words of this chapter and those words yet to be read in the remainder of this book. Indeed, the life of the reader and of the movement rests squarely in your hands. If both are handled with care, faith and commitment, the ultimate outcome for all will be "the best that can be!"

Suggested Readings

Ardell, D.B. *High Level Wellness: An Alternative to Doctors, Drugs and Disease*. Emmaus, PA: Rodale Press, 1977.

Ardell, D.B. *The History and Future of Wellness*. Dubuque, IA: Kendall/Hunt Publishing Company, 1985.

Hahn, D.B. and W. A. Payne. *Focus on Health*. St. Louis: Mosby-Year Book, Inc., Chapters 1 and 3, 1991.

Hales, D.R. *An Invitation to Health: Taking Charge of Your Health*. Redwood City, CA: The Benjamin/ Cummings Publishing Company, Chapters 1 and 7, 1989.

Kemper, D.W., J. Giuffre, and G. Drabinski. *Pathways: A Successful Guide for a Healthy Life*. Boise, ID: Healthwise, Inc., 1985.

Ryan, R.S. and J. W. Travis. *The Wellness Workbook*. Berkeley, CA: TenSpeed Press, 1981.

Smith, S.F. and C. M. Smith. *Personal Health Choices*. Boston: Jones and Bartlett Publishers, Chapters 1 and 9, 1990.

CHAPTER 2

THE LIFE-STYLE DISEASES

Judith S. Hurley
Richard G. Schlaadt

Learning Objectives

- Learn the aspects of lifestyle which are associated with diseases.
- Understand the risk factors associated with cardiovascular disease.
- Determine the role of exercise and proper diet in preventing lifestyle diseases.
- Comprehend the various forms of cancer and their major risk factors.
- Know the causes and prevention strategies for osteoporosis.
- Learn the factors which are associated with injuries and prevention strategies.
- Prescribe behavior modifications which will help reduce the occurrence

Important Terms

adrenal glands
aerobic exercise
anxiety
atherosclerosis
calcium
carbon monoxide
cardiovascular disease
cerebrovascular disease
cholesterol
cirrhosis (of the liver)
coronary artery disease
esophagus
HDL cholesterol
heart attack
hypertension
LDL cholesterol
melanoma
menopause
nicotine
obesity
osteoporosis
pancreas
pathologist
resting heart rate
saturated fat
sodium
stress
thrombosis

INTRODUCTION

Most Disease that kill Americans prematurely today are not caused by foreign organisms, such as viruses and bacteria, and they are not sudden in onset - they are caused, slowly but surely, by the way we live. Our inactivity, fatty diets, smoking and drinking habits, and nonchalance about routine safety matters take their toll in early disabilities and deaths, which are unnecessary, tragic, and costly. The number of common diseases, illnesses, and injuries influenced by our daily lifestyle choices are many: heart disease, cancer, stroke, lung disease, diabetes, osteoporosis, motor vehicles and other accidents, and **cirrhosis of the liver**, among others. Most of these are on the "top 10" list of leading causes of death. But, as one observer puts it, "the American way of life need not be hazardous to your health." Simple changes that lead to feeling better in the short term and reducing the likelihood of disease in the long term are within easy reach.

Live and Let Die

CARDIOVASCULAR DISEASE

Cardiovascular disease, disease of the heart or its blood vessels, is the leading cause of death in industrialized countries, killing close to 1 million people annually in the United States alone. An additional 42 million have some form of cardiovascular disease, and 1.5 million Americans suffer nonfatal heart attacks each year (1,200 people each day).

Coronary artery disease is the most common type of cardiovascular disease. Gradually and silently over the years, the arteries that supply blood to the heart become narrowed by deposits of fatty material in their walls. When an artery becomes clogged with debris to the point that blood cannot reach a portion of the heart muscle, a **heart attack** occurs, the result of the heart tissue being deprived of oxygen.

Heart Attack is #1

Men are over twice as likely to develop coronary artery disease as women, although the incidence in women has been steadily rising in recent years; it is the number one killer of women as well as men. The likelihood of developing coronary artery disease also increases with age for both men and women. Once women reach **menopause**, changes in the production of sex hormones cause women's chances of suffering cardiovascular disease to catch up with those of men. Genetics plays role, too; some families have a higher-than-average incidence of cardiovascular disease.

Atherosclerosis

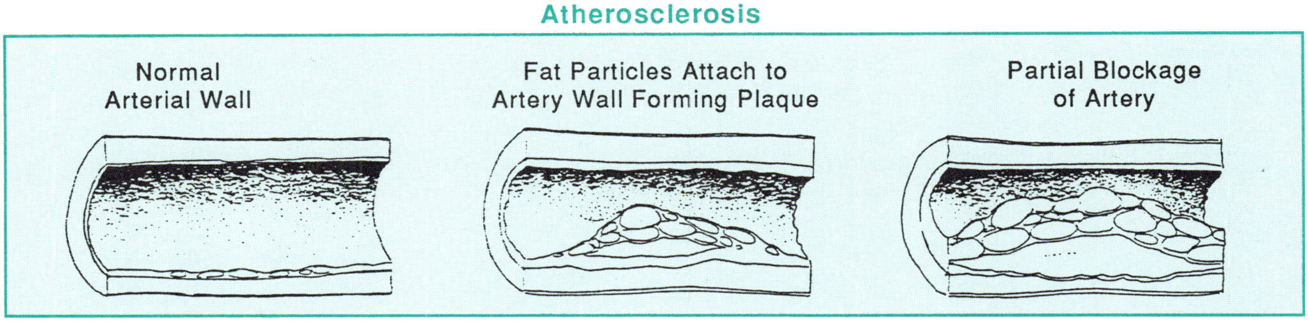

Figure 2.1. Atherosclerosis occurs when fatty substances such as cholesterol build up inside the coronary arteries. When the flow of blood to portions of the heart is restricted or blocked, a heart attack occurs.

Estimated Percentage of U.S. Population Having Selected Risk Factors for Coronary Heart Disease

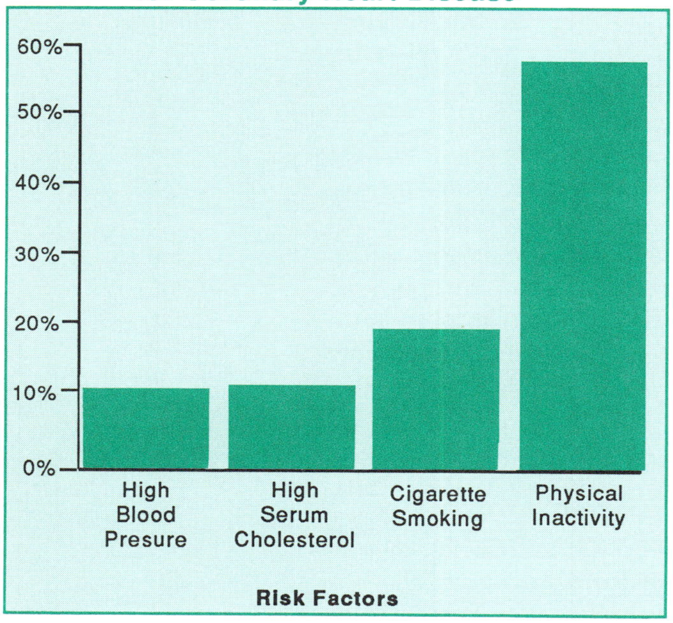

Figure 2.2. More Americans are at risk for heart disease because of physical inactivity than because of any other manageable risk factor. Source: "Protective Effect of Physical Activity on Coronary Heart Disease," *Mortality and Morbidity Weekly Report*, Vol. 36, No. 26, 10 July 1987, p. 429.

Although gender, age, and genetic makeup influence susceptibility to cardiovascular disease, they are obviously factors one cannot do much about. Other major risk factors are within control, however; smoking, high blood **cholesterol**, hypertension (high blood pressure), and lack of exercise. Other factors that increase risk are being overweight, having diabetes, drinking alcohol excessively, taking birth control pills, and having high levels of unmanaged stress. One eminent cardiologist feels the evidence is strong enough to say unequivocally, "Heart disease before [age] 80 is your own fault."

Having one of these risk factors present increases risk, but having more than one factor present dramatically increases the likelihood of developing cardiovascular disease. For example, smokers have 3 times the nonsmokers' risk of developing heart disease, but women who both smoke and take birth control pills are up to 39 times more likely to have a heart attack than women who do neither according to the American Heart Association. Even if a risk factor is present that cannot changed, such as a genetic predisposition, research shows that the change of developing cardiovascular disease can be greatly reduced by taking charge of the manageable risk factors. Three of these factors deserve a closer look - smoking, blood cholesterol, and exercise.

SMOKING

Smoking one pack of cigarettes a day triples the risk of death from cardiovascular disease. A single cigarette reduces the amount of blood the heart pumps with each beat, causing it to work far harder than necessary to pump blood through 60,000 miles of blood vessels in the body.

Cigarettes are a Downer

Smoking damages the cardiovascular system by raising blood pressure and cholesterol, changing factors in the blood to cause increased clotting, constricting blood vessels, and speeding the heart rate. Smokers have elevated **carbon monoxide** levels and carry 20 percent less oxygen in their blood than nonsmokers, a factor that affects the functioning of all organs, not just the heart. On the other hand, once a smoker quits, the damaged cardiovascular system repairs itself within 5 to 10 years, and heart disease risk is cut in half.

CHOLESTEROL

Pathologists at the turn of the century noticed a common condition in the bodies of heart attack victims - their blood vessels were clogged with a yellowish substance, and arteries were hard and calcified. The predominant ingredient in the yellowish substance? Cholesterol. Much research has gone on since then to clarify the role of this fat-like compound in heart disease.

Several major studies and numerous smaller ones have clearly shown that elevated blood cholesterol increases the risk of cardiovascular disease. A small percentage of the population has a genetic predisposition to develop high blood cholesterol. For the majority of the population, however, manageable life-style factors are the main cause of elevated blood cholesterol. The most prevalent are smoking, not exercising, and consuming a diet high in **saturated fats** and cholesterol. Of the two dietary factors, saturated fats are the biggest contributor - they raise blood cholesterol levels even more than the cholesterol in food does. These and other dietary factors are discussed in chapter 9.

Life-Styles and High Cholesterol

The cholesterol picture is complicated by the fact that two major forms of cholesterol occur in the blood, **LDL cholesterol** and **HDL cholesterol**. LDL cholesterol is the "bad" kind, on its way to being deposited in the arteries. HDL cholesterol is the "good" kind, a scavenger compound carrying cholesterol out of the arteries. A low level of HDL cholesterol is thought by some cardiovascular researchers to be the most significant risk factor for disease because it indicates that the body is not able to clear cholesterol from the arteries adequately.

Harmful LDL cholesterol is raised by saturated fat and cholesterol in the diet. Beneficial HDL cholesterol is raised by exercise but lowered by smoking. To have an optimum ration of "good" to "bad" forms of cholesterol, one needs to eat a diet low in fat and cholesterol (to keep the "bad" LDL cholesterol low) and obtain regular exercise and forgo smoking (to keep the "good" HDL cholesterol high).

LDL vs. HDL

Vigorous exercise alone, although very important, may not protect one from heart disease, since a low-fat diet is equally important in order to keep LDL cholesterol low. The exerciser who says "I don't need to worry about what I eat, I burn it off" is hanging onto potentially harmful misconception.

The process of **atherosclerosis**, the buildup of fatty deposits in arteries, begins as early as age 15. Healthy habits are thus as important in the teenage years, twenties, and thirties as they are during middle age and older years.

EXERCISE

"Did you brush your teeth today? Did you exercise? How long can you live without your teeth? How long can you live without your heart?" So begins a lecture by one fitness expert. The heart, the most important muscle in the body, is the muscle most ignored by people in industrialized nations.

Health Benefits of Exercise

1. **Heart** - Aerobic exercise increases the size and stamina of the heart muscle, conditioning the heart to circulate a great volume of blood with each beat, lowering the risk of heart disease and heart attack.

2. **Circulation** - Exercise increases the amount of oxygen in the bloodstream, and the level of HDL cholesterol in the blood. It lowers blood pressure, which helps prevent stroke and heart attack.

3. **Muscles** - Exercise increases the oxygen supply to muscles while strengthening and toning them, and increasing coordination.

4. **Joints** - Exercise keeps the joints supple and prevents joint disorders by thickening the cartilage.

5. **Bones** - Regular exercise thickens the bones and inhibits loss of calcium from the bones, preventing osteoporosis.

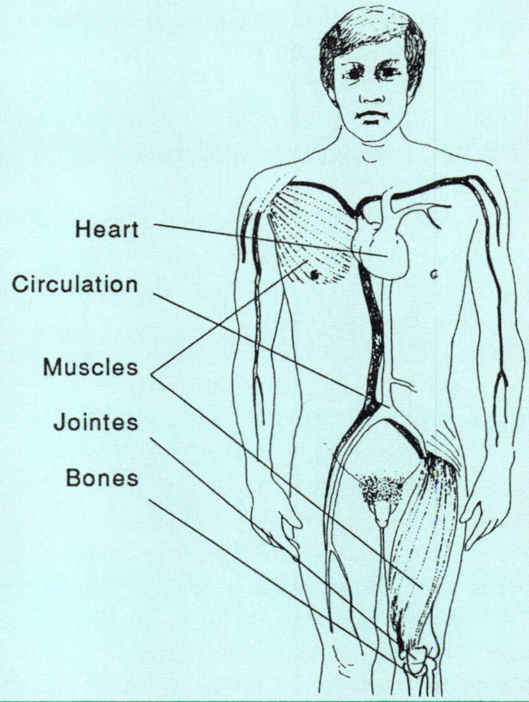

Figure 2.3. Besides tightening and toning muscles, aerobic exercise also strengthens the heart, stimulates the building of new blood vessels which promotes better circulation, and often reduces the level of fat in the blood.

Men who are sedentary have twice the risk of heart attack as men who are moderately active and triple the rate of heart attack compared to men who are vigorous exercisers. In addition,when heart attacks do occur in nonexercisers, they are three times more likely to be fatal than when they occur in exercisers.

Less than half the population in the United States is regularly active, and it is estimated only 10 percent of the population engages in the type of exercise that strengthens the heart muscle and prevents heart disease.

Aerobic Exercise and the Heart

The type of exercise that makes the heart more fit is termed **aerobic exercise**. Examples of aerobic exercise are brisk walking, jogging, swimming, cycling, and rowing. These activities share in common the ability to raise the heart rate to a necessary threshold zone and maintain it there for a sustained period of time (15 to 20 minutes or more). These activities also work the large muscle groups of the body. They are not "stop and go" activities, such as baseball, and they can be carried out at a level of intensity that does not cause huffing and puffing, as more vigorous sports do. The details of aerobic exercise are discussed further in chapter 6.

Aerobic activities condition the heart to pump more blood with each beat. Weight-lifting, calisthenics, and stretching do not have this effect. After a few weeks of regular aerobic exercise, the **resting heart rate** goes down (the heart beats per minute while the body is at rest), one indication that the heart has become stronger. The heart can now beat fewer times per minute to accomplish the job of pushing blood throughout the body. If, through exercise, one's heart rate decreases by 2 beats per minute (for example, from an initial resting rate of 72 beats per minute to 70 beats per minute, this amounts to 2,880 fewer beats each day, 20,160 fewer beats per week, and 1,048,320 less per year!

The wear and tear saved on the heart is considerable. Aerobic exercise also stimulates the building of new blood vessels, which promotes better circulation of blood and oxygen, providing alternative pathways to organs, especially the heart, sold a blood vessel become clogged. Exercise also helps control blood cholesterol levels by raising the cholesterol-scavenging capabilities of the blood, the beneficial HDL cholesterol.

CANCER

Cancer is the second leading cause of death in the United States, responsible for approximately 22 percent of deaths. Cancer of the lung is the most frequent type (440,000 deaths yearly), followed closely by colon, breast, and prostate cancer.

As many as 75 percent of cancers are life-style related caused primarily by tobacco use, dietary fat, obesity, and alcohol. The degree of known cancer risk because of food additives, industrial pollutants, pesticides, and other environmental factors, although of great concern, appears small in comparison to these major risk factors.

American Cancer Society's Guidelines to Reduce Risk for Cancer

1. Eat more cabbage family foods (broccoli, cauliflower, brussels sprouts, cabbage, kale).
2. Eat more high-fiber foods.
3. Choose fruits and vegetables with vitamin A (beta-carotene).
4. Choose foods with vitamin C.
5. Control body weight.
6. Trim fat from the diet.
7. East salt-cured, smoked, and nitrite-cured foods only occasionally or not at all.
8. Stop cigarette smoking.
9. Go easy on alcohol.
10. Avoid exposing your skin to too much sun and wear sunscreen.

Source: Adapted from Taking Control: 10 Steps to a Healthier Life and Reduce Cancer Risk (New York: American Cancer Society, 1985).

TOBACCO

Not smoking is the single most effective step one can take to lower cancer risk. Lung cancer accounts for 15 to 25 percent of all cancers, and smoking is clearly the most frequent cause. Not breathing second-hand smoke is important, too. Research now shows that people exposed to the smoke of others have increased rates of lung cancer and respiratory infections. The children of smokers with lung cancer, if they go on to become smokers themselves, have a 15 to 25 times higher likelihood of developing lung cancer than if they do

Risk of Lung Cancer After Smoking Cessation

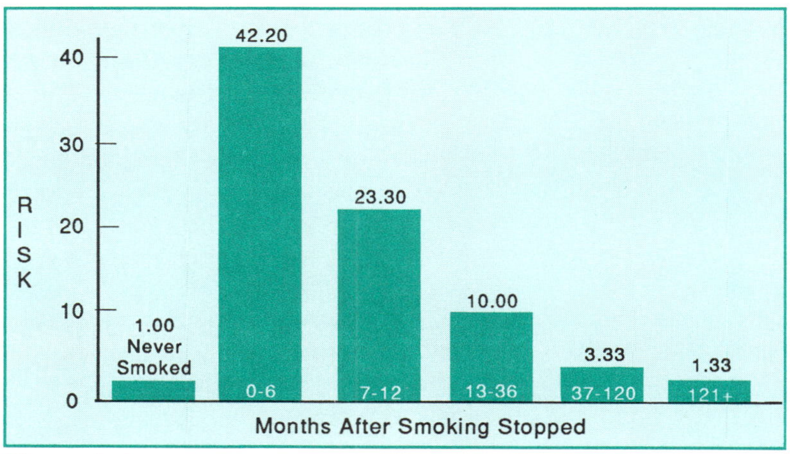

Figure 2.4. Quitting smoking eventually lowers lung cancer risk almost to that of a nonsmoker. Source: Donald M. Vickery, M.D., Lifeplan (Reston, VA: Vickson, Inc., 1990), p. 151.

not become smokers. Smoking is also associated with cancers of the **esophagus**, stomach, and **pancreas**, especially in heavy drinkers.

Smokeless tobacco use (snuff and chewing tobacco) has increased among people under age 24, and although many harmful chemicals present in smoke are absent when this form of tobacco is used, risk of cancer of the mouth, stomach, and esophagus remains. The **nicotine** is still present, increasing heart disease risk. Addiction to tobacco occurs just as with smoking and, in fact, many smokeless tobacco users go on to become smokers.

DIET AND EXERCISE

Fat and Cancer

Excessive intake of any type of dietary fat, whether saturated or unsaturated, is associated with increased cancer risk, particularly of the breast and colon. Most Americans need to reduce fat intake by approximately 25 percent to meet current guidelines for a diet containing no more than 30 percent of calories from fat. In addition, the fiber found in whole wheat and other whole grains may be beneficial in preventing cancer of the colon.

Some research, most notably the study of 17,000 Harvard alumni who were followed for several years, indicates that regular exercise reduces deaths from cancer as well as from heart disease.

SUN WORSHIPING

Sun and Cancer

Too much time in the sun without adequate protection significantly adds to the threat of skin cancer. This disease is on the increase, in part because of the thinning of the earth's protective ozone layer, and in part because of the whims of fashion - the popularity of the dark tan. Incidence of malignant **melanoma**, a very deadly form of cancer, has risen alarmingly in recent years. At highest risk are those with fair skin and blonde or red hair, and those who freckle easily, live at high altitudes, or spend a lot of time outdoors.

Simple steps to take to prevent skin cancer are using sunblock, wearing hats, and limiting exposure to sun, especially during the middle of the day. In particular, sunburns should be avoided. Severe sunburns in children are associated with development of skin cancer later in life. Even without the skin being visibly burned, the more time one spends in the sun, the higher the risk.

CEREBROVASCULAR DISEASE

Cerebrovascular disease, or stroke, is brain damage that occurs when blood vessels in the brain hemorrhage or when a blockage or blood clot called a **thrombosis** occurs. Control of hypertension (high blood pressure) over the last two decades has resulted in a remarkable decrease in occurrence of cerebrovascular disease. Since 1972, deaths due to stroke have dropped 48 percent. It remains the third leading cause of death, however, and is largely preventable.

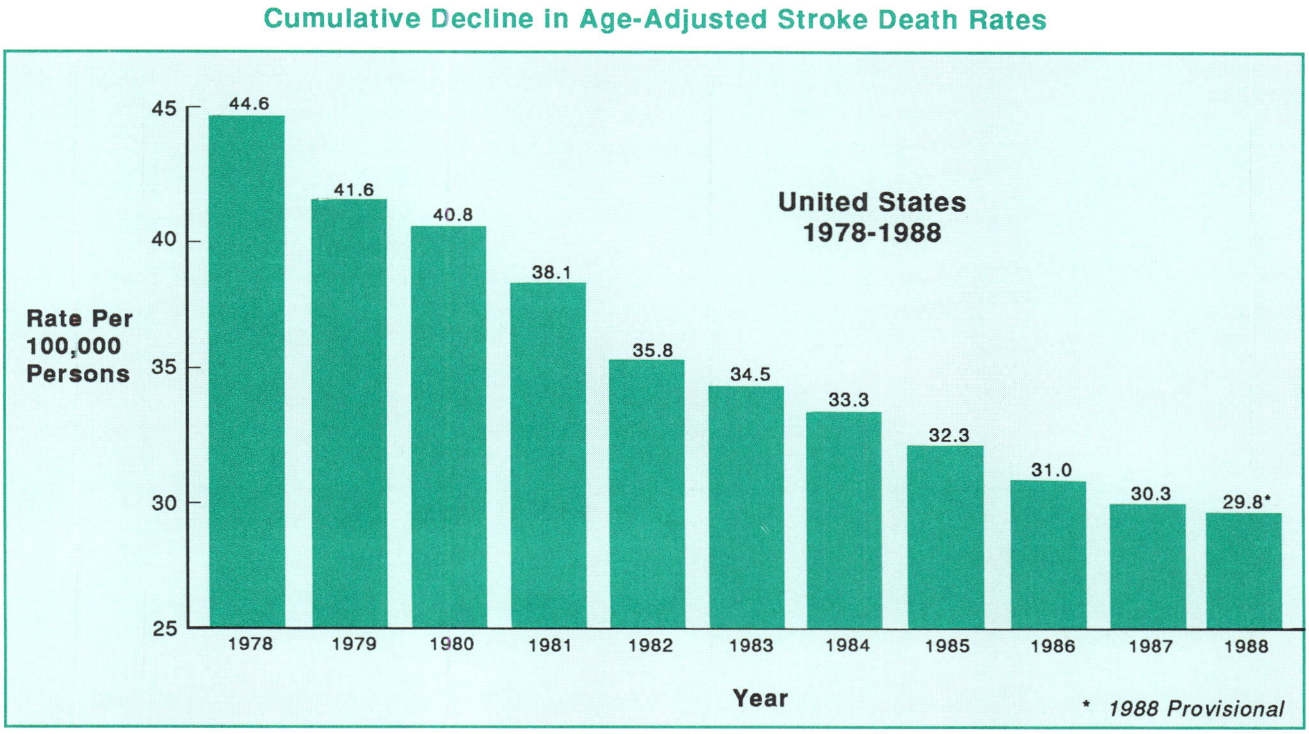

Figure 2.5. Control of high blood pressure over the last two decades has resulted in a remarkable decrease in stroke death rates. Source: National Center for Health Statistics, Public Health Service, Department of Health and Human Services, and the American Heart Association.

Factors that increase risk of stroke include **hypertension** (by far the most significant), overweight, diabetes, and birth control pills. In addition, the factors that increase risk of cardiovascular disease are major risk factors for stroke as well - a high-fat diet, smoking, and lack of exercise can result in clogged blood vessels in the brain as well as the heart.

HYPERTENSION

Only a small percentage of people with hypertension suffer strokes, but hypertension is the leading risk factor. Hypertension can occur as a result of other diseases, such as kidney disease, but it more commonly develops in the absence of disease. One-third to one-half of all cases of hypertension have developed in response to **sodium** intake, so limiting salt and other sources of sodium in the diet is important. Other factors include the consumption of too much alcohol. Too little **calcium** (found primarily in milk and milk products) or too little potassium (found in fruits and vegetables) also appears to increase the likelihood of hypertension. Exercise can effectively lower both blood pressure and stress levels. Unmanaged stress levels are thought to be a significant factor in high blood pressure, since release of stress hormones by the **adrenal glands** causes an increase in blood pressure.

Exercise Lowers Hypertension

OSTEOPOROSIS

A total of 15 million people (25 percent of women over the age of 65 and nearly 13 percent of men over the age of 65) have **osteoporosis**, a painful condition in which bones become thin and porous with age. Of the 2,000,000 hip fractures in the United States each year, 160,000 are due to osteoporosis. All too often, a bone fracture in an older person leads to infection, poor healing, lengthy hospital stays, and a downward spiral in health. An estimated 32,000 deaths occur each year from the complications that follow a hip fracture in older adults.

Osteoporosis and Spinal Deformity

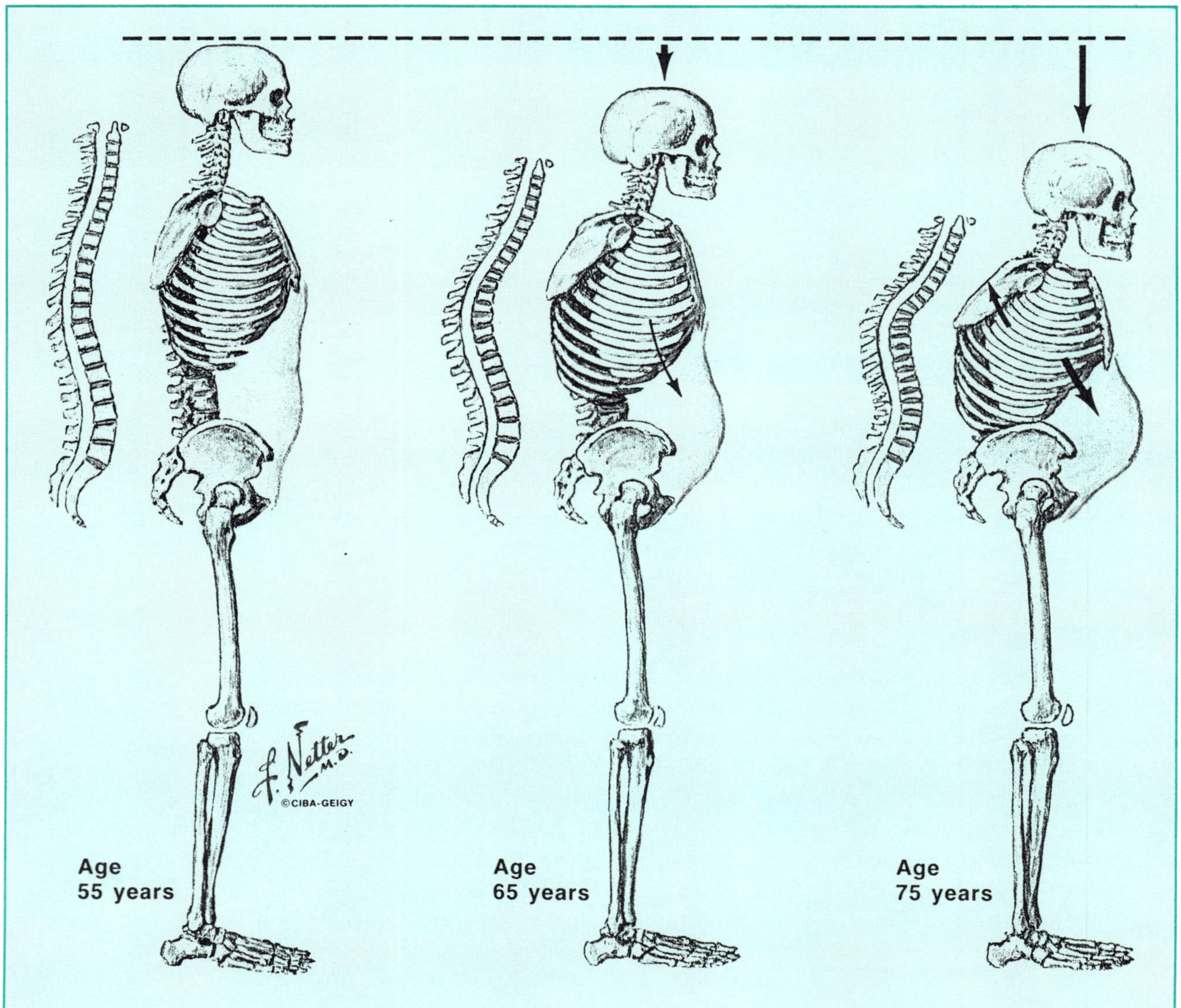

Figure 2.6. More frequent among women than men, osteoporosis is characterized by a continuing loss of bone mass. It can produce severe spinal deformity as shown here. Source: F. Kaplan, "Osteoporosis," Clinical Symposia/CIBA, Vol. 35, No. 5 (1983).

We tend to think that becoming shorter and bent over is an inevitable part of aging, but this is not so. Bone health in the later years depends considerably on life-style habits throughout life. Although bones stop growing in length in the late teens or early twenties, growth in bone density or hardness continues through the mid-30s. Minerals move in and out of bones on a daily basis, making the replacement through diet of the lost minerals important throughout life.

Exercise is a crucial factor in bone health. The ones in the right arm of a right-handed tennis player may be 15 percent denser than those in the left arm. Bones steadily lose calcium when one is inactive. Much calcium from their bones while in a zero-gravity environment. Astronauts now perform special exercises to put pressure on bones while in flight.

Several alcoholic drinks a day, smoking, eating too much protein, and consuming too much phosphorus (found in soft drinks, processed foods, and protein-rich animal foods, and protein-rich animal foods) are factors that increase risk by causing a greater loss of calcium from bones.

Developing strong, dense bones before the age of 35 is thought to be the most important way to prevent osteoporosis. A diet providing calcium from low-fat milk products or other sources and regular, weight-bearing exercise result in healthy bones with large amounts of minerals in them. Vitamin D, obtained from sunlight or through food, is also required for calcium use in the body. Research indicates that adults over age 50 may not get enough vitamin D. At least fifteen minutes outdoors each day and consumption of vitamin D-fortified milk are ways to obtain this nutrient. Adequate calcium and vitamin D intake and regular exercise remain important after age 35 as well. Swimming, though beneficial for the heart, by itself does not place enough pressure on bones to maintain their health, but a 30-minute daily walk, jog, or other weight-bearing activity will contribute significantly to bone health.

Calcium in Foods

Food	Amount	Milligrams of Calcium
whole milk	1 cup	290
skim milk	1 cup	302
yogurt	1 cup	270
cheddar cheese	1 ounce	213
cottage cheese	1/2 cup	100
ice cream	1 cup	194
canned salmon	3.5 ounces	225
sardines	3 ounces	375
tofu	2 in. x 1 in. piece	154
spinach, cooked	1/2 cup	116
broccoli, cooked	1/2 cup	68
okra, coked	1/2 cup	147
lentils	1/2 cup	25
lima beans	1/2 cup	40
orange	1	70
cornbread	2 in. square	133
blackstrap molasses	1 tbs.	137
raisins	3 tbs.	54

Recommended daily allowance for males and females age 15-24: 1200 mg, age 25 and older: 8000 mg

Table 2.1. The best way to avoid osteoporosis is to eat foods rich in calcium on a regular basis. Source: U.S. Dept. of Agriculture. Handbook No. 456.

OVERWEIGHT

Being overweight is not uncommon in our sedentary society. As many as 20 to 30 percent of adults are 10 percent or more above their recommended weight. Overweight is a concern primarily because it increases the likelihood of developing several common diseases, including heart disease, cancer, hypertension, and diabetes. Having excess weight puts extra strain on joints, can aggravate arthritis, and can make any necessary surgery more difficult and risky. Being overweight also leads to lethargy and low self-esteem, conditions that affect how one feels day in and day out.

The cause of **obesity** (excess body fat) are complex and for some people may involve difference in fat cells, genetics, metabolic factors, and brain regulatory functions. But for most, the cause is far simpler: a sedentary life-style and a diet too high in concentrated calories from fat, sugar, or alcohol.

STRESS

Stress Can Be Controlled

Stress is an aspect of life difficult to measure and research, but one that appears to affect our health as much as diet, exercise, or cigarettes, events that have the potential to cause stress are unavoidable. How strongly we react to the events determines the impact on our cardiovascular, nervous, and immune systems. When a situation is perceived as stressful, changes occur in hormones, nerves, blood pressure, breathing, and muscles. Either chronic low-level stress or a sudden, major stress can be a factor in hypertension, depression, **anxiety**, heart disease, some cancers, and lowered resistance to colds and infections. Some experts estimate that as may as 85 percent of illnesses are stress-related and that the degree of absenteeism in work sites is a reflection of stress more than any other factor.

Anything that brings change can cause stress - whether it is a negative event or a positive one. Being late for work, having a flat tire, losing a loved one, or having financial difficulties can produce stress. Similarly, being promoted to a new job, getting married, or retiring can be stressful events.

Many early warning signals of stress can occur, including headaches, muscle tension, allergies, nervous tics, anxiety, fatigue and frequent colds. If stress is not coped with when these early signs appear, possible results include ulcers, high blood pressure, depression and other mental health problems, and an increased likelihood of major disease.

INJURIES

Accidents kill more young people than any other cause, accounting for 50 percent of fatalities that occur between the ages of 15 and 24. By age 44, accidents drop into fourth place as a cause of death. Motor vehicle accidents are by far the leading culprit, killing more than 140,000 Americans each year. Drownings, poisonings, and falls together account for 33 percent of fatal accidents, less than two-thirds as many deaths as motor vehicles accidents.

About two-thirds of states have mandatory seat belt laws. The resulting decrease in fatalities is as much as 33 percent. All 50 states now require that infants and young children be in child safety restraints while in vehicles. Individuals who choose not to wear seat belts are far more likely to die in a crash than those who wear them - it is estimated that seat belt use can prevent 50 percent of motor vehicle deaths.

Fifteen percent of accidental deaths occur on the job (approximately 14,000 deaths each year). An additional 2.5 million disabling injuries occur in work sites yearly. Among those age 75 and older falls are the most frequent type of accident. The death rate from injures in older adults is more than 2 1/2 times that of teenagers and young adults. Deaths because of injury are really only the tip of the iceberg - an estimated 75 million serious or disabling injuries occur each year.

Seat Belt Use

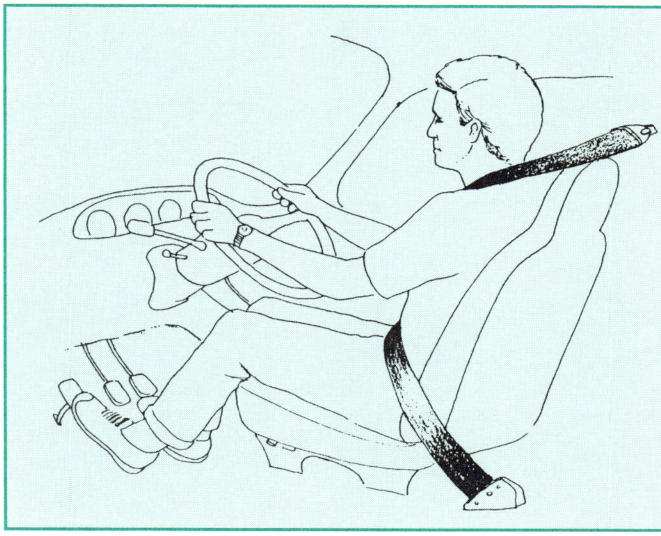

Figure 2.7. It is estimated that seat belt use can prevent 50 percent of all deaths resulting from motor vehicle accidents.

Perhaps the word "accident" is a misnomer because it implies an occurrence of freak change or something unavoidable. The most important factor in accidents, however, is something over which one does have control - alcohol use. Alcohol is involved in over half of motor vehicles injuries and close to half of motorcycle injuries. Alcohol is a major factor in injuries to pedestrians, drownings, and job injuries as well.

Alcohol is a Killer

Although wellness and personal health promotion often center upon changing fitness, nutrition, and other lifestyle habits, accidental injury remains a common threat to health and one fairly easy to control. Simple steps for preventing injuries are discussed in the next chapter.

CHOICE IS YOURS

Staying fit and healthy gives us the means to enjoy each day and be able to pursue and accomplish our goals over the course of a lifetime. In the next chapter, you will see that the life-style patterns that improve energy and wellbeing and that prevent major disease are one and the same - and, the daily choices one needs to make, relatively simple and rewarding.

Suggested Readings

Donatelle, R.J., L.G. Davis, and C.F. Hoover. *Access to Health.* Englewood Cliffs, NJ: Prentice Hall, 1991.

Hurley, J.S. and R.G. Schlaadt. *The Wellness Life-Style.* Guilford, CT: Dushkin, 1992.

Ornish, D. *Dr. Dean Ornish's Program for Reversing Heart Disease.* New York: Random House, 1990.

Roberts, S.W. *Health Wellness.* Dubuque, IA: eddie bowers publishing, inc., 1989.

CHAPTER

3 CHANGING PERSONAL LIFE-STYLE BEHAVIORS

Parris Watts

Learning Objectives

- Describe at least five barriers which get in the way of effectively changing life-style behaviors.
- Define the five major steps of the health behavior change process.
- Discuss reasons why maintaining altered health behaviors is both difficult and complex.
- List the important questions needed to be asked by an individual who is planning to initiate a health behavior change program.
- Describe the models and theories that have been developed to illustrate how health behavior change typically occurs.

Important Terms

cues
enabling
health behavior change
human wholeness
personal wellness assessment
predisposing
reinforcing
self-image
significant emotional event (SEE)
wellness
wellness lifestyle

INTRODUCTION

In February of 1968, an article written by a man named Bob Hoke was published in the *Archives of Environmental Health.* Almost obscurely hidden within that highly specialized professional journal was Hoke's gem of an article titled "Promotive Medicine and the Phenomenon of Health." Nestled among other statements of professional value were the following ones which are profound.

> *"Being healthy is having confidence in the future. The healthy man's future does not happen passively to him; it is an active extension of his life. For him the future is created by his choices and decisions Instead of the future coming to him, he takes himself to it and his living becomes a joint creation. Health is a participation in that creation, a participation in one's own being, a commitment to one's living in the world. To be healthy is to celebrate one's life."*

Create a Personalized Approach

Long before the days of wellness as a common term, Bob Hoke's words appear to have been precocious, if not prophetic. Nevertheless, even more remarkable than Hoke's foresighted vision of wellness was his conceptualization of health related behavioral change. His statements about internal locus of control, choices, decisions and participation in the "creation" of a personalized wellness life-style are consistent with some of the most highly regarded behavioral change theories currently being applied in the health education discipline.

Ironically, the choices and decisions associated with living a wellness life-style are matters of common sense.

Activities Promoting Wellness

1. Exercising regularly
2. Eating a balanced low fat diet
3. Becoming aware of stressors in daily life and learning how to manage them effectively
4. Using positive self-talk
5. Enhancing personal self-image
6. Wearing seatbelts
7. Avoiding risk taking behaviors such as smoking and driving too fast

Practice What You Know

Frequently the following question is asked, "What can people be taught about wellness that they do not already know?" An appropriate answer to that question is, "They can be taught to put into practice what they already know." At first, such an answer may seem flippant. Teaching people how to apply more healthful behaviors within their daily lives is perhaps the most important thing a health educator does. In essence, the "calling" of all health educators is to help people SEE — that is, to have a **significant emotional event (SEE)** — before it is too late. For too many individuals their SEE comes in the form of a survived heart attack, malignant results of a lung or breast biopsy or word that they have a peptic ulcer. It is unfortunate that it takes such dramatic "events" to motivate people to take control of their health behaviors and to become active participants in the creation of more healthy life-styles.

BARRIERS TO CHANGING LIFE-STYLE BEHAVIORS

Why is it that humans have little or no motivation to make wellness life-style choices, changes, and sacrifices necessary to be healthy UNTIL they are almost forced to do so? As discussed previously in Chapter 1, much of this phenomenon can be traced to taking one's health for granted and to failing to assume responsibility for one's personal wellness. Following are the major contributors to persons falling short of enjoying the optimal level of wellness they could achieve if they would only strive to live more healthfully.

Why Wellness Fails

Some people subconsciously do not want to be healthy. For certain individuals, being ill enables them to receive the care and attention they do not get when they are well. For others, being healthy just takes too much effort they are unwilling to exert. Regularly exercising, shopping for and preparing low fat meals, and doing progressive muscle relaxation and deep breathing/meditation exercises daily require a lot of time and energy.

Another group of persons do not believe they can be healthy. They are convinced that it is their fate to have a heart attack, a cancer condition, a stroke, or adult-onset diabetes. They will even cite family history, poor medical services, and environmental factors out of their control as supportive evidence to substantiate their beliefs. They fail to understand that life-style factors are more important than are all the other determinants of their health COMBINED. Furthermore, they do not realize that perhaps the reasons for generations of chronic health problems in their families are related more to life-style than genetics. Likewise, their criticism of medical services might be more a function of failure to apply preventive health care practices or waiting too long to seek treatment for a serious medical condition. In terms of environmental factors, people will sometimes allow themselves to be routinely exposed to health damaging and life threatening elements, hoping that they will be lucky enough to escape their deleterious effects.

It Can't Happen to Me

The delusion of invulnerability, or false belief that "it cannot happen to me," is an additional contributor to taking one's health for granted or not assuming responsibility to protect it. Although people will smoke, drink and then drive and/or place themselves at risk for AIDS and other sexually transmissible diseases, they somehow believe they will be spared the consequences of their negative health practices. When their day of health behavior accountability eventually arrives, they blame heredity, the medical care system, or the environment for their problems. They seem to be totally oblivious to the fact that if they had only considered the consequences of their actions in advance and had acknowledged the stewardship of their health, they could have made much better health related choices and decisions.

Another factor which lulls humans into complacency regarding their wellness is that health problems are generally the result of an accumulation of abuses. Behaviors which may not cause harm if done only a few times can become dangerous and even life threatening if repeated for several years.

Classic examples of this are high dietary fat consumption and overreacting to stressors in the workplace and/or at home. The cumulative effects of these and other similar actions insidiously take their toll over a period of time without the individual being aware of the gradual erosion of his/her wellness state. Because of their lack of a realization of what is happening, they continue the behaviors unaware that they are on a collision course with health problems, which in many instances, could have been avoided.

Still another barrier to following a wellness life-style is the unrealistic dependence of some persons on medicine and technology. It is as though they believe that no matter how much they abuse their bodies, minds, and spirits, there will always be a medical doctor, a counseling professional, or a "person of the cloth" to save them. Because of this way of thinking, many individuals will ultimately face a rude awakening. Undoubtedly the constant health related research being done and the scientific breakthroughs which occur periodically only further encourages such a mindset. Perhaps the most effective way to remove this barrier is to convince the people who tend to adopt this philosophy that the old saying, "an ounce of prevention is better than a pound of cure," is a far more sensible approach to living.

An Ounce of Prevention

PRECURSORS TO HEALTH BEHAVIOR CHANGE

Many people find it hard to alter deeply rooted health behaviors. The process involved in changing anything is a difficult one for most human beings. The transition through adolescence, getting married, moving to a new residence, beginning a new job, having an addition to the family, or going through a divorce are common examples of life changes which create considerable discomfort. Changes in health habits are really no different. Many of the same discomforts associated with the life changes listed previously are felt when one starts an exercise routine, begins a body fat reduction program, or tries to stop smoking.

Physical discomfort related to sore muscles from exercising, hunger pangs from reduced caloric consumption, and nicotine withdrawal from cessation of smoking are all very real results of health behavior changes. Other dimensions of the whole person also may have to endure discomfort. For example, intellectually the person may seriously question whether the change is worth the time, effort, and pain involved. Social resistance and even ridicule from family members and friends may have to be experienced by the person trying to change a behavior. As irrational as it may seem, the people closest to the individual attempting to change a health practice may be the greatest stumbling block. This can also spill over into the vocational dimension of the person's life. The point to be made here is that health behavior changes will not come easily. If people want to alter their wellness life-styles with as much ease as possible, they need to consider the following questions prior to initiating such a program.

Change Takes Effort

Questions for Health Behavior Change

1. **How positive is my self-image?**
Self-image includes how one sees oneself and how he/she believes others perceive them. This may be the most crucial precursor to health behavior change of all. If a person does not feel good about himself/herself, they will need to work harder on positive self-talk and on developing strategies for intrinsic motivation in order to improve their chances of making successful and lasting life-style changes.

2. **Why do I need to make this *health behavior* change?**
Here the person must candidly face facts regarding blood cholesterol, body fat percentage, blood pressure, and other indices correlated with current and projected health status. Then they must acknowledge the need to make the changes required to improve or protect their personal wellness.

3. **Why do I want to make this health behavior change?**
This is more a matter of personalizing the need to change a health behavior. In response to this question, the individual should research the action required to determine the pros and the cons of the change for them. The extent of their willingness to change a behavior is often identified as a part of this process.

4. **Do I possess the willingness to make this health behavior change?**
The person not only has to be able to change one's life-style, they must be willing to make the sacrifices which are necessary to successfully complete the process. That process is often quite complex and may require much patience and even numerous attempts before real success is experienced. Cessation of smoking or discontinuing the use of smokeless tobacco are health behavior changes which often require many repeated attempts in order to succeed.

5. **How much do I love my old health habits?**
Health habits which have been formed and reinforced over a period of many years will die hard. Breaking old habits and making new ones is possible, but it will require much time, effort and discipline. Behavior change experts believe that in order to form a new health habit, such as regular aerobic exercise, a person must repeat the act a minimum of 40 times!

6. **How much reinforcement will I get from others as I make this health behavior change?**
People working on health behavior changes may receive positive feedback in the form of compliments and encouragement from supportive family and friends. On the other hand, they may get negative feedback characterized by the lack of cooperation or even resistance from others. Being prepared to counteract negative feedback with positive self-talk and a keen awareness of the benefits already experienced up to that point in time, are secrets to success in this critical realm of behavior change.

7. **Do I view this health behavior change as apart of a new and permanent wellness life-style?**
It is of paramount importance for the individual working on a health behavior change program to perceive that what they are doing comprises merely a thread in the fabric of a life which will become more healthful and fulfilling in the end. Although care must be taken not to broaden the horizon to the extent that the value of the one behavior being altered is minimized, the person must at least be aware that their concentrated efforts will ultimately contribute to a greater, everlasting outcome.

HEALTH BEHAVIOR CHANGE: MODELS AND THEORY

It has already been established by leading wellness researchers that there is clearly a relationship between health and life-style. Preventive health behaviors and even health behavior changes which enable people to enhance and/or maintain their wellness states have been studied rather extensively. Various models and theories have been developed in recent years to better illustrate the dynamics of health behavior change. Three of these, A) Precede Model, B) Health Belief Model and C) Social Learning Theory are worthy of at least brief discussion in this chapter.

Planning and Promoting Wellness

A. **The Precede Model** was developed during the 1980s by Lawrence Green, who is still a prominent public health education leader. Green's Precede Model is well suited to planning for and promoting improved wellness states among individuals and groups who will apply its principles. In Figure 3.1, a version of the Precede Model, which has been adapted to include the previously discussed "Health for **Human Wholeness**" concept, is presented.

Precede Model and Health for Human Wholeness Model Combined

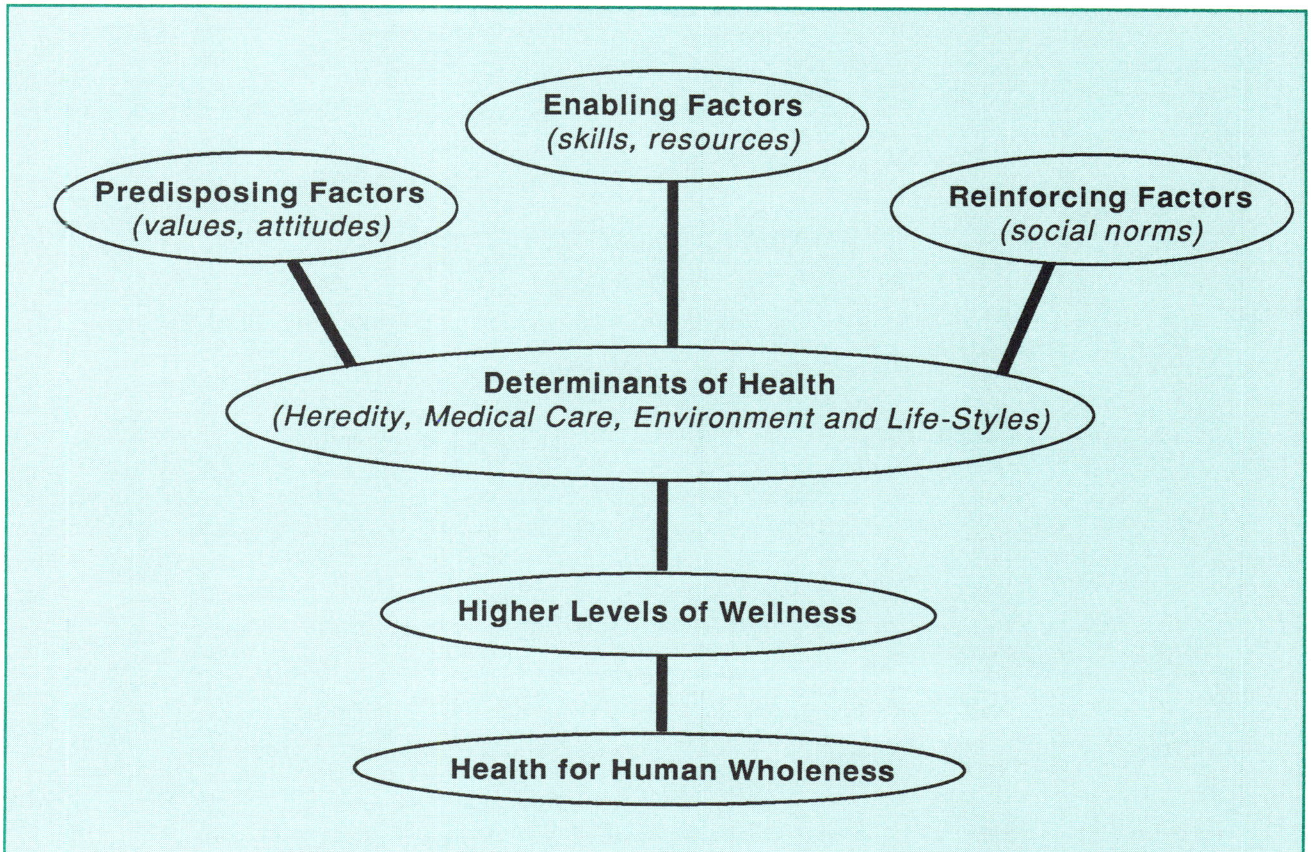

Figure 3.1.

The Precede Model divides the factors which affect environment and behavior into three categories - predisposing, enabling, and reinforcing.

Precede Model Dynamics

1. **Predisposing** - Included among the predisposing factors are priorities, values, attitudes, and knowledge. They are dynamic and are impacted by the cultural and familial backgrounds of individuals.

2. **Enabling -** These factors are skills and resources. Learning how to exercise safely within one's target zone, how to lower one's body fat percentage sensibly, and how to become aware of and manage stress effectively are all examples of enabling skills. A supervised exercise class, a registered dietician, a smoking cessation seminar, stress management, progressive relaxation, or mental imagery audio tapes, and even this book are resources.

3. **Reinforcing** - The health attitudes and behaviors of persons with whom one lives and works are the vitally important reinforcing factors in the Precede Model. The reinforcement of health attitudes and behaviors by family and friends can greatly influence the determinants of our health, the level of wellness we eventually attain/maintain and our ultimate achievement of Health for Human Wholeness.

B. **The Health Belief Model** is based on the premise that life-style behaviors are more likely to be positive when:

Health Belief Model Principles

1. Individuals perceive that if they fail to apply wellness principles in their lives, they will be more susceptible to disease.

2. The consequences of their failure to apply wellness principles will be serious.

3. They perceive that there are benefits associated with applying wellness principles.

4. The perceived benefits of a wellness life-style are greater than the required expenditure of time, energy and money.

5. There is a belief that the application of wellness principles will be successful.

6. One or more health related factors catalyze and/or reinforce the behavior being considered.

The Health Belief Model is valuable because it explains not only why individuals begin to practice preventive health behaviors but also why they often fail in some of those practices. If a person has tried unsuccessfully for a considerable period of time to reduce high total cholesterol levels through dietary modification and exercise, the lack of positive expectations may cause the individual to discontinue their dietary modification and exercise program. On the other hand, if another person with a similar problem has experienced success in reducing total blood cholesterol as a result of decreased saturated fat consumption, body fat percentage reduction and accompanying aerobic exercise, their belief in the efficacy of the program will reinforce its continuation.

Positive Life-Style Behavior

C. **The Social Learning Theory** as applied to health behavior change stresses that an individual's behavior is closely correlated with expected outcomes and their anticipated effectiveness over time. It is tied to the theory that what one gets from changing a health behavior is what one expects to get. Also involved is a related theory that if a person believes a health behavior change will be effective, chances for its success are improved. Thus, in a nutshell, Social Learning Theory is based on perceptions of outcome expectations and self efficacy expectations. It should be emphasized that social learning theorists believe that efficacy expectations are learned from personal experiences, role modeling and verbal persuasion. The extent to which these three factors have influenced previous health habits must be determined and appropriately addressed if life-style changes are to become successful and maintained.

Get What You Expect

HEALTH BEHAVIOR CHANGE: GOALS AND OBJECTIVES

Now that the precursors to health behavior change are clearly understood, the next logical step involves preparing to alter selected health practices. Health behavior change seldom comes overnight or without considerable effort. A plan for change needs to be formulated and sincere commitment to that plan is vital to its success. Later in this chapter a suggested personal wellness plan will be presented. However, prior to presenting that suggested plan, a hierarchy of personal wellness program goals and objectives needs to be established.

Set a Plan

Without the hierarchy of goals and objectives, persons preparing to change health behaviors have no concise meaningful overview of all the key elements of a wellness life-style. On the following page is an example of a hierarchy of goals and objectives to assist the reader to conceptualize a possible sequence and recognize the inherent value of such a plan (Table 3.1).

Hierarchy of Health Behavior Change: Goals and Objectives

Goal

Improved levels of physical, intellectual, emotional, social, spiritual and vocational dimensions of health experienced by responsive individuals as a result of health related knowledge acquired, attitudes changed and behaviors modified in all six dimensions of their lives.

Sub-Goal

Establishment and/or reinforcement of positive health behaviors in the lives of persons who have a desire to achieve human wholeness.

Outcome Objective

To reduce, over time, health risks associated with the lack of regular aerobic exercise, excessive body fat, improper eating habits, poor stress awareness and management practices, and a negative self-image.

Primary Educational and Behavorial Objectives
(Involving knowledge acquired, attitudes changed, and behaviors modified)

- To lower resting heart rate
- To lower exercise heart rate
- To lower total cholesterol
- To lower systolic blood pressure
- To lower diastolic blood pressure
- To achieve maximal participation in selected program interventions
- To attain optimal adherence to selected program intervention strategies
- To promote improvement in personal self-image

Secondary Educational and Behavioral Objectives
(Involving knowledge acquired, attitudes changed, and behaviors modified)

- To reduce consumption of sodium, dietary cholesterol, saturated fat, sugar, and excessive calories
- To increase consumption of complex carbohydrates and dietary fiber
- To reduce percentage of body fat
- To assist in the improvement in time management skills, identification of stressors, and development of relaxation techniques

Educational and Behavioral Change Interventions

- Moderate Exercise
- Body Fat Management
- Dietary Modification
- Stress Awareness and Management
- Positive Self-Image Enhancement

Table 3.1.

HEALTH BEHAVIOR CHANGE: STRATEGIES

Develop Strategies

Many people in today's society would like to improve their health by changing certain behaviors. Throughout America there are countless thousands who recognize the benefits of exercising more, reducing their percentage of body fat, lowering their blood cholesterol levels, quitting smoking cigarettes, managing stress more effectively, and/or enhancing their self-image. Most of these individuals will fail UNLESS they develop effective **health behavior change** strategies and learn to apply the skills needed to make and maintain those changes. Without clearly defined behavior change strategies and the development of accompanying skills needed to break old habits and form new ones, they will almost certainly be doomed to failure.

In spite of what many people believe, most of our **health behaviors** are learned. We are not born into this world with appetites for high fat, high cholesterol and high sodium diets—we learn to eat that way, unfortunately at an early age. We are not born smoking or misusing and abusing alcohol and other drugs. Although the birth process is stressful if not traumatic, we are born with the potential to manage stress and for developing a positive self-image. No matter how long we live, we never lose the ability to reinforce positive health behaviors previously learned or to "rehabit" negative ones which must be altered if we are to live the "wellness life-style."

Behavior Is Learned

Reinforcement or alteration of health behaviors does not occur by chance, based on some vague goals like "I want to get in shape" or "I want to lose weight." Effective and lasting health behavior change is a result of conscious effort built on a foundation of a well designed plan of action. Such a plan is a systematic, step-by-step process for which the individual who is committed to making behavior changes is ultimately responsible. On the following page is an outline of a process which has been used by health educators in their own lives, in counseling their wellness program participants, and in teaching their students who have in turn, successfully applied its principles personally and professionally as health promotion and wellness education specialists (Table 3.2).

STIMULATING MOTIVATION

There are several points which should be clarified and a few that need to be amplified related to the Health Behavior Change Process outlined above. It cannot be emphasized too much that the best motivation for changing health behaviors comes from within the individual. Until a person reaches a point where they acknowledge the need to reduce body fat, to manage stress more effectively, or to quit smoking, they will not be very likely to make a lasting health behavior change. Often a significant emotional event will create a spark which ignites an inner desire to alter a behavior. In some instances, listing behaviors to be changed and their accompanying benefits can be effective motivational factors. The key to success is that the lists and benefits must be specific, relevant, and achievable.

Change Comes From Within

Health Behavior Change Process

1. **Stimulate Motivation**
   a. Capitalize on "significant emotional events" (SEEs).
   b. List desired health behaviors to be changed.
   c. Make a list of long term and short term benefits for changing each behavior.

2. **Formulate Objectives**
   a. State specific objectives for each behavior to be changed.
   b. Specify steps to be taken to achieve objectives.
   c. Establish specific "checkpoint" dates to evaluate progress toward achieving those objectives.
   d. Prepare and sign a health behavior change contract. (Ask a "witness" to also sign the contract).
   e. Tell others about your objectives and progress.

3. **Implement an Action Plan**
   a. Identify triggers and avoid them.
   b. Substitute positive, competing behaviors.
   c. Break negative behavior chains.
   d. Reward yourself.
   e. Plan small steps/Strive for gradual, steady progress.
   f. Use mental imagery/Alternative thinking/ Positive self-talk.
   g. Get help from others — Use social support/Buddy system.

4. **Keep Records**
   a. Use an exercise log.
   b. Use a fat, fiber, and sodium log.
   c. Keep personal stress management and positive self-image enhancement diaries.
   d. Develop your own record keeping process.

5. **Maintain New Behavior**

Table 3.2.

FORMULATING OBJECTIVES

Plan Is Specific

Objectives to be pursued, steps to be taken, and checkpoint dates which are established to serve as benchmarks in the behavior change process must all be as specific as possible. If any of these three elements are stated vaguely, they will reduce the likelihood of successfully altering health habits and practices. Preparing and signing a health behavior change contract, asking someone to witness that commitment by also signing, and telling others about the objectives and progress will help in the achievement of expected outcomes.

IMPLEMENTING AN ACTION PLAN

Be Aware of Negatives

Identification of triggers and obstacles is an important aspect of any health behavior change action plan. Recognizing that sitting at the dinner table after a meal can create an urge to smoke in a person trying to quit or that hectic schedules can crowd out plans to exercise are examples of triggers and obstacles, respectively. Substituting positive, competing behaviors is an effective strategy to use in avoiding triggers. Getting up from the table immediately after eating and going for a leisurely walk or working on a favorite hobby instead of smoking a cigarette are examples of positive, competing behaviors. Breaking negative behavior chains is also a key to the successful implementation of a healthful action plan, and in the process, overcoming obstacles. Breaking away from a sedentary pattern of living by scheduling aerobics into the Monday, Wednesday, and Friday lunch periods of one's monthly calendar is an example of a technique to use in implementing an action plan which addresses the obstacle of a busy daily schedule in the planning process.

Need For Rewards

Rewards are also extremely important aspects of a health behavior change action plan. They need to be both short term and long term in nature. Rewarding oneself for exercising, for staying within the daily fat budget or for not smoking a cigarette during the past 24 hours by setting aside time to read the newspaper or a good novel at the end of the day are all examples of short term rewards. Setting aside one dollar for every mile walked or jogged, for any fast food meal avoided or for each pack of cigarettes not smoked and then buying a new outfit of clothing or some other item wanted for a considerable time, are examples of long term rewards.

Slow But Sure

Perhaps the secret to successfully implementing a health behavior change plan is to make small changes—slowly, yet steadily. One of the world's great sayings is "by small and simple things, great things come to pass." If small behavior changes are gradually, but continuously made over time, the results become cumulative and often quite significant. As a case in point, if a person will alter their milk drinking behavior from whole milk to 2% to 1% to $^1/_2$% and finally to skim milk, over a period of weeks or even months, the fat content of that person's milk consumption can be reduced by a whopping *20 times* for *each* eight ounce glass. An eight ounce glass of skim milk contains only .4 of a gram of fat whereas the some amount of whole milk has 8 grams of fat.

Think Positive

The use of mind imagery, alternative thinking, and positive self-talk are other important strategies to employ when designing a health behavior change action plan. Imagining doing positive things which will enhance one's personal health can create a "success pattern" in the mind. In essence, this is simply an application of Robert Rosenthall's psychological theory commonly known as the Pygmalion effect. That theory essentially states that what we expect in life is usually what we will get. Alternative thinking and positive self-talk produce better decision making abilities and a more upbeat psychological mind set, respectively. As a result, success cycles replace old failure patterns which previously characterized health life-styles. In short, the individuals making health behavior changes realize that if they continue to do what they have always done, they will get what they always have gotten in the past—a level of health lower than that which they are capable of achieving.

An additional and vital factor in successful action planning for health behavior change involves support from significant others in one's life. The use of a support system of family members, friends, and co-workers has proved to be extremely valuable for the majority of people who have used this approach (Figure 3.2). Social reinforcement of new or rehabited forms of health behaviors often tip the scales in favor of their continuation. A buddy system, wherein one's success is tied in some way to the success of another person, is also a highly positive health behavior change reinforcer. Many people would be much less likely to get out of bed at 6:00 a.m. to go walking or to play racquetball if their buddy were not expecting to meet them for their scheduled exercise session together.

Partner Activity

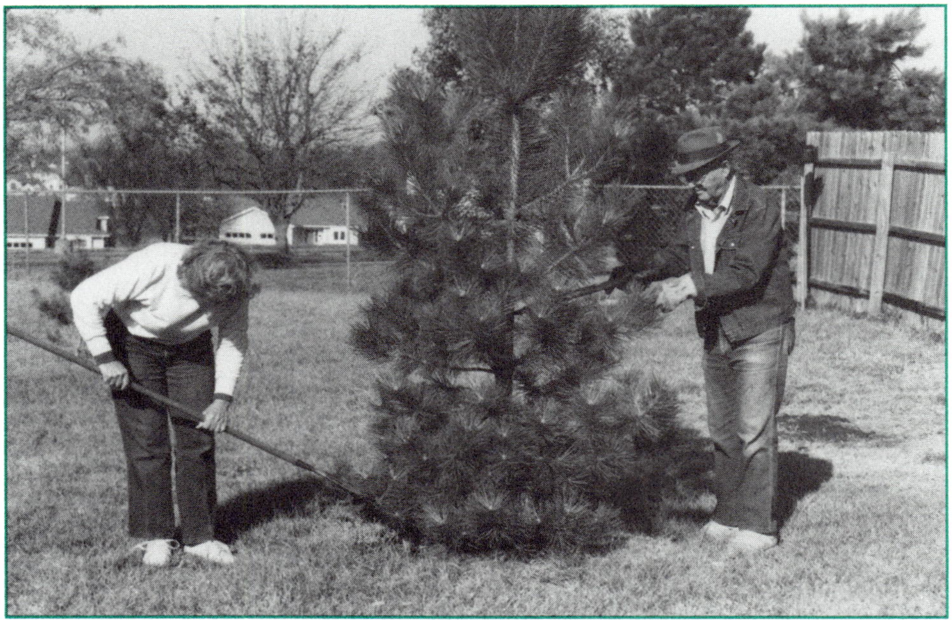

Figure 3.2. Support of spouse and friends influence life-style behavior.

KEEPING RECORDS

Keep a Log

Perhaps one of the most important contributors to successful health behavior change is record keeping. There are numerous ways to keep records and two examples are offered. In Inventory #28, on page 277, a log is provided for a fast and simple way to keep track of physical exercise activities. The exercise log also can be used to identify progress being made and patterns of activity emerging during a given period of time in which the exercise occurs.

A quick and easy approach to keeping records for uses in modifying the diet can be found in Inventory#30 on page 281. Notice that there is no calorie counting involved. The exclusion of counting calories is based on the belief that doing so becomes a laborious and often counterproductive task. Furthermore, emphasis on tracking fat (particularly saturated fat), fiber, and sodium is far more important as a health related focus than is calorie counting for the vast majority of the population.

Fat Tracking

In health behavior interventions associated with stress management and self-image, logs do not appear to be conducive to effective record keeping. In those realms, using diaries to monitor progress toward managing stress or enhancing self-image should prove to be more effective. Of course, in all of the interventions mentioned as well as others which could be included in health behavior change programs, the option of developing other record keeping techniques best suited to the needs of the individual is a viable one.

MAINTAINING NEW HEALTH BEHAVIORS

Because the final segment of this chapter will be devoted to the maintenance of health behavior change, that aspect of the process being discussed herein will be mentioned only in passing. However, an important point related to maintaining new health habits that are formed or those which are "rehabited" should be made. If and when one stumbles and falls along the pathway toward the ultimate goal of human wholeness, he/she should get up as soon as possible and start down the path again.

Stumble But Don't Fall

ASSESSING PERSONAL WELLNESS

Prior to stepping onto the pathway toward human wholeness, the individual must assess the status of his/her personal health. Although there are numerous ways this objective may be accomplished, the following **Personal Wellness Assessment** (Table 3.3) is perhaps the most efficient and effective means available. It employs a set of questions whose answers provide a general overview of the health status frame of reference for the person to consider while preparing to begin the quest for a higher level of wellness.

Begin the Quest

Personal Wellness Assessment

1. **Wellness Inventory** - What are my strengths and weaknesses? What are my "good" and "bad" health habits?
2. **Personal Growth** - What information do I need to acquire in order to improve and/or maintain my health?
3. **Life-Style Risks** - Current health related behaviors—smoking, over-weight, not exercising often enough or hard enough, overeating, and not controlling fat and/or sodium intake, etc.
4. **Current Emotional Condition, Past Family Health History, Past Personal Health History, and Current Personal Health Status**

Table 3.3.

FORMULATING A PERSONAL WELLNESS LIFE-STYLE PLAN

The "bottom line" on the contract for a healthier life—one that has the achievement of human wholeness as its ultimate goal—requires a plan. To some extent, that plan must be well structured and will essentially synthesize what has been presented within this chapter up to this point. For the most part, it is up to the individual to initiate those behaviors to enhance his/her well-being. The more the person wants to make behavior changes and the more they believe that those changes will positively impact their health, the more willing and capable they will be to take the action required. However in spite of the best of intentions, without a systematic plan, the probability for successful health behavior change will be reduced. Therefore, with this thought well in mind, the following Personal Wellness Life-Style Plan (Table 3.4) is offered as an example of a means through which health behavior changes are more likely to be successfully made. It is intended to be readily adaptable to individual needs, and it is believed that it provides the basic structure necessary to guide its user to formulate a personal wellness life-style plan for himself/herself.

MAINTENANCE OF HEALTH BEHAVIOR CHANGE

Maintenance of improved health behavior is a highly complex process. Some behavior change experts believe that one must repeat or abstain from a given activity at least 40 times in order for the change to become a new habit.

Successful Maintenance of Health Behavior Change is Dependent on the Following

1. Formulating realistic expectations
2. Using rewards to reinforce motivation
3. Continuing commitment to alter the behavior
4. Employing self-controlling strategies which include self-monitoring and self-evaluation.

Be Realistic in your Expectations

As previously discussed, realistic expectations are vital to the success of health behavior change. The same is true of maintaining behavior changes which are intended to improve health status. For many people in today's society, living a healthy life-style is associated with "suffering" through regular, vigorous exercise; "depriving" themselves of eating foods they love, and generally feeling "guilty" if they indulge in anything pleasurable. Behavior change strategies which employ what could best be termed the "traditional approach" are often based on fear of disease, competitive themes, and punitive approaches with an external control orientation. A more realistic approach to health behavior change involves developing expectations which are kinder and gentler and which emphasize self-trust and self-esteem instead of self-deprivation and self-control. Such expectations are based on the joy of living, cooperative themes, and the development of behaviors which evolve from an internal cue system.

Positive Approach

Such an internal cue system relates closely to the use of rewards to reinforce motivation, which in turn, is vital to the success of health behavior change. **Cues**, which are also known as antecedents, manifest themselves in the form of environmental factors which trigger given behaviors. Rewards, which are also known as consequences, more often than not need to be short term or they will lose their effectiveness. In essence, the relationship between cues, behavior, and rewards is best characterized by the diagram on page 44.

Personal Wellness Life-Style Plan

The following completed plan is an example for your review . Please turn to Inventory #26 on page 271 and detail "your" Personal Wellness Life-Style Plan.

1. **Specific** wellness life-style intervention objectives I would be realistically able and willing to work on are as follows:
   a. **Moderate Exercise** - Complete my three exercise sessions per week and participate in at least one other weekend aerobic activity.
   b. **Body Fat Management** - Reduce my DAILY caloric intake by at least 500 calories (100 calories/day maximum reduction).
   c. **Dietary Modification** - Reduce my sodium, sugar, and saturated fat intake and increase my consumption of complex carbohydrates.
   d. **Stress Management** - "Rebalance" my autonomic nervous system three times each day through aerobic exercise, meditation, prayer, relaxation techniques, mind imagery, etc.
   e. **Smoking Cessation** - Not applicable to me.
   f. **Positive Self-Image Enhancement** - Use positive self-talk and "I Am Loved and Capable Thoughts" throughout the day.

2. Of the above wellness life-style interventions, the ONE I will select as my PERSONAL HEALTH BEHAVIOR CHANGE is: Dietary Modification

3. Specific steps I will take to achieve the objectives in my chosen health behavior changes are:
   a. Determine what my DAILY total fat and saturated fat "budgets" should be.
   b. Start using my fat "budgets."
   c. Begin to substitute complex carbohydrates for high fat foods.

4. Dates by which I plan to achieve:
   a. February 27
   b. February 28
   c. March 1

5. Rewards (specify LT for long term and ST for short term) I will give myself for completing each step are:
   Celebrate my first day of controlled consumption of high fat foods by going to a movie (ST). Buy a new clothing/hobbie item on the 30th day of sustained control of dietary fat consumption (LT).

6. Following are some of the benefits (specify LT for long term and ST for short term) I expect to gain from my Personal Wellness Life-Style Plan:
   Better health from reduction of dietary fat intake (LT). Improved self-image because of improved "life control" (ST and LT).

7. Obstacles that might get in the way of my success are:
   a. Friend says "programs" like this one never work.
   b. "Slip" and have a Snickers candy bar for afternoon snack.
   c. Over consume fat on a given day and exceed my daily budget.

8. Ways I can avoid or remove these obstacles:
   a. Use positive self-talk to counteract doubt.
   b. Adjust fat budgeting for remainder of day.
   c. Alter fat budgeting for the rest of week.

9. I will keep track of my progress by:
   Entering relevant behavior change activities and fat amounts (in grams) consumed daily in my health behavior modification log.

10. I will commit myself to this Wellness Life-Style Plan by signing below:

____
("Life-Style Changer")

____
(Date)

____
(Witness)

____
(Date)

Table 3.4.

Cues	⇒	Behavior	⇒	Rewards

Cues

In such a relationship, each health related behavior is activated in response to one or more cues. The more numerous or powerful the cues, the greater the likelihood that the behavior will be activated. The behavior can then be tracked to the rewards associated with it. The more immediate and meaningful the reward, the more likely the behavior will be repeated in the future.

Continuing the commitment to altering health behavior change is often the most difficult aspect of the process. Because people soon forget the negative consequences associated with the previous health behaviors they are attempting to change, they often fail to maintain their commitment.

Strategies designed to enhance adherence to exercise and other positive health behaviors must stress that instant health gains without effort are not realistic. "Diet pills" or other rapid weight loss programs may appear to be the answer, but in reality, permanent behavior alterations such as switching from whole to skim milk products are the only kinds of changes which will be effective over time. Such a health behavior change will have a much better chance of becoming permanent because a lasting commitment to maintaining the change will have been made.

Self-image Is Key

Individuals who develop an internal locus of control relative to their health behaviors experience greater success in behavioral changes. Because they take better care of themselves, they feel better about themselves. The better they feel about themselves (measured by improvement in self-image), the more they want to take better care of themselves. Such a pattern becomes a cycle which enhances all dimensions of the person's health and total being. Individuals who begin to feel they have greater self worth and who value themselves enough to commit the expenditure of time and effort to improve their own wellness, are more apt to maintain healthy behavior changes. This is especially true if they continually monitor and evaluate their progress. The end result of the health behavior change and maintenance process is a feeling of being in control of and effectively managing one's life. It is no coincidence that such a result is also the reward of the health for human wholeness life-style previously discussed in

Suggested Readings

Ardell, D.B. and J. Langdon. *Wellness: The Body, Mind, and Spirit.* Dubuque, IA: Kendall/ Hunt Publishing Company, 1988.

Donatelle, R.J., L. G. Davis, and C. F. Hoover. *Access To Health.* Englewood Cliffs, NJ: Prentice Hall, Chapter 1, 1991.

Girdano, D.A. and D. E. Dusek. *Changing Health Behavior.* Scottsdale, AZ: Gorsuch Scarisbrick Publishers, 1988.

Hales, D. *An Invitation To Health.* Redwood City, CA:The Benjamin/Cummings Company, Chapter 1, 1992.

Roberts, S.W. *Health Wellness: An Introductory Approach.* Dubuque, IA: eddie bowers publishing, inc., Chapter 1, 1992.

CHAPTER 4

SPECIFICITY OF EXERCISE TRAINING

Tom Thomas

Learning Objectives

- Describe the metabolic energy sources for aerobic and anaerobic activity.
- Comprehend the role of physical activity in gaining and maintaining health and fitness.
- Describe the cardiovascular response to a single bout of exercise.
- Determine the time frame for losing the effects of training due to inactivity and lay-offs.
- List factors which dictate what fuels are used for exercise energy.
- Become familiar with the components and concepts related to oxygen consumption.
- Know terms and concepts which are associated with exercise training for specific personal goals.
- Understand the adaptation of the cardiovascular system to exercise training.

Important Terms

adenosine triphosphate (ATP)
aerobics
aerobic training
anaerobics
atherosclerotic plaque
blood glucose
carbohydrate (CHO)
cardiac output
contractility
creatine phosphate (CP)
detraining
exercise training
fast-twitch fibers
free fatty acids (FFA)
glycogen
hypoxia
lactate threshold
maintenance training
maximal oxygen consumption (VO_2 max)
oxygen consumption (VO_2)
recovery energy
slow-twitch fibers
triglycerides (TG)
type I fibers
type IIa fibers
type IIb fibers

SPECIFICITY OF EXERCISE TRAINING

The physiological and biochemical systems of the body adapt to the stress of exercise in different ways depending upon the type of activity which is performed. Physical activity can be divided basically into two categories: anaerobic and aerobic. A single bout of activity is called acute exercise while repeated bouts of exercise over a period of time is called exercise training.

ANAEROBICS

Key is Producing ATP

Anaerobics refers to high intensity, short-burst activity in which the muscles rely heavily on the production of energy without adequate oxygen. **Adenosine triphosphate (ATP)** is a key substrate for this high intensity activity. ATP is the only immediate source of energy for muscular contraction. Other energy sources must be converted to ATP for use by the muscle. **Muscle creatine phosphate (CP)** and stored **carbohydrate (CHO)** called glycogen are utilized to replenish ATP during vigorous exercise (Table 4.1). The anaerobic use of glycogen produces lactic acid, a metabolic end product which can cause fatigue. High intensity activity cannot be sustained for very long periods because anaerobic metabolism is very inefficient, and the contracting muscle fibers generally do not tolerate the increased acidity caused by the buildup of lactic acid.

Energy Sources

Anaerobic Activity	Aerobic Activity
Adenosine Triphosphate (ATP)	Muscle Glycogen
Creatine Phosphate (CP)	Adipose Triglycerides (TG)
Muscle Glycogen	Liver Glycogen and Blood Glucose
	Muscle Triglycerides

Table 4.1.

Plus and Minus of Hard Exercise

Anaerobics make the heart and cardiovascular system work very hard. In the trained individual, this has little adverse effect and may at times be beneficial to the total physiological fitness of the individual. For example, high intensity activity enhances muscular strength, improves anaerobic performance, and stimulates energy use during exercise and in recovery. For the older individual, especially those out of condition, high intensity activity may do more harm than good. Atherosclerotic plaque in coronary vessels and other arteries may produce sufficient constriction to prevent adequate blood flow to the hard working skeletal muscles and the heart and brain. The result can be a serious hypoxia or lack of oxygen to these vital organs.

Fast and Slow Twitch

Anaerobic exercise utilizes primarily **fast-twitch muscle fibers** and especially Type IIb, the most anaerobic fibers (Table 4.2). These fibers are very adept at producing large amounts of anaerobic energy. Thus, they can work very hard for short periods of time, but **Type IIb fibers** fatigue relatively quickly. **Type IIa fibers** also are used in short-burst work, but they have less anaerobic capacity than the IIb fibers. Even the slow-twitch or **Type I fibers** are involved in anaerobic activity. Because these fibers have a lower threshold for stimulation than fast-twitch fibers, they are recruited in high intensity activity, but they provide only a little help since **slow-twitch muscle fibers** cannot produce large amounts of anaerobic energy. Only when the fast-twitch muscle fibers begin to fatigue, do the slow-twitch fibers play a significant role in performing anaerobic work. At this time anaerobic performance declines. These principles indicate, however, that both fast and slow-twitch fibers can be affected by anaerobic training.

Basic Differences Among Muscle Fiber Types

Characteristics	Fiber Type		
	Slow Twitch I	***Fast-Twitch IIa***	***Fast-Twitch IIb***
Animal Nomenclature	SO*	FOG	FG
% in Typical Muscle	50	34	16
Twitch Time	slow	fast	fast
Color	red	white	white
Fatigue	slow	fast	fast
Motor Neuron Size	small	large	large
Stimulation Velocity	slow	fast	fast
Threshold:Ease to Stimulate	low:easy	high:harder	high:harder
Aerobic Capacity	high	medium	low
Oxidative Enzymes	high	medium	low
Mitochondria Number	high	medium	low
Anaerobic Capacity	low	medium	high
Lactate Production	low	medium	high
Fat Stores	high	low	low
Glycogen	high	high	high

*SO = slow twitch oxidative FOG = twitch oxidative and glycolytic FG = fast twitch glycolytic

Table 4.2.

AEROBICS

Activities which are low enough intensity so that they can be prolonged and thus use large amounts of oxygen are called **aerobics**. The majority of the scientific research indicates that this type of exercise produces the most beneficial overall effects on the body and especially on the cardiovascular system. As with anaerobic exercise, stored ATP is the immediate source of energy for aerobic muscular activity. But these supplies last only a few seconds. Thus, other energy sources must be converted to ATP. **Muscle glycogen** provides a primary energy source for aerobic activity (Table 4.1). In addition, fat stored in muscle and adipose tissue (around stomach, thighs, etc.) also is a valuable source of aerobic energy. This stored fat is called **triglycerides (TG)**. TG are broken down to **free fatty acids (FFA)** prior to use by muscle. Carbohydrate in blood is called blood glucose. This energy source originates from a recently ingested meal or from the liver which can release glucose when the muscles need energy.

Burning Stored Fat

Aerobics depend primarily on slow-twitch fibers which are capable of producing large amounts of aerobic energy because of their numerous cellular mitochondria (Table 4.1). Fast-twitch muscle fibers are not recruited in low intensity activity until the slow-twitch muscles are very fatigued. Type IIa fibers have some aerobic capabilities and thus are able to assist to some degree late in the aerobic workbout. Type IIb muscle fibers have little aerobic capacity and thus cannot sustain aerobic activity for very long. Therefore, aerobic exercise training primarily affects slow-twitch fibers, with some carry-over effect on IIa fibers, but little effect on IIb fibers.

CARBOHYDRATE AND FAT AS ENERGY SOURCES

ATP, CP, and muscle glycogen are the primary fuel sources for anaerobic activity. Muscle glycogen is the primary carbohydrate source of energy during prolonged activities, but some energy also is derived from stored liver glycogen, which is transported to the working muscle in the blood as glucose. The primary source of fat for aerobic exercise is TG stored in adipose tissue such as the stomach and buttocks. This energy is transported to the muscle in the blood, and thus there is a time lag before adipose TG can be used in exercise. Once at the muscle, TG are taken up and degraded to free fatty acids which are then used by the muscle mitochondria to produce aerobic energy.

Key Fuels of Activity

TG stored in skeletal muscle also can be utilized as energy in aerobic activity. However, this source of FFA does not appear to be as important for aerobic metabolism as adipose tissue TG. Trained individuals rely more on TG from muscle than untrained individuals.

Although glycogen is a very effective form of stored energy, most energy in the body is stored as fat. Fat depots are efficient methods of energy storage because fat does not require large quantities of water in storage as does CHO and protein. A gram of stored fat will yield 9 kilocalories (Cal) while a gram of CHO will yield 4 Cal of energy. Body fat stores probably could provide close to 75,000 Cal as energy while CHO only about 2000 Cal. Thus, the supply of CHO is relatively limited and can be depleted in prolonged vigorous work. On the other hand, CHO provides more energy per liter of oxygen (5.0 vs 4.7 kcal/l O_2) and thus is slightly more efficient as an energy source than is fat.

Fat is Where It's At

Because of this greater efficiency, CHO is often mistakenly considered the preferred energy source for all types of activity. Muscle glycogen is a very important fuel and is probably used to some degree in all activities lasting longer than a few seconds. However, the extent that fat or carbohydrate is used as energy depends primarily on the intensity and duration of the exercise bout.

Figure 4.1 illustrates that the body's use of fat is slightly higher than the use of CHO at rest. This illustration assumes that the use of protein for energy is negligible. This assumption is probably accurate except at times when CHO stores are very low such as after very prolonged exercise or in starvation. When an individual works very mildly, up to about 50% of maximal capacity, the extent of fat utilization increases while the use of CHO decreases. At the beginning of light exercise, stored ATP, CP, and CHO are the most important energy sources, but after sufficient FFA mobilization occurs and a steady metabolic rate is achieved, fat becomes the primary energy source. Therefore, fat is the principle energy substrate, providing up to 75% of the total energy requirement after 15-30 minutes of light exercise (50% **maximal oxygen consumption, VO_2 max,** heart rate about 130 bpm).

Use of Fat and Carbohydrate as Energy Sources During Exercise of Different Intensities

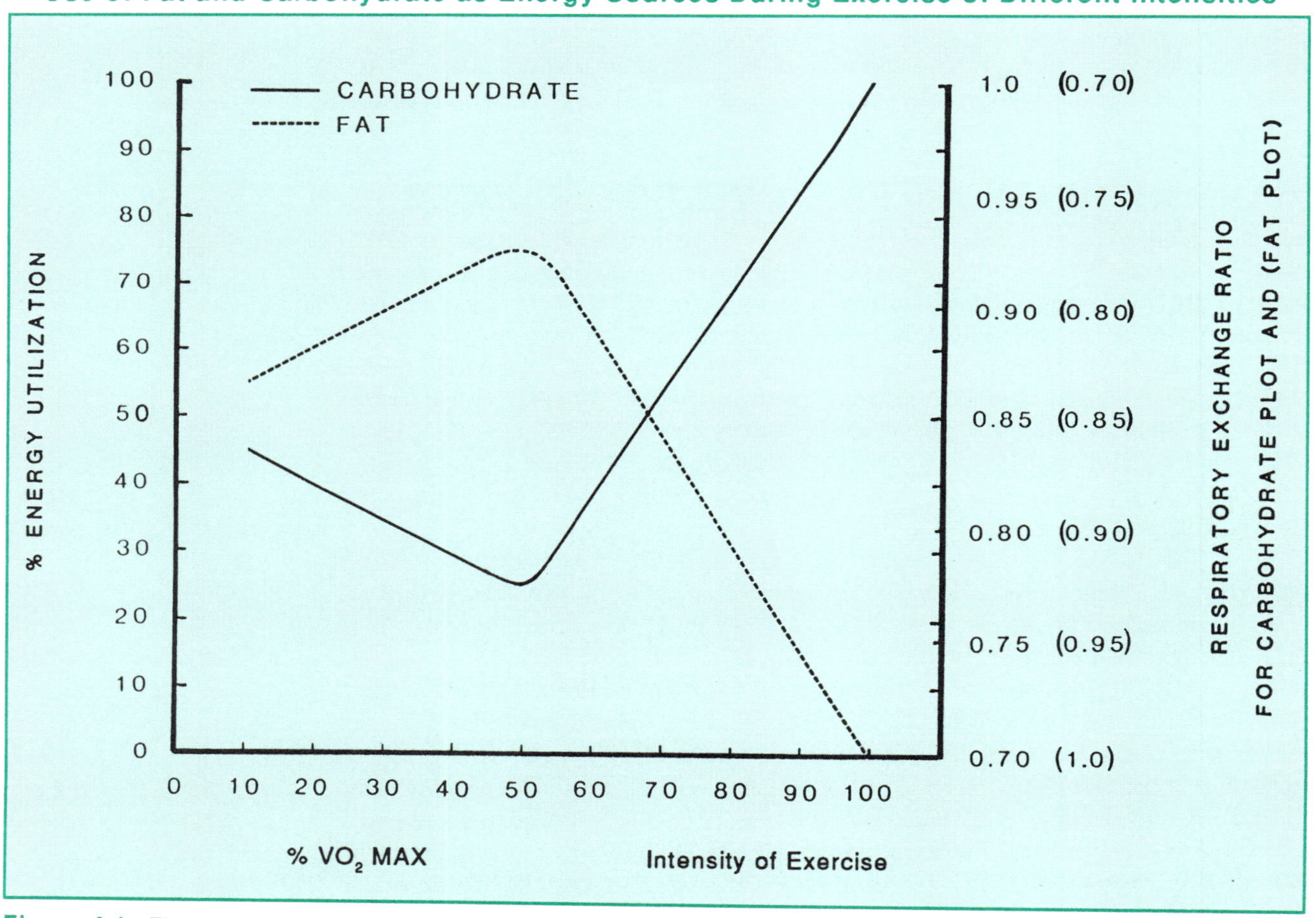

Figure 4.1. The respiratory exchange ratio (RER) is the relationship between the carbon dioxide produced and the oxygen consumed by the body. The RER provides an estimate of the relative contribution of fat and CHO to the total energy cost.

From 50-100% VO_2 max, the use of CHO increases with the exercise intensity, while the use of fat is decreased as the work gets harder. Fat and carbohydrate are used equally for energy at about 60-70% VO_2 max (heart rate about 150 bpm). Lactic acid from anaerobic CHO metabolism in high intensity exercise inhibits fat utilization. At 100% maximal capacity, CHO provides nearly 100% of the required energy if stored ATP and CP supplies are depleted.

Use of Fat as an Energy Source at Different Exercise Durations and in Recovery

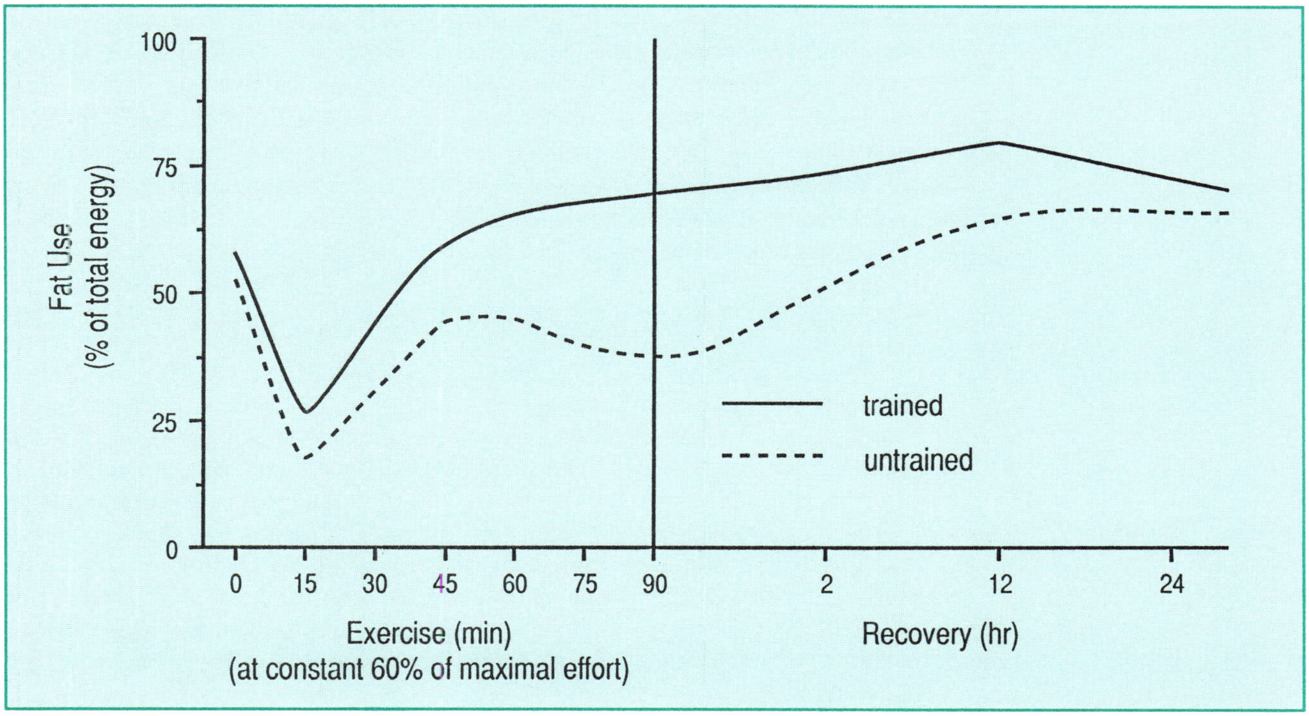

Figure 4.2.

Another factor which is a critical determinant of energy utilization is the exercise duration (Figure 4.2). Very little fat is used for energy during the initial 15 minutes of exercise. After 20 minutes, fat begins to be burned and contributes an increasingly greater proportion of the energy as exercise is prolonged. As the figure indicates, an aerobically trained individual utilizes more fat during exercise than an untrained person.

When exercise ends, the body's increased metabolic rate does not stop immediately but gradually slows down. This recovery energy use can be very small and last only a few minutes or may be large and continue for several hours after the exercise bout. Recovery energy use is especially high after prolonged, high intensity exercise. However, even following moderate exercise for 45-60 min, recovery may continue for about 12 hours and account for an additional 100 kcal. In contrast, recovery energy use may be only 2-3 kcal after a low intensity 20 min walk. In either case, fat provides the majority of the energy for fueling the recovery process (Fig. 4.2).

An
Hour
a
Day

Slow-twitch fibers are very adept at using both CHO and fat as energy sources. The aerobic metabolism of these foodstuffs depends on the number and efficiency of the fiber mitochondria. The aerobic slow-twitch fibers have more mitochondria with enhanced aerobic enzyme activity. In contrast, fast-twitch fibers utilize CHO better than they use fat, although the intermediate IIa fibers can utilize fat better than the anaerobic IIb fibers.

Training the Fat

The curves in Figures 4.1 and 4.2 are shifted in certain conditions. Endurance trained individuals utilize fat better than untrained or anaerobically trained persons. This allows distance athletes to utilize more fat during prolonged exercise and conserve the limited CHO energy. Exercise in hot temperatures stimulates greater use of CHO, while work in the cold causes a greater use of fat than in a temperate environment. Diet also affects the energy substrate used during exercise. Increased dietary fat intake enhances the utilization of fat during exercise, while diets high in CHO stimulate the use of CHO during exercise. This phenomenon probably relates to the availability of these substrates for muscular uptake as they are carried in the blood after digestion and absorption.

PHYSIOLOGICAL EFFECTS OF EXERCISE

Exercise causes the physiological systems of the body to respond in a unified way in order to increase the oxygen supply to working muscles. The cardiovascular effects of a single maximal exercise bout are summarized in Table 4.3. Resting values are contrasted with maximal values to illustrate the magnitude of change for each CV variable. **Oxygen consumption (VO_2)** is enhanced about 12-16 fold from rest to maximal exercise. This response is possible due to the large increases in heart rate and stroke volume. Also improved is the tissue uptake of oxygen as indicated by the arterial and venous O_2 difference (A-VO_2). Elevations in muscle blood flow, blood pressure, and ventilation also support the enhanced delivery of oxygen to working tissues.

Cardiovascular Response to Acute Maximal Exercise in Healthy Young Adults

CV Parameter	Rest	Maximal Exercise
O_2 Consumption (l/min)	0.25	3.5*
O_2 Consumption (ml/kg/min)	3.5†	50.0*
Heart Rate (bpm)	72	190
Stroke Volume (ml)	70*	120*
Cardiac Output (l/min)	5*	23*
Arterial-Venous O_2 (ml%)	5	15
Blood Pressure (mm Hg)	120/80	180/80
Blood Flow to Working Muscles (l/min)	1	20
Blood Lactic Acid (mg%)	15	100
Respiratory Ventilation (l/min)	6	100*

* Female values are about 10-20% lower   † 1 MET

Table 4.3.

Repeating the exercise bouts over several months or years is called exercise training, and this causes changes in the way the cardiovascular system meets the oxygen requirements of the body at rest, during submaximal exercise, and during maximal exercise. Perhaps the most significant alteration induced by aerobic training is the ability of the heart to pump more blood with each stroke while maintaining a lower heart rate at all levels of work. CV parameters at rest and maximal exercise before and after a training program are contrasted in Tables 4.4 and 4.5. At rest, the heart maintains a constant cardiac output of about 5 liters per minute before and after a training program. However, in the trained state the cardiac output is obtained with a larger stroke volume and lower heart rate than before training. This is due in part to the myocardial hypertrophy and improved contractility induced by chronic aerobic activity.

You're All Heart

Cardiovascular Adaptation to Aerobic Exercise Training—Rest

CV Parameter	Rest	
	Before Training	After Training*
O_2 Consumption (l/min)	0.25	0.25
O_2 Consumption (ml/kg/min)	3.5	3.5
Heart Rate (bpm)	72	60
Stroke Volume (ml)	70	84
Cardiac Output (l/ml)	5	5
Arterial-Venous O_2 (ml%)	5	5
Blood Pressure (mm Hg)	120/80	120/80
Blood Flow to Muscles (l/min)	1	1.5
Blood Lactic Acid (mg%)	15	15
Respiratory Ventilation (l/min)	6	6
Heart Size		increased
Myocardial Thickness		increased
Myocardial Contractility		increased
Myocardial Capillary Supply		increased
Parasympathetic Influence		increased
Sympathetic Influence		decreased

* Before and after one year of aerobic training

Table 4.4.

Cardiovascular Adaptations to Aerobic Exercise Training-Maximal Exercise Response

CV Parameter	Maximal Exercise	
	Before Training	After Training*
O_2 Consumption (l/min)	3.5†	4.4†
O_2 Consumption (ml/kg/min)	50†	60†
Heart Rate (bpm)	190	188
Stroke Volume (ml)	120†	150†
Cardiac Output (l/min)	23†	28†
Arterial-Venous O_2 (ml%)	15	16
Blood Pressure	180/80	190/80
Blood Flow to Working Muscles (l/min)	20†	25†
Blood Lactic Acid (mg%)	100	150
Respiratory Ventilation (l/min)	100†	120†

* Before and After one year of aerobic training.
† Female values are 10-20% lower.

Table 4.5.

Metabolic Adaptations to Exercise Training*

Metabolic Parameter	Effect
Total Body Fat	Decreased
Muscle Fat Stores	Increased
Muscle Glycogen Stores	Increased
Blood Triglycerides	Decreased
Fat Utilization	Increased
Fat Cell Size	Decreased
Fat Mobilization Enzymes	Increased
Aerobic Enzymes	Increased
Anaerobic Enzymes	Little Effect
Mitochondria	Increased
Lactate Threshold	Increased
Lactic Acid Production	Decreased
Lactic Acid Tolerance	Increased
Insulin Sensitivity	Increased
Catecholamine Sensitivity	Increased
Heat Tolerance	Increased

* After one year of aerobic training

Table 4.6.

After training, the CV adaptation to maximal exercise is characterized by an enhanced stroke volume and slight improvement in A-VO_2. Blood flow to working muscles and respiratory ventilation also are increased as a result of consistent aerobic training. The net result is an increased maximal oxygen consumption of about 20% compared to before training. The ability of the body to take in and utilize oxygen during maximal work may be the single best measure of overall cardiorespiratory fitness. Numerous tests have been developed to estimate VO_2 max and one such test is described in Inventories #24 and 25 on pgs. 267 and 269.

In addition to cardiovascular changes induced by aerobic training, numerous metabolic alterations occur in skeletal muscle which improve the efficiency of energy production (Table 4.6). Most of these changes enhance the aerobic capacity of muscle and its ability to utilize fat. Since the muscles of the trained individual rely more heavily on aerobic metabolism, they can work harder before requiring substantial anaerobic energy metabolism and the production of lactic acid. The intensity or pace of the exercise which causes a significant lactic acid accumulation in blood is called the lactate threshold. If an individual exercises beyond this intensity, lactic acid accumulates, breathing becomes labored, and the exercise gets uncomfortable. If the exercise is kept below the lactate threshold, the workbout can be prolonged and still be comfortable. Therefore, it is important for each individual to estimate the lactate threshold. One simple way is to note the exercise intensity which causes hard breathing or the inability to talk during exercise. At the beginning of a training program, the exerciser may be able to work at only 50-60% VO_2 max before substantial anaerobic metabolism is required (Figure 4.3). As a result of chronic aerobic training, the lactate threshold may be elevated to 65-70% VO_2 max. Elite distance athletes can exercise at 75-85% VO_2 max before significant amounts of lactate accumulate. This allows them to maintain a much faster pace for a longer time than individuals with lower anaerobic thresholds.

Don't Cross the Threshold

Aerobic exercise may also help relieve tension, promote improved feelings of well-being and self concept, and improve productivity. Some information from epidemiological research indicates that aerobic exercise training may improve longevity. However, this hypothesis needs further research. It may take several decades, when the participants of the current aerobic fitness boom reach old age, before the effect of chronic activity on longevity can be determined. In the meantime, exercisers can take heart because research evidence suggests that they have healthier, more productive lives than non-exercisers. Chronic exercisers have fewer absences, less time in the hospital, and fewer illnesses than sedentary populations. Thus, it may be unwise to wait until the final answer on exercise and longevity is determined before instituting an exercise training program.

Lactate Threshold Untrained and Trained

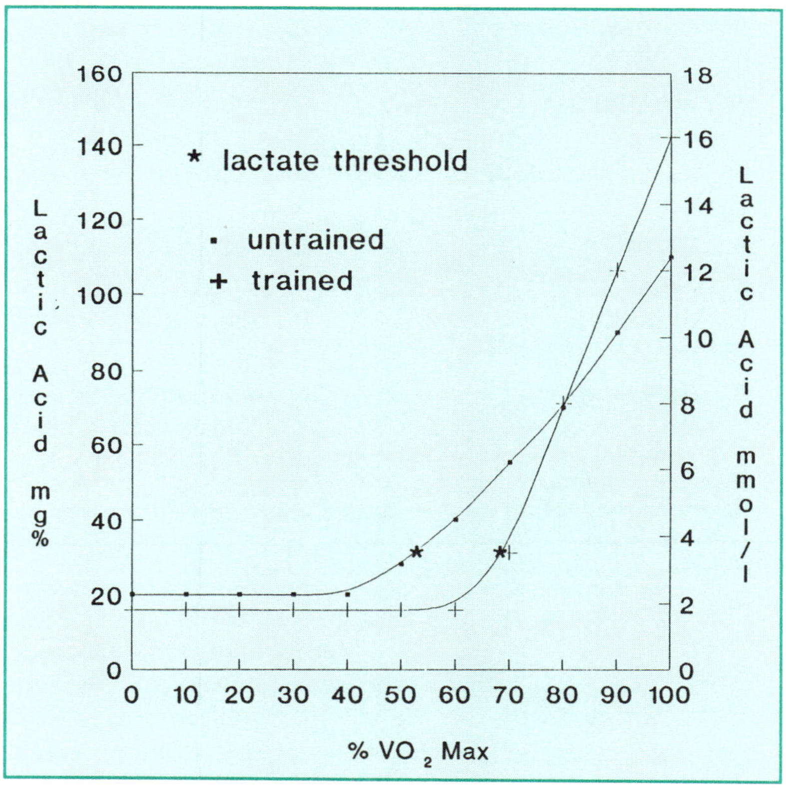

Figure 4.3. The difference in the lactate threshold between untrained and endurance trained individuals. The endurance athlete is able to work at a higher exercise intensity before lactic acid accumulates in blood.

EXERCISE AND CARDIOVASCULAR FITNESS

A physically active life-style is an important component in CV health. But some types of exercise are better for the heart than others (Table 4.7). CV activity is aerobic and causes the heart to work moderately for a prolonged period of time. Anaerobic activities are not as effective as aerobic in producing beneficial CV adaptation. Sometimes these short-burst activities can be detrimental to the heart.

Characteristics of Cardiovascular Exercise

1. **Moderate Intensity**	60% maximal oxygen consumption or 75% maximal heart rate (140-160 beats per min) or 60% heart rate reserve or 12-15 RPE or 6-8 METS
2. **Prolonged**	At least 30 minutes of continuous activity
3. **Continuous**	Non-stop activity
4. **Frequent**	3-5 times per week, alternate days
5. **Large Muscle Groups**	Total body activity, especially the legs
6. **Calorific**	Burn 300-500 kcal/session
7. **Extended**	At least one year program duration
8. **Relaxing**	Non-competitive enjoyable activity

Example activities: *jogging, brisk walking, stepping, swimming, level cycling, skilled rope jumping, hiking, rowing, cross country skiing, some types of aerobic dancing.*

Table 4.7.

Many of the cardiovascular variables such as the lipid profile (Table 4.8) and body fat require an extended exercise training program (~one year) to be affected. Therefore, rapid reduction in CV disease risk cannot be expected to occur. Rather, exercise should become part of the total long-term life-style. The characteristics in Table 4.7 are not meant to be starting points. The CV exercise training program should progress to these goals. Any type of exercise which can meet these criteria should be considered appropriate for CV fitness. It is likely that any low-moderate intensity activity will benefit the overall health of an individual even if the activity does not meet all the CV exercise characteristics.

Values for Blood Lipids and Lipoproteins in Young Adults

Variables (mg%)	Men		Heart Disease Patients	Women	
	Healthy	Endurance Trained		Healthy	Endurance Trained
Total Triglycerides	90	80	180	80	70
Total Cholesterol	190	180	240	185	180
HDL-Cholesterol	45	60	39	60	75
HDL_2-Cholesterol	12	18	8	18	22
LDL-Cholesterol	125	110	160	115	100
VLDL-Cholesterol	20	10	40	10	5
Total Cholesterol / HDL-Cholesterol	4.2	3.0	6.0	3.0	2.5
Apoprotein A-1	120	160	110	135	180
Apoprotein B	110	90	150	100	90

Table 4.8.

CARDIOVASCULAR DETRAINING

Exercise programs are invariably interrupted, sometimes due to illness or injury and sometimes due to other job and family priorities. Withdrawal from training initiates a reversal process called detraining in which benefits from exercise begin to decline. Many of the physiological and psychological gains from training recede rapidly. The rate of this decline and the amount of loss due to inactivity may depend on the fitness level of the individual. Persons who have been chronic exercisers for at least one year seem to lose fitness rather slowly. In one research study, habitual exercisers lost only 16% of their endurance capacity after three months of detraining. Likewise, heart function, body composition, and blood lipids are only little changed in exercisers following several weeks of detraining. Even after several months, detrained exercisers have much higher CV fitness levels than untrained people. Many trained individuals notice the psychological detriments of a layoff much more quickly. They recognize that something is missing from their life-style and report sluggishness and decreased performance after missing only a few exercise sessions.

Dangers of Reversal

On the other hand, individuals without an extensive training base seem to lose CV fitness very rapidly. Following short-term training, such as a 12 week aerobic dance class, most of the fitness gains are lost in four weeks. This loss can be offset by maintenance training in which the aerobic exercise is performed only one or two days per week. This theory suggests that even periodic exercise can be helpful if some exercise sessions must be missed. Fitness also may be maintained by reducing exercise duration, e.g., from 40 minutes to 20 minutes, while continuing to exercise three to four times per week. However, the intensity of the training must be continued if complete CV fitness is to be maintained. That is, if less frequent training is performed, the target heart rate of the initial training program must be maintained in the reduced training workouts.

Intensity is the Key

Long-Term Fitness Base

Thus, the key to preventing CV detraining is establishing a long-term (one to two years) fitness base. In addition, maintenance exercise of once or twice per week for 30 to 40 min duration *or* three times per week for 15 to 20 minute duration can prevent the loss of CV fitness. These principles illustrate the importance of developing a long-term exercise training program. The exercise must be enjoyable and convenient so it can become part of the life-style. But even if several exercise sessions must be missed, it is important to realize that reduced aerobic exercise can help maintain CV fitness. In addition, activity sessions of even shorter duration and lower intensity may not develop CV fitness but can have other important health benefits. Healthy activities are discussed in Chapters 5 and 6.

Aerobic Dance

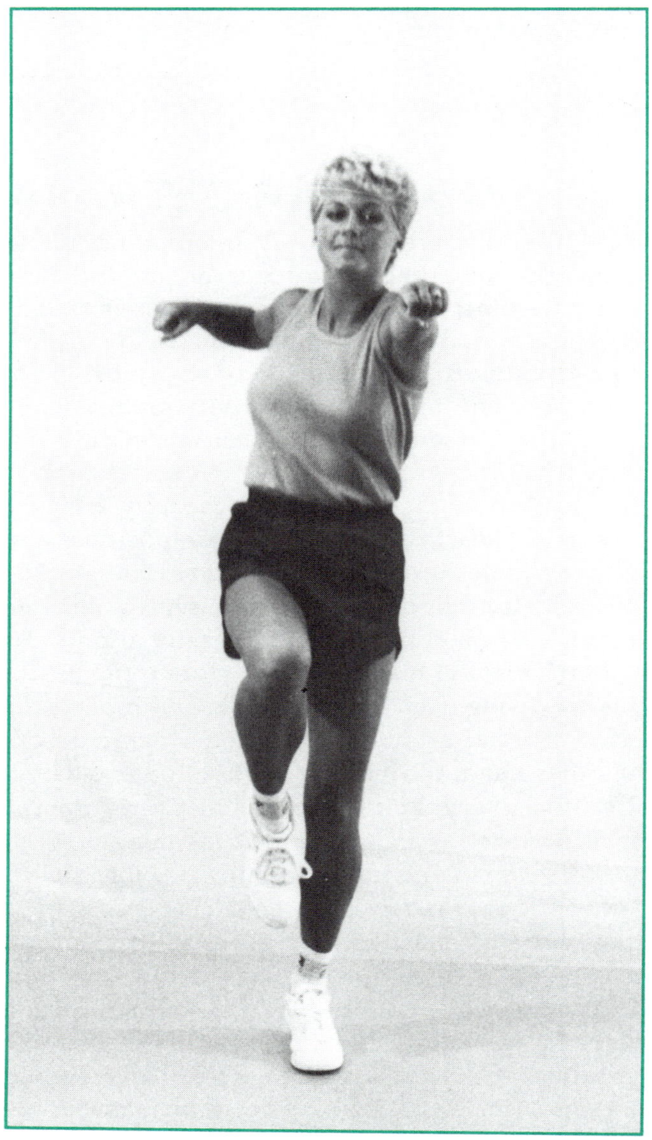

Suggested Readings

American College of Sports Medicine. The recommended quantity and quality of exercise. *Medicine and Science in Sports and Exercise* 22:265-274, 1990.

Fox, E.L., R.W. Bowers, and M.L. Foss. *The Physiological Basis of Physical Education and Athletics*. Philadelphia: Saunders, Chapters 2, 3, 13, and 15, 1988.

LaPorte, R.E. and S.N. Blair. Physical activity or cardiovascular fitness: Which is more important for health? *Physician and Sportsmedicine* 13:145-157, March, 1985.

This chapter is adapted from a chapter which first appeared in T.R. Thomas and C.J. Zebas. *Scientific Exercise Training*. Dubuque: Kendall/Hunt, 1987. Reprinted with permission.

CHAPTER 5

STARTING AND MAINTAINING ACTIVITY

Tom Thomas

Learning Objectives

- List guidelines and strategies for those people just beginning an exercise program.
- Understand the discomforts associated with an exercise program and know precautions to help prevent them.
- Describe the exercise target heart rate and know how to estimate and monitor it.
- List strategies to use for staying with an exercise program.
- Know guidelines for appropriate exercise prescription for persons seeking cardiovascular fitness.
- Describe potentially dangerous physical activities and guidelines to decrease the danger.
- Outline clothing strategies to use during exercise in hot and cold weather.

Important Terms

adherence

angina pectoris

breathholding

catecholamines

cool-down

dehydration

heart rate reserve (HRR)

hyperventilation

metabolic equivalent (MET)

myocardial oxygen consumption

rating of perceived exertion (RPE)

talk test

target heart rate (THR)

INTRODUCTION

One of the problems associated with increasing the activity level is that it is easy to start-off too rigorously, to do too much too quickly. It may have taken years to get out of shape, and it is important to allow plenty of time to get back into shape. Perhaps the most important consideration early in an exercise program is personal comfort. It is important that an individual really enjoy the activity being performed. You say there is no activity that you enjoy? Then fitness will be a long uphill battle! Nearly everyone can find some form of movement that is enjoyable and/or relaxing, even if it is a casual walk around the block. Be open to trying new activities, new exercise equipment. You might discover just the right mode for you. But if the activity causes pain or if it is a real chore to perform, it is very likely that it will not be continued. All the reports about how good an activity is for you does not matter, if you will not do it.

Too Much Too Quick

PRINCIPLES OF COMFORTABLE EXERCISE

GETTING STARTED

A list of some items to consider when exercising is presented in Table 5.1. Initiating the activity may be the hardest part of any conditioning program. If progression is too rapid, aches and pains may arise in previously unheard from places. The key to starting to exercise is to begin at a very low volume and progress very slowly. How slow should one progress? It is not possible to progress too slowly. Add to the exercise load by increasing the intensity or duration but not both simultaneously. For example, go from 120 to 130 THR one week and add 5 min duration at 130 bpm the next week. Progress in this manner until you achieve your THR goal and target exercise duration (discussed later in this chapter). Many factors are involved in a decision to exercise, but the key is not to overdo early. The exercise must also be convenient; that is, a person should feel that it does not take too much away from the day's responsibilities. Therefore, exercising at the worksite, at home, or at a conveniently located fitness center usually works best.

Factors for Comfortable Exercise

	Factor	Behavior
1.	**starting**	start at low intensities, short duration
2.	**progression**	progress slow with intensity ***or*** duration
3.	**convenience**	quick to get into and out of, easy to use equipment, showers available
4.	**time to exercise**	comfortable stomach, before meals, not before sleep
5.	**clothing**	proper shoes, dress for weather
6.	**warm-up**	mild intensity at beginning before stretching
7.	**stretching**	static (not bouncing), before and after exercise
8.	**cool-down**	progressively decreasing intensity at end
9.	**breathing**	natural and rhythmic, no breath-holding
10.	**stitch-in-the-side**	empty stomach, stretch torso, warm-up

Table 5.1.

TIMING

Before Not After Eating

The timing of the exercise is an important consideration. It may be uncomfortable for some people to exercise in the early morning. Before breakfast, blood glucose levels are low from the long overnight fast. Although the muscles can use more fat in these early morning workouts, the brain needs glucose; thus the exerciser may not feel quite right. If early morning time is the most convenient, eating a light carbohydrate breakfast (e.g., one bowl of cereal or one breakfast bar) 60-90 min prior to exercise may help you feel better during the exercise. On the other hand, exercising just prior to a meal may inhibit caloric intake. **Catecholamines** (epinephrine and norepinephrine) are released during exercise, and these hormones have an inhibitory effect on appetite. They also cause arousal, and so it may be difficult to sleep after exercising.

CLOTHING

Clothing is another consideration related to comfortable exercise. Obviously the exerciser should dress for the environment. A description of clothing recommended for hot and cold weather exercise is presented later in this chapter. However, some general principles relate to most exercise conditions. For example, proper footwear is one of the most important clothing considerations, especially if the exercise is weight-bearing. Sales personnel at fitness shoe stores usually can provide advice on the shoes most suited for your feet and your activity. Socks which have a high sweat absorbing capacity (cotton blends) and a tight fit are helpful in preventing foot blisters. On the other hand, cotton and polyester blends in shorts can cause friction on the legs. Loose fitting nylon shorts are often better for activities such as jogging and walking. A cotton blend T-shirt is recommended for exercise in a temperate climate.

WARM-UP

Start Slow -- End Slow

Other factors associated with comfortable exercise relate to the individual exercise bouts. For example, it is important to stretch before and after an exercise session. If the activity is mild enough, e.g., slow walking, it is probably useful to stretch only after the exercise. Some exercise scientists believe it is most beneficial to stretch after the muscle has undergone a warm-up. Therefore, prior to a hard aerobic exercise session, it may be best to do five minutes of mild aerobic exercise, such as walking, and then stretch. Stretch again after the higher intensity portion of the exercise session. For more information on flexibility and warm-up, see Chapter 7.

COOL-DOWN

As with warm-up, physiological systems operate more efficiently with a **cool-down** period. After vigorous exercise, the intensity should be gradually decreased. This strategy allows lactic acid to be removed more rapidly from muscle and blood. More importantly, the continued elevation of cardiac output and blood flow allows the heart to pump more blood out to the recovering muscles and up to the brain. If the exercise is abruptly stopped, blood pools in the active muscles, especially in the legs. Less blood, therefore, is available to get back to the heart and its output is diminished. The lower cardiac output results in a decreased blood flow to the muscles and heart as well as the brain. Dizziness, fainting, or even heart ischemia could result.

BREATHING

Breath Naturally

Breathing during exercise should be a very natural process. The exerciser should not need to concentrate on the sequence or depth of breathing. A critical guideline related to exercise is never to hold the breath. This is especially important when exerting against a load, such as with push-ups, sit-ups, or weight lifting. **Breathholding** increases the pressure in the chest and decreases the amount of blood which can get into the heart plus makes the heart push harder against this resistance. Air should always be exchanged when performing any type of exercise.

Stitch-in-the-Side

Getting Blood to the Stomach

Finally, the stitch-in-the-side can be very painful and cause an individual to avoid exercise. This pain is thought to be caused by lack of blood flow (ischemia) to the abdominal or respiratory muscles. This ischemia may cause metabolic by-products to accumulate and stimulate pain receptors. This stitch can usually be prevented by ensuring that no food or stomach gas blocks flow to the trunk area. Therefore, the stomach should be relatively empty during exercise and gas producing meals avoided, even for several hours prior to exercise, in people who have predictable pain. In addition, the trunk area can be stretched (e.g., side bends) prior to vigorous exercise to stimulate blood flow to the stomach area. Slow progression of the intensity during the exercise bout also may help prevent the stitch. Once the pain is present, it is difficult to alleviate without completely stopping the exercise. It may even be necessary to stretch the area throughout the day if the pain persists. Fortunately, the stitch-in-the-side presents no real physiological danger to the exerciser.

DETERMINING EXERCISE INTENSITY

TARGET HEART RATE

THR

Monitoring the exercise intensity can be valuable regardless of the goals of the exercise program. Even when performing low intensity activity it is useful to determine the difficulty of the work. When performing moderate intensity aerobic CV exercise, it is even more critical to monitor the intensity because exercise at the **target heart rate (THR)** will have the most beneficial effect on the CV system. For CV exercise, the THR should be around 75% of maximal heart rate (HRmax).

Determining Exercise Intensity

HRmax = 220 - age (yrs)
THR = HRmax x .75

Example

HR max = 220 - 40 yrs = 180 bpm
THR = 180 x .75 = 135 bpm
Use a range of ~5 bpm around the THR, 130-140 bpm.

The THR can also be determined by the **heart rate reserve (HRR)** method which includes the use of resting heart rate (HRrest):

220 - 40 =	180 bpm
HRrest =	70 bpm
HRR =	180 - 70 = 110 bpm
THR =	HRR x 60% + HRrest
THR =	110 x .60 + 70
THR =	136 bpm
Range =	131 - 141 bpm

The use of resting HR should be used with caution since this variable can be easily affected by such factors as stress, previous exercise, diet, etc.

The Beat Goes On

The exercise HR should be monitored by counting the pulses at the radial artery (behind the thumb in the wrist) or counting the heart beats with the hand over the heart. Some researchers have determined that palpating the carotid artery in the neck can slow down the HR and cause an underestimation of the actual HR. If the carotid artery must be used, apply only light fingertip pressure. Count the beats during exercise or immediately after stopping. Quickly locate the pulse and begin counting with the number "1" and count for six seconds. Simply add a "0" to this count and this is the exercise HR. The pace can be increased or decreased to achieve the THR.

A variety of electronic HR monitoring devices are available. Most are easy to use and some are relatively inexpensive. Many of these, however, are movement sensitive and do not give accurate HR measurements during exercise, especially during bouncing movements used in jogging or stepping. If you desire to obtain an accurate HR measurement *during* exercise, be sure to check whether the instrument is intended for such use.

METABOLIC EQUIVALENTS

Some individuals find it too difficult or time consuming to monitor exercise HR, and so other monitoring systems for exercise intensity have been developed. In the **metabolic equivalent (MET)** system, exercise intensity is estimated based on the metabolic cost of an activity as previously tested in a laboratory. For example, jogging at a 10 min/mile pace has an energy cost of about 10 METS. Tables of MET values for various activities can be found in a number of exercise science books, such as the **ACSM Guidelines** manual listed in the Suggested Readings at the end of the chapter. MET values around 6-10 usually provide an appropriate stimulus to the CV system.

6-10 METS

RATING OF PERCEIVED EXERTION (RPE)

Another method of monitoring exercise intensity is by using the **rating of perceived exertion (RPE)** scale. This scale is shown in Table 5.2. When beginning an exercise program, a person should perceive the effort between 7-11. The perception of effort can progress up to 15-16 for CV benefit. Efforts beyond this are for athletic populations and can lead to injury. Some individuals interested in relaxing, healthy activity may not need to go beyond 10 on the RPE scale. In untrained individuals, this "comfort index" can be a very easy and practical method of monitoring exercise intensity. Some exercise scientists have shown that the numbers on the RPE scale correspond to the exercise HR less the "0", e.g., 140 bpm = 14 RPE.

RPE Scale

Rating of Perceived Exertion

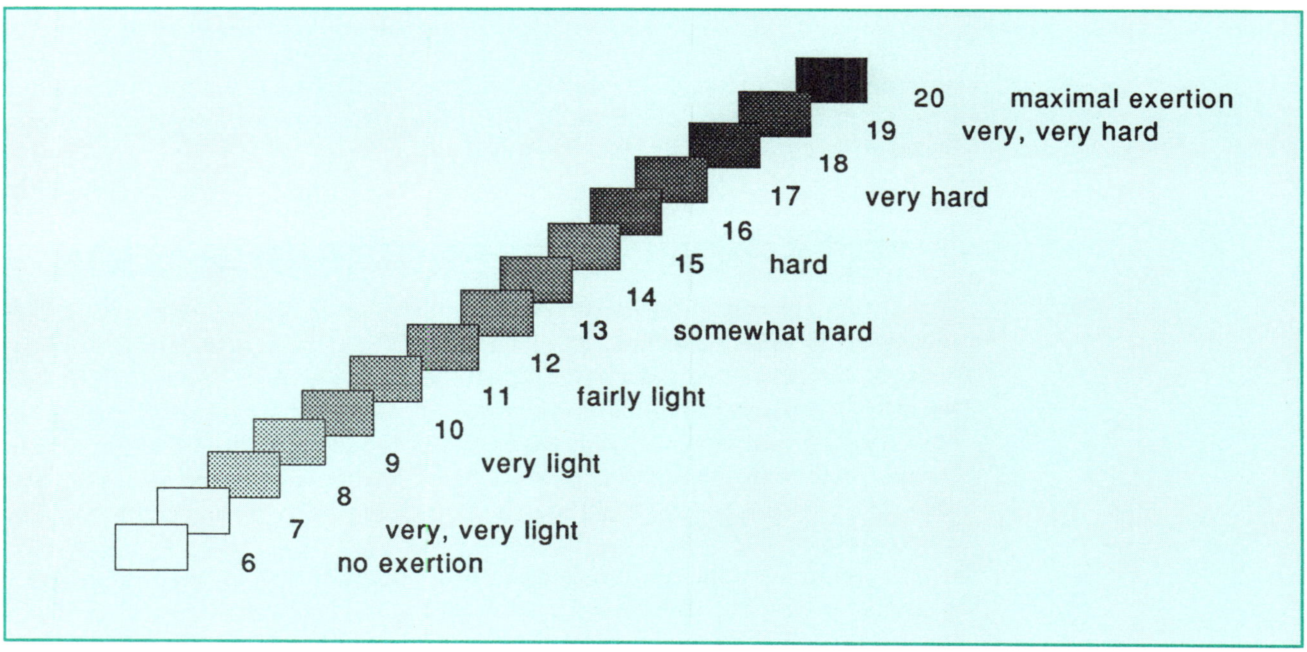

Table 5.2. From G. Borg and B.J. Noble. Perceived exertion. *Exercise and Sport Sciences Reviews*. 2:131-151, 1974.

TALK TEST

Another practical method of monitoring exercise intensity is called the **talk test**. This technique is based on the association of lactic acid accumulation to **hyperventilation** (greatly increased breathing). This point of increased breathing is called the ventilatory threshold. If one is breathing so hard that talking is difficult, then the intensity is too high. Beginners should control exercise intensity so that very little hard breathing occurs. The exercise should progress just up to the point where talking is difficult. Periodic "harder breathing" is appropriate after fitness levels are improved.

LACTATE THRESHOLD

Key to Advanced Training

Although the talk test is a good indicator of ventilatory threshold, for more serious aerobic training, one can more accurately measure or estimate the lactate threshold. In a laboratory setting, this threshold is measured by analyzing blood lactate at several different exercise intensities (Figure 4.3). Training at the pace which produces slight lactate accumulation in blood may increase the CV and metabolic gains of the exercise. Distance athletes use this pace for their "quality" training sessions. Analysis of blood lactate is not usually possible, so other simpler estimates of this training pace have been developed. One technique uses an all-out 2-mile run. Another field test estimate of lactate threshold pace was developed by Conconi in Italy. In this procedure, the athlete increases the pace of running or cycling every 200 yds up to maximal effort, and HR is measured with a watch monitor. The speeds and HR's are plotted on a graph, and the speed at which HR plateaus or levels off is close to the lactate threshold pace. Once this training pace is determined, it is used once or twice per week for hard training sessions.

DETERMINING EXERCISE DURATION

Like exercise intensity, the duration of an exercise session should be increased in small increments. To achieve CV fitness, the duration of the exercise eventually should extend to 40-60 min. The primary reason for this length is to ensure that substantial amounts of stored fat are used during the activity. In addition, prolonged exercise causes additional energy to be burned after the work in recovery. (See Chapter 4.) Exercise sessions of shorter durations will benefit health status, especially if the brief exercise is performed each day.

Increase HR First

In an unfit individual, the starting duration may be very short and at a low intensity, e.g., 5 min at a HR of 100 bpm. The intensity and duration should be increased each week, but only one at a time. Once the HR has gradually been increased to near the target zone, the duration should be increased 5-10 min each week until a duration of 40-60 min is achieved. It is acceptable to perform exercise of 20-30 min duration. However, longer exercise sessions are more beneficial and worth the extra time for the additional weight control and physical fitness that is gained.

STAYING POWER

Many of the factors which make starting exercise easier (Table 5.1) also make it easier to sustain an activity habit. Exercise scientists use the term **adherence** (or compliance) in addressing the problem of drop-out. No one knows for sure why some people can stick with activity and some cannot. Enjoyment is one factor that seems to be important. It is critical that an individual choose an activity which he or she likes. If you dislike jogging but take it up because it is "good for you," the chances of adhering to the jogging program are very slim. In fact, at least half of all people who begin an exercise program stop after a few weeks. Not only is enjoyment important, it is also necessary that you feel confident about performing the chosen activity (self-efficacy). If you cannot learn an activity quickly and feel confident in performing it, try a different activity.

Pick an Enjoyable Exercise

It may be wise to find out what you like about the exercise sessions. Is it the social aspects? If so, try to exercise with a partner or group. Is it the setting (environment)? If so, be sure the setting is pleasing to you. Is it the post-exercise stretching or relaxation period? If so, be sure to allow enough time for this phase of the session.

Perhaps one of the most discouraging aspects of any exercise program is the slow and subtle pay off. Most people expect too much too quickly. It may take time for exercise to affect your metabolism, your energy level, and your weight. But nearly everyone who has maintained a program for at least one year has exhibited desirable effects in any number of body systems. The goal should be a lifetime change, so short-term effects cannot become a major focus. In addition, incorporation of extra activity into one's set life-style may take time. Be ready to start again after an unexpected layoff or unmotivated time period. Even when you miss, some of the built-up benefits last a long time and will continue to improve when you get back to the activity.

POTENTIALLY DANGEROUS ACTIVITIES

For most individuals any form of movement is better than being sedentary. If a person enjoys an exercise, it may be a valuable activity even if the activity has a dangerous element. Regardless, it is important to recognize that some activities carry greater risks for injury and illness than others. The exerciser may want to avoid these dangers completely or when performing a certain activity, be more cautious.

HOT WEATHER EXERCISE

Hot, humid weather is one of the most hazardous conditions for exercise. The body's ability to cool itself is drastically decreased because evaporation of sweat is inhibited by the high water content of the air. In addition, the hot air prevents cooling the skin by convection. Under such conditions, the core or internal temperature of the body can rise very high.

Hazard Warning

Several strategies can decrease the risk of running in hot weather. If the daytime temperature is higher than 85°F, exercise in the early morning or night time is a wise choice. Exercise in the shade will help but sometimes not provide enough protection from the heat. Exercising in an air-conditioned room is the most obvious solution to the heat problem, but this strategy is not always available, and it may increase the inconvenience of the exercise session.

Fluid Intake

If hot weather exercise is necessary, the most critical strategy is to maintain fluid intake. Large amounts of water loss during exercise in hot weather can lead to **dehydration**. Therefore, fluid replenishment is generally the most important aspect of safe and comfortable exercise in the heat. During brief exercise bouts, cold water is an appropriate replacement fluid because energy replenishment is not necessary for such brief exercise periods. As the sessions increase in duration, intensity, or frequency, carbohydrate (CHO) and minerals become more important in the drink. Solutions of 7-10% CHO (7-10 g of CHO per 100 ml of fluid) appear to be optimal for replacing fluid as well as providing an energy source during exercise. For comparison, most soft drinks are 11-12% CHO solutions. As the weather cools down and the duration increases, the concentration of CHO can be increased up to 12%. Solutions closer to 7% should be used during prolonged exercise in very hot weather. Use of glucose polymers such as polycose may allow greater fluid absorption from the stomach than simple sugars such as glucose or sucrose. Most sport drinks now use polycose solutions. Rehydration breaks should take place approximately every 15 min when exercising in hot weather. Drink as much as possible during each break without causing stomach discomfort during the succeeding exercise.

Stop and Have a Drink

The use of minerals in exercise drinks has been controversial. Although salt (NaCl) may inhibit water emptying from the stomach, it may stimulate water and CHO absorption from the small intestine to the bloodstream. Thus NaCl should be used in small amounts (0.5% solution, not salty tasting) in exercise drinks. Other minerals, such as Mg^+ and K^+, which are often found in sport drinks, also may be advantageous to fluid absorption. It is unnecessary, however, to take mineral supplement tablets except under extreme conditions such as working all day for several days in the heat. Fluid intake should be continued for several hours after exercise in hot weather because the thirst drive lags behind the actual fluid loss. Usually more fluids should be taken in than one feels is necessary; i.e., overdrinking is beneficial following exercise in hot weather.

Sugar and Salt

Never wear heavy or insulated clothing during physical activity in hot weather. Rather dress lightly wearing a mesh type shirt to allow air flow next to the skin and decrease the amount of sun radiation to the skin. Likewise, a billed or brimmed cap can prevent overexposure of the face and neck to the sun.

COLD WEATHER EXERCISE

Clothing

Exercise in cold weather usually does not have the degree of danger as that associated with exercise in hot weather. The increased muscle metabolism keeps the core of the body warm. In fact, heat buildup can be a major danger if heavy, insulated clothing is worn. Clothing should be light enough to prevent profuse sweating, which can cause the body to cool too rapidly during recovery in the cold air and cause chills. Wearing layers of clothing can be an effective strategy because it allows the body to stay warm as metabolism gets started, and then by taking some clothes off, it allows cooling as the core temperature increases with exercise duration. It may be necessary to cover all parts of the skin to prevent frostbite when exercising in very cold, windy weather. Clothing should be lightweight, loose fitting and absorbent. With shorter bouts in the cold, a light nylon jacket provides a shield against the wind and helps prevent the loss of upper body heat. However the jacket may provide too much insulation in longer exercise bouts. On cold, windless days, only light clothing is necessary after warm-up. Military research indicates that running an 8:00/mile pace in -5°F weather requires only the amount of clothing necessary to be comfortable sitting indoors at 70°F. Sweat rate and comfort can be used as guides in determining the amount of clothing necessary for exercising in the cold.

Dress Right

Hypothermia and Frostbite

Cold wind increases the danger of cold injury, but a greater danger lies in wetness. Body heat and dryness must be maintained. In extreme cold, wet conditions, hypothermia risk is greatly increased, and exercise outdoors should only occur in sheltered areas. A useful strategy is to move with the wind late in the exercise bout to lessen the cooling effect of cold wind on sweating skin.

The risk of hypothermia and frostbite is also increased if an individual is working at a low intensity which may occur due to fatigue and injury. In such cases, additional clothing would be necessary to maintain body heat.

Exercise in cold weather has some known metabolic benefits and may be advantageous for conditioned individuals. However, outdoor activity in the cold is generally not recommended for cardiac patients or the elderly. Cold air can cause constriction of blood vessels in the skin which increases the resistance against which the heart must work. Vigorous outdoor activities such as snow shoveling increase the work of the heart. In addition, muscular straining against a heavy load (isometric work) increases the resistance in blood vessels and causes a rapid elevation in blood pressure. The rise in HR and increased vascular resistance in heavy arm exercise increases the demands on the heart and thus the **myocardial oxygen consumption**. Expiratory strain or breathholding (Valsalva maneuver) causes abrupt increases in heart work. This increased chest pressure is magnified by a full stomach.

Run Into the Wind

Cold air inhalation poses no danger for the healthy lungs and heart. The air passages in the sinuses and chest warm and moisturize the cold air to near body conditions by the time it reaches the lungs. Any slight burning sensations in the chest are probably caused by the dryness of the cold air. However, the inhalation of cold air may cause reflex constriction or spasms of the coronary arteries. If a person's coronary circulation is already compromised by atherosclerosis, the combination of the CV effects of the cold can have serious consequences. **Angina pectoris** (chest pain) and irregular heart beats (arrhythmias) are more common during activity in cold weather than in warm weather.

Cold Alert

Exercise in cold weather can be healthy and invigorating. However, the increased demands on the CV system mean that an individual should have some degree of CV fitness before performing vigorous activities in this environment. In addition, lifting light loads and breathing throughout the movement are helpful. No muscular straining while breathholding should be performed. Large meals, caffeinated beverages, and cigarette smoking should be avoided prior to activity in cold weather. Individuals with diagnosed heart disease or with any two cardiovascular disease risk factors (Chapter 3) should avoid heavy, high intensity arm exercise in general, but especially in cold weather.

PROBLEM PRACTICES

Dangerous Exercises

Several types of specific exercises are potentially dangerous. Several calisthenics/stretching exercises are not recommended by sports medicine and physical therapy specialists. Some of these exercises, e.g., supine leg lifts, put the lower back at risk for injury. Others, such as the hurdlers' hamstring stretch, are potentially dangerous for the knee. Calisthenics which place the back or knee in an awkward position or cause too much tension in these areas should be avoided. A complete list of potentially dangerous calisthenics/stretching exercises is presented in Chapter 7.

Exercise in a Rubber Suit

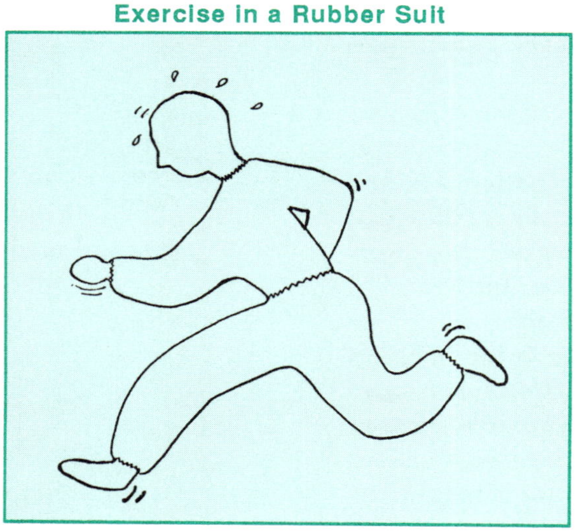

Figure 5.1. Potentially dangerous practice of exercising while wearing an insulated suit.

Dehydration

Besides the flexibility and strength activities, other exercise practices carry increased risk. Using plastic suits or insulated clothing to increase the loss of water weight can be extremely hazardous, especially in hot weather (Figure 5.1). Any additional weight loss is only temporary, and no legitimate reason exists for using this strategy. Likewise, use of a sauna can exaggerate water weight loss. The relaxation effect of the sauna may be of some benefit, but this procedure should not be used after vigorous exercise, especially in hot weather, when cooling and rehydration need to be the primary concerns.

Static (isometric) and heavy resistance exercises (Figure 5.2 and 5.3) usually are not necessary activities for individuals with general fitness goals. Both types of exercise are associated with the contracting muscles occluding blood flow which leads to additional strain on the heart and acute elevations in blood pressure. This response is compounded by breathholding during these exercises. The increase in chest pressure allows less blood to return to the heart. HR must increase to compensate and maintain cardiac output. This CV response is not as efficient or as beneficial to the heart as that associated with aerobic activity in which cardiac output is maintained with comparable elevations in HR and stroke volume. Breathing during the activity can help alleviate some of the risk, and the use of lighter resistance also is a wise strategy. For more information on resistance training, see Chapter 8.

Isometric Exercise

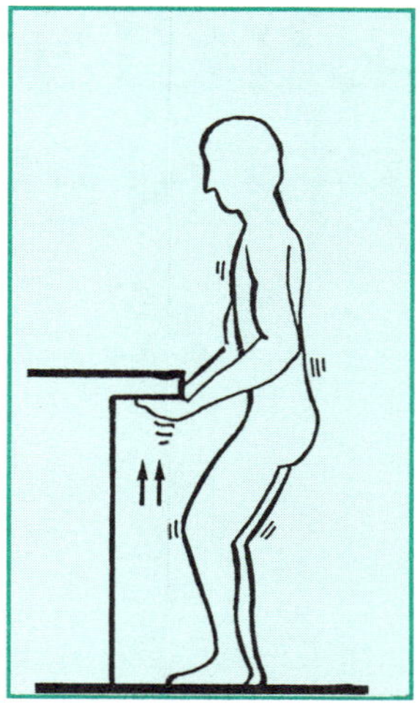

Figure 5.2. Potentially dangerous exercise of vigorous isometric contractions.

Heavy Weight Lifting

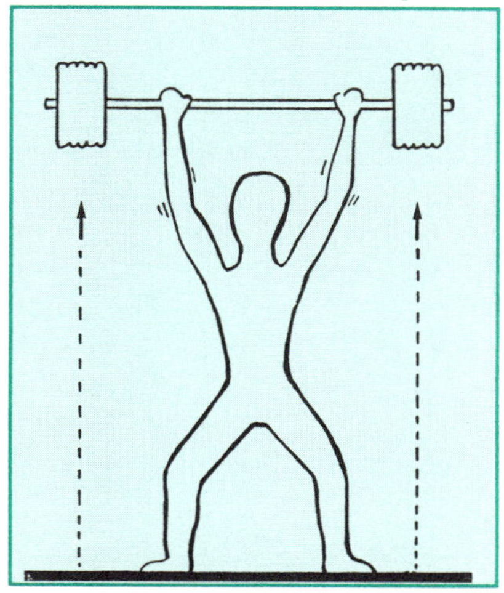

Figure 5.3. Potentially dangerous exercise of heavy resistance lifting.

Short-burst, very high intensity exercise is another practice that deserves cautious use (Figure 5.4). Such activity is vital to athletes training for sports competition, but should not be used in the beginning of an exercise training program. In these anaerobic activities, the unconditioned heart is caused to work too hard and recover too rapidly. After some degree of fitness is attained, "speed work" or vigorous sport contests can be used to add diversity to the program. Prior to participating in high intensity games such as racquetball, basketball, etc. the sedentary individual should undertake a mild, preparatory aerobic program for at least one month. A benefit of high intensity activity is to magnify a person's caloric expenditure during exercise as well as during recovery. However, these activities should not constitute the primary emphasis of the fitness/health program.

Short Burst, Strenuous Exercise

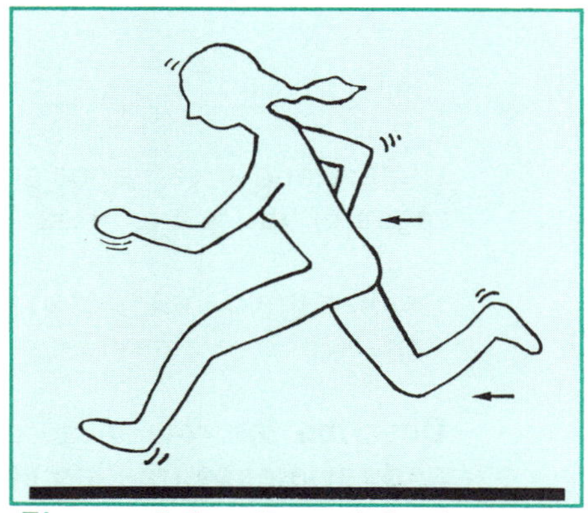

Figure 5.4. Potentially dangerous practice of very high intensity training or game contests prior to establishing some level of fitness.

Suggested Readings

American College of Sports Medicine. The recommended quantity and quality of exercise. *Medicine and Science in Sports and Exercise.* 22(2):265-274, 1990.

Browder, S. Don't be an exercise dropout. *Readers Digest.* 139:168-172, Aug., 1991.

Claremont, A.D. Taking winter in stride requires proper attire. *Physician and Sportsmedicine.* 4:65-68, December, 1976.

Cooper, K.H. *Running Without Fear.* New York: M. Evans, 1985.

CHAPTER 6

EXERCISE FOR FITNESS AND HEALTH

Tom Thomas

Learning Objectives

- Understand advantages and disadvantages of various exercise modes.
- Realize the benefits of experiencing a variety of exercise modes.
- Describe the role of aerobic training and resistance training in fitness and health promotion programs.
- Distinguish between activities for cardiovascular fitness and those for health improvement.
- Describe a variety of healthy physical activities.
- Know techniques of increasing the caloric use during various activities.

Important Terms

cardiovascular fitness

circuit resistance training (CRT)

health status

high impact

low impact

podiatrist

weight-bearing

GENERAL CONSIDERATIONS

Several population studies indicate that virtually any type of activity performed routinely improves health status. Activity can be of very mild intensity, e.g., gardening, slow walking, etc., and it can be performed only briefly, but it must be performed consistently to obtain a health benefit. On the other hand, aerobic activity at moderate intensities may be the best kind of exercise because it not only improves **health status** but also enhances **cardiovascular fitness**. Improved health status means that some aspect of a person's well-being is changed. Such changes could be greater immunity to sickness, greater bone strength and prevention of osteoporosis, and improved emotional health. Increased health status also indicates protection against all-cause mortality, i.e., a decreased risk of dying soon. On the other hand, CV fitness implies improved aerobic capacity (VO_2 max), a variable which is associated with improved function of the heart, lungs, blood vessels, and muscles. Exercise which affects CV fitness also affects health status, but mild or brief activity which affects health status, generally will not improve CV fitness.

All aerobic activities basically have two common denominators: they are prolonged and are low to moderate intensity. Characteristics of cardiovascular exercise are presented in Table 4.7. Virtually any activity which can be performed continuously for at least 30 min can be called aerobic. Therefore, the list of potential aerobic activities is very long, but the extent that each exercise is aerobic depends on the manner in which it is performed. Generally, all types of aerobic activity are beneficial to the heart, but more calories are used during exercise which uses a large proportion of the muscle mass and is **weight-bearing**, i.e., the body weight is supported by the legs as in jogging.

Jogging Outdoors

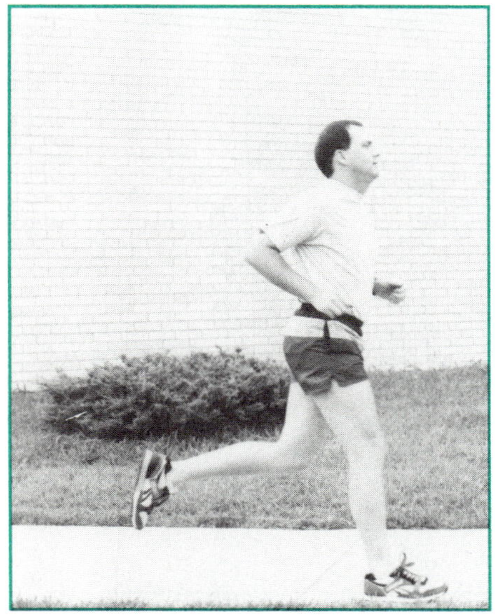

Figure 6.1. This activity is one of the most widely used aerobic exercises. It can be performed in nearly any location.

Jogging Indoors

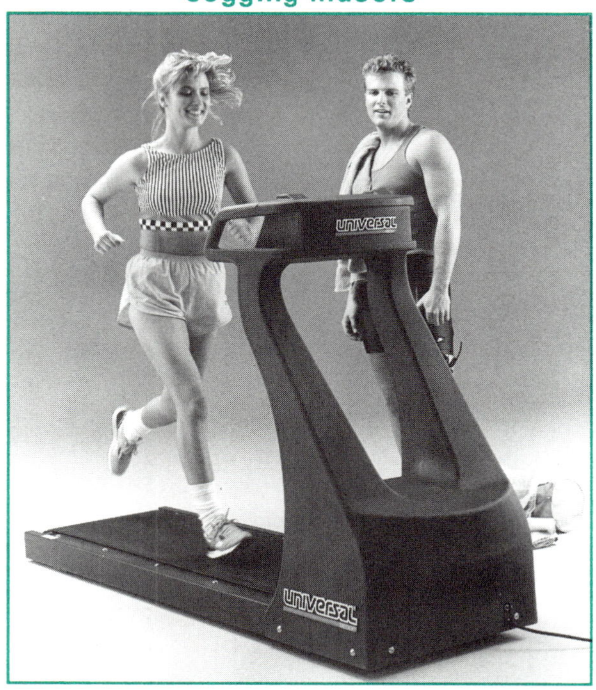

Figure 6.2. Motorized treadmills like the Tredex provide walking or jogging activity in the home or fitness center. Photo was provided by Universal Gym Equipment, Inc.

JOGGING/RUNNING

Jogging and running are the most widely used types of aerobic activity. These are activities which nearly everyone can perform and thus the exercises which initiated the fitness boom (Figures 6.1 and 6.2). This mode of physical activity requires more energy to be used than most types of aerobics. One reason for the increased caloric cost is that a person is likely to "self select" a relatively vigorous intensity when jogging or running. In other words, it is difficult to exercise at a mild intensity with this exercise. Research studies also indicate that jogging stimulates body fat utilization better than many other activities. Jogging or running can be per-

Aerobic Dance

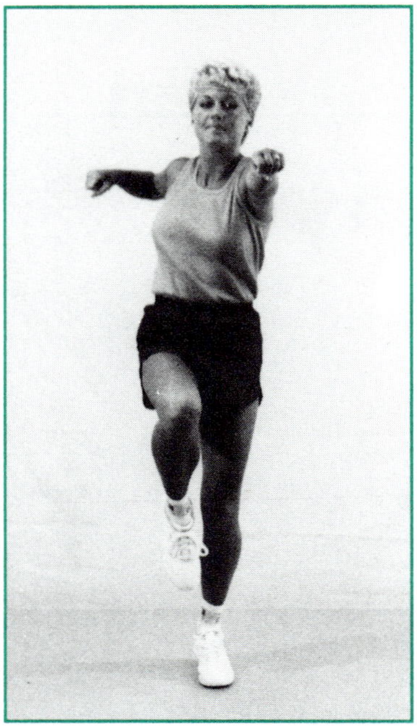

Figure 6.3. This aerobic activity is rapidly growing in popularity. Supporting the body weight increases calorie burning.

Aerobic Dance with Wrist Weights

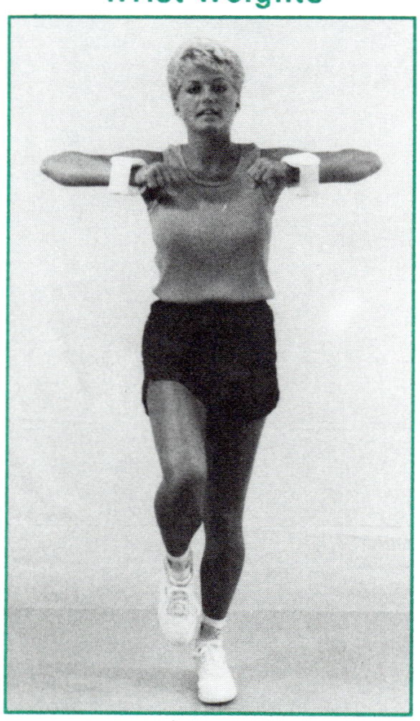

Figure 6.4. Using hand or wrist weights can increase caloric expenditure.

formed in almost any location at any time of day with little or no assistance and very little equipment. The full body weight is supported and lifted during jogging/running, which increases energy use, but leg injuries are common. Thus, it is important that proper precautions be followed. Shoes are the most critical aspect of safe, comfortable jogging. Proper running form, surface considerations, and stretching also are keys to comfortable exercise and injury prevention during jogging.

AEROBIC DANCE

Aerobic dance is one of the most widely used modes for organized group activity. Some of the national organizations, such as the YMCA, attract over 150,000 participants each year. Aerobic dance videos commonly are found on best seller lists. A portion of this recent growth stems from the many modifications available in aerobics-to-music programs which make such routines attractive to a greater variety of people.

PRECAUTIONS AND BENEFITS

Aerobic dance or aerobic rhythms potentially has the same benefits as jogging. It is usually weight-bearing, thus stimulating increased energy expenditure (Figure 6.3). Major advantages also include the variety of exercises and intensities performed and the social aspect of exercising with other people. Like jogging, aerobic dance can produce injuries, especially to the legs. But with proper precautions and wise shoe selection, this form of exercise can be very effective.

The great interest in aerobic dance classes has spurred research into the effects of this activity. Generally moderate intensity classes have produced increases in maximal oxygen consumption, which is the single best measure of aerobic or CV fitness. The extent of the improvement depends on keeping the HR in the target zone for 30 min, the frequency of the program, and the length of time spent in the program. Caloric expenditure and upper body muscle tone can be enhanced with the use of hand-weights or wrist-band weights (Figure 6.4). However, this practice also can elevate blood pressure and increase the risk of injury. Therefore, the use of limb weights should be handled with caution and probably used only periodically in the aerobic routine and only after some degree of fitness has been obtained (Table 6.1).

Besides the CV and muscular benefits, some research suggests that aerobic dance, like other forms of aerobic activity, can enhance or maintain bone mineral content. In the elderly, who are more susceptible to osteoporosis, this exercise can be especially beneficial.

Use of Hand/Arm Weights with Aerobic Dance Routines

1. Use only after one month in the exercise program. Never in the beginning unless in good aerobic condition.
2. Use no more than 2 pound weights on each wrist or hand.
3. Do not use weights on upper arms or legs.
4. Use only periodically during the aerobic exercise period.
5. Do not hold weighted hands over the head. This increases the strain on the heart.
6. Avoid firm grasping of the weight. It is best if the weight can be attached to the limb. Tight grasping is an isometric contraction which can elevate blood pressure.

Table 6.1.

SELECTING CLASSES

Because of the great variety of activities and intensities offered with aerobic dance classes, the matching of personal goals with those of the exercise classes must be carefully considered. Some dance activities involve primarily stretching and strengthening exercise. The popular Callanetics by Callan Pinckney is such a routine. Pinckney's exercises are not performed to music. The cardiovascular response to this routine would be minor, and thus it is not truly an aerobic activity. However, it would be an appropriate choice for individuals with primary goals of improving muscular tone and flexibility. But this routine would not be appropriate for individuals seeking improvement in CV fitness.

In a Class by Yourself

On the other hand, some aerobic dance routines can be too strenuous for the heart. Heart rates near maximal frequently have been recorded in aerobic dance classes. Such high intensity may help burn calories but is not beneficial for the heart. In fact, heart rates over 80% of maximal can be dangerous to out-of-shape or older individuals. Guidelines for determining your personal maximal and target heart rates are described on page 64.

Although low intensity activity, such as stretching, is not usually beneficial for improving the aerobic and CV systems, it can be beneficial in other ways. Nearly any kind of movement is more beneficial to the body than sitting or lying. Health status is improved by consistently participating in even low intensity exercise. In addition, enhanced flexibility and muscle tone as well as a feeling of well-being can be important benefits of low intensity exercise.

General Questions

1. Is the instructor properly trained in aerobic dance, exercise physiology, anatomy, and emergency procedures?
2. Is the space adequate for each participant?
3. Is the room well ventilated?
4. Is the floor surface appropriate? The surface should "give" but not be too soft; avoid concrete surfaces or unpadded tile or carpeting over concrete.
5. Is the exercise intensity appropriate?
6. Can your target HR be maintained for at least 30 min? The routines should not be interrupted by extended rest periods.
7. Can the routines be used at home?
8. Will the program continue for at least one year?

Each participant must judge an aerobic dance class based on their exercise goals, but some general questions should always be explored.

Specific Guidelines

1. Always prepare for aerobic exercises with a warm-up and static stretching.
2. Always end class with static stretching.
3. The aerobic period should be maintained at least 25 min.
4. Always follow aerobic exercise with a cool-down period.
5. Always stretch muscles which have been involved in the aerobic or strengthening routine.

The entire routine,including stretching and cool-down, may take 50 to 75 min. the activities within this sequence can vary, but the order should follow specific guidelines.

LOW IMPACT

Lift Those Knees

One of the newest and most beneficial practices in aerobic dance is individualized pacing to the same music. This personalized intensity has been termed low and high impact. Basically, the intensity is controlled by the height which the knees are lifted and the extent of the arm movement. By modifying the extent of the leg and arm actions, the target HR can be maintained regardless of the speed or beat of the music. In addition, individuals of vastly different ages or fitness levels can exercise together to the same music. Injured individuals also may be able to perform low impact exercise without aggravating the injury or necessarily withdrawing from the program. Low impact or low effort movements are appropriate for warm-up and cool-down activities and are ideal for the elderly or beginning exercisers. It seems important to utilize the **low** and **high impact** method of movement in aerobic dance classes with different levels of participants.

WALKING

Walking is one of the fastest growing fitness activities in America (Figure 6.5). Although this is a weight-bearing activity, the impact on the legs is not as great as in jogging or aerobic dance. Still, proper form, shoes, and precautions are necessary. Walking technique should be natural and rhythmic. Very little instruction is necessary. However, if leg pains result from low intensity walking, the feet and the walking stride should be examined by a **podiatrist** or foot doctor. This specialist can determine if the anatomy of the fore-foot allows appropriate heel strike and foot take-off. Slight alterations in the shoe, such as shims and soft orthotics, may provide more comfortable and effective walking.

Walking is an excellent way to incorporate some activity into the regular daily routine. One can walk to and from work or errands, up and down stairs, or around the block with a friend (Figure 6.6). Healthy walking does not require a fitness center or exercise equipment.

Although walking is weight-bearing, the impact forces against the ground are not as great as in jogging. Thus injuries are not as prevalent in walkers. This weight-bearing difference, however, also causes walkers to utilize fewer calories. Most individuals can achieve an appropriate target HR by walking. Certainly sedentary or unfit or elderly populations may find walking to be the ideal exercise. On the other hand, as the fitness level progresses, the target HR is more difficult to achieve by walking. In one study, only about half of fit middle-aged males could achieve their target HR, even when they were walking as fast as possible.

Research studies indicate that walking burns as many calories as jogging at speeds above 5 mph. While this speed is not achievable by most walkers, it is possible to increase the caloric cost of walking by speeding up the pace. On the other hand, individuals who use a "self selected" comfortable walking pace burn only about half the calories as when using a "self selected" comfortable jogging pace. However, the slower walking pace may have greater relaxation value. At an "easy" pace, a walker uses a little more than half the body weight (in kcal) per mile and a jogger uses a little less than the total body weight per mile. For example, a 150 lb person uses about 85 kcal per mile when walking and about 140 kcal per mile when jogging. The caloric expenditure of walking increases closer to that of slow jogging if the individual "walks as fast as possible."

Walking

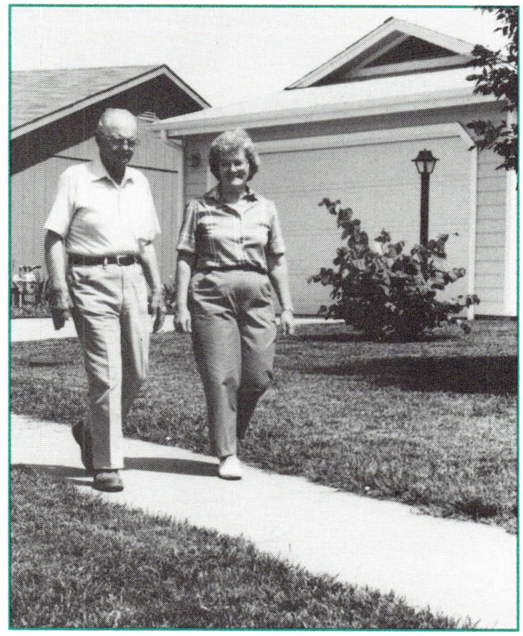

Figure 6.5. This exercise is a healthy habit, indoors or out.

Walking

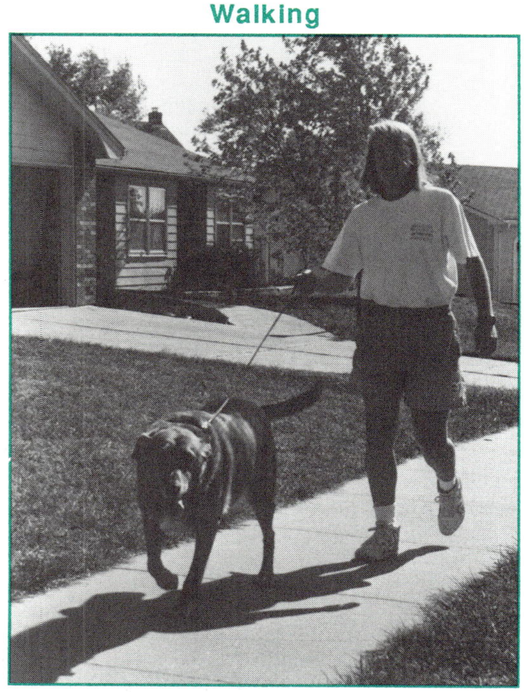

Figure 6.6. Strolling with a pet is an excellent way to include exercise in the daily routine.

Swing Those Arms

Another method of increasing the exercise intensity is to use hand, wrist, or ankle weights while walking. In addition, the arm swing can be exaggerated to increase the involvement of the upper body muscles. Adding weights of 3 lbs. on each arm and exaggerating the arm swing can nearly double the caloric cost of walking. The added arm involvement also enhances upper body muscle tone. Blood pressure elevation caused by the limb weights is the major disadvantage. (See Table 6.1 for other precautions.) Therefore, a conservative recommendation is to use 1-2 lbs. per limb and move the hands no higher than shoulder height. This strategy will increase calorie burning during walking by about 20%. In walking, the use of ankle weights causes stride changes which could cause leg muscle soreness or injury. Thus, the advantage of burning extra calories when using weights must be weighed against some increased risks.

STAIR CLIMBING/STEPPING

Burn Calories

Walking or running stairs has been a popular method of training athletes and is frequently used in home exercise programs. Until recently, this mode has been limited by access to appropriate stairways. This was a problem, particularly for those who lived in ranch style houses (with no basement). Recently, equipment manufacturers have developed portable in-home stairclimbing devices. The exercise devices are actually stairway treadmills, and the movements are a little like going up a down escalator (Figure 6.7). The foot impact forces are lower than jogging but the caloric cost is still high. A handrail can be used, or the caloric use can be increased by swinging the arms during the exercise. This activity is an excellent alternative to jogging to periodically reduce the impact forces on the legs.

Stairclimber Machine

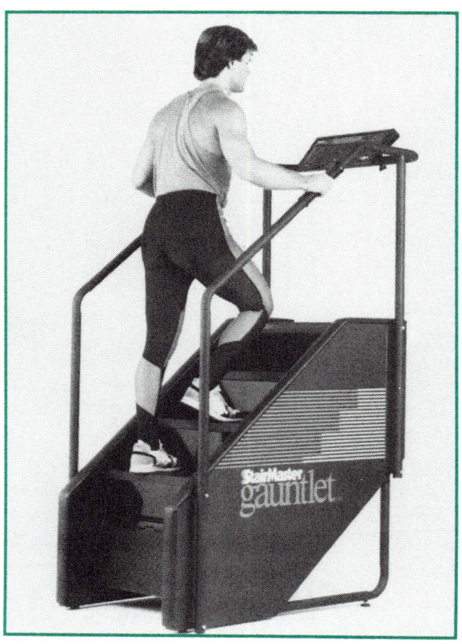

Figure 6.7.

Stairclimbing exercise can be performed at various intensities. The photo of the Stairmaster Gauntlet was provided by Randal Sports Medical Products, Inc.

Stepping Machine

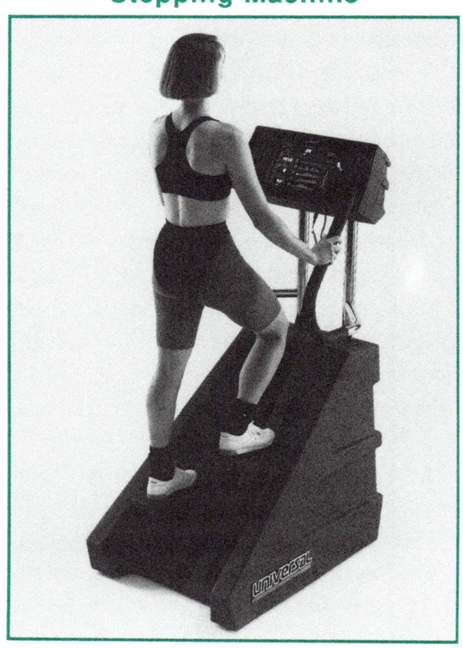

Figure 6.8.

This instrument provides exercise at various intensities with or without hand support. Photo was provided by Universal Gym Equipment, Inc.

Other devices called steppers have a slightly different action than the stairs (Figure 6.8). Some steppers are more like climbing devices and offer adjustable resistance for both the legs and arms (Figure 6.9). For those steppers which do not provide resistance for the arms, the upper body can be used by swinging the arms during the stepping activity. Jarring of the legs is very minimal with stepping exercise. At high resistance settings, the climbing machine also can be used as strength exercise for the upper and lower body. At low resistance settings, a beginner can perform this type of exercise. By increasing the repetition rates on the steppers, the energy expenditure can be very large. However, such high intensity exercise should be reserved for fit individuals. This type of equipment can provide excellent diversity and overload for those individuals with training experience.

Stepping/Climbing Machine With Arm Exerciser

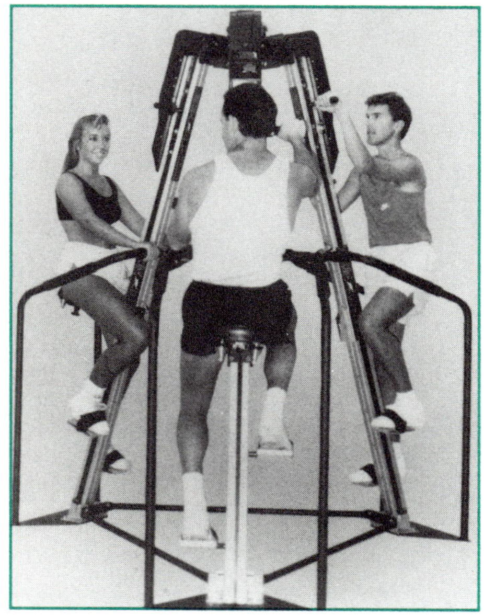

Figure 6.9. The Versa Climber provides intensity settings for arm and leg activity. Photo was provided by Heart Rate, Inc.

CROSS-COUNTRY SKIING

The cardiovascular and muscular benefits of cross-country skiing have been known for many years. Scandinavian skiers have exhibited some of the highest maximal oxygen consumption values on record. Until recently, snow skiing was reserved for individuals living in cold climates. Modern fitness equipment has changed that, and exercise machines are available which simulate cross-country skiing (Figure 6.10). This type of activity provides excellent total body muscle utilization. Energy expenditure generally is high during skiing exercise because it is weight-bearing and upper and lower body muscles are used. Another caloric advantage of the ski simulator is that individuals "self select" a fairly high intensity on this activity. It is difficult to select a mild pace on this total body exercise. In addition, the jarring associated with jogging/running activities is reduced. The adjustable resistances should be kept low for beginners (especially the arm resistance) but can be increased as fitness level increases. A person may need patience when learning to use the ski simulator, but the results are generally worth the effort. As with all vigorous aerobic exercise, HR should be monitored. Rather than stopping to count pulses, it is safer and more effective to use an accurate HR monitor, which often can be purchased with the machine. It is wise to purchase a monitor which is not movement sensitive so that HR can be assessed during the exercise.

Cross-Country Skiing

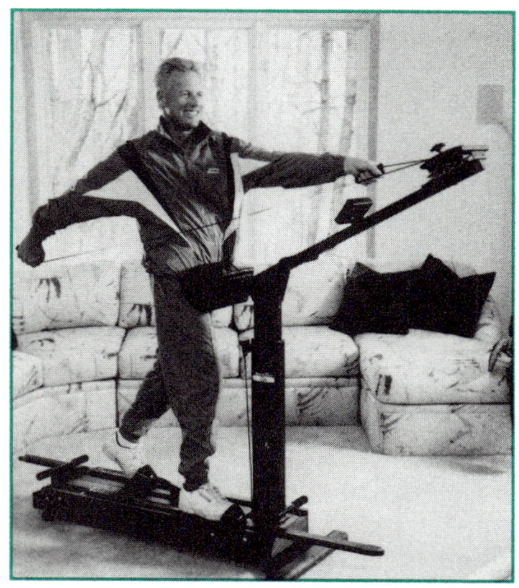

Figure 6.10. The NordicTrack provides an aerobic activity which utilizes the total body musculature. Photo was provided by NordicTrack.

REBOUNDING

Give a Little

One of the most inexpensive exercise instruments is the rebounder. Like the traditional trampoline, the rebounder allows a bouncing exercise with cushioning of the weight support through the "give" of the springs. Less joint stress is encountered than jogging in place on non-giving surfaces. Jogging in place on the rebounder has been shown to be effective CV exercise if the target HR is maintained for at least 30 min. Boredom has been a complaint by some users, but this problem can be overcome with the use of music, videos, etc. This exercise is most useful in adding diversity to the aerobic exercise program.

CYCLING

Maintain Target HR

Like most forms of aerobic activity, cycling with a regular bicycle or stationary cycle is an effective form of CV conditioning. Many people prefer the outdoor scenery associated with bicycling (Figure 6.11). In addition, this mode of exercise can serve as an inexpensive means of transportation. For some, indoor cycling is more feasible, and the stationary cycle provides an effective mode of aerobic exercise. If the target HR is maintained, then indoor and outdoor cycling will produce similar CV benefits. Since cycling is nonweight-bearing, the caloric expenditure is often less than some other forms of aerobic exercise. However, joint and muscle trauma are much less than in typical weight-bearing exercise. Most cycles provide exercise primarily for the legs (Figure 6.12). However, a few of the stationary cycles provide arm exercises as well (Figure 6.13). Implementing arm exercises with cycling not only enhances energy expenditure, but also increases the effect on upper body muscle tone.

Bicycling

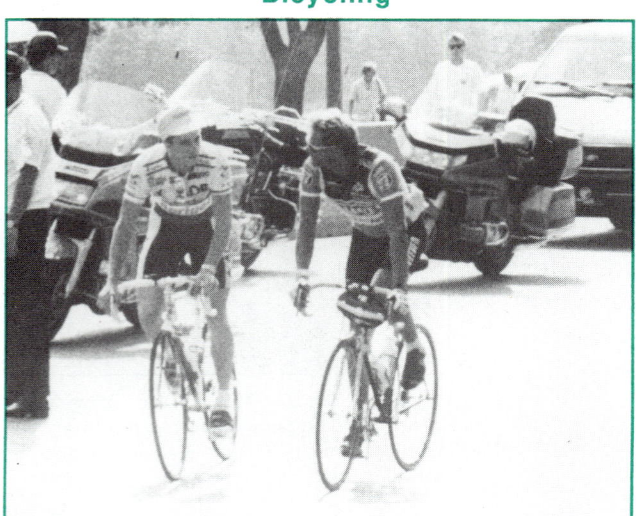

Figure 6.11. Outdoor scenery and fresh air are advantages of bicycling.

Cycling

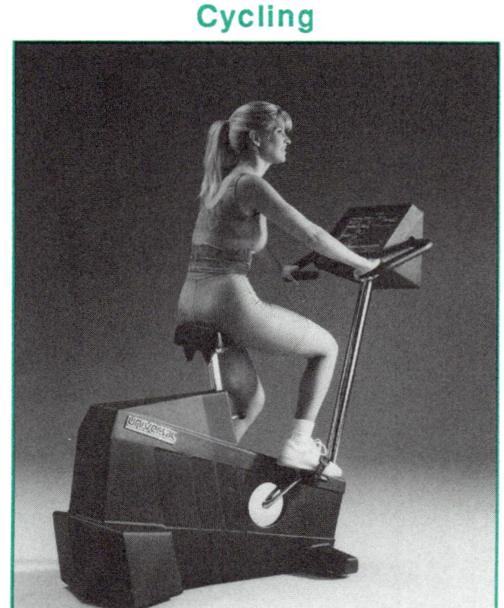

Figure 6.12. Stationary cycling is a very popular aerobic exercise in the home and in fitness centers. Photo was provided by Universal Gym Equipment, Inc.

As in all CV exercise, it is important that the age-adjusted target HR be maintained for at least 30 min. Most cycles provide easily adjustable leg workloads, and thus the HR can be controlled within a narrow target zone.

Research studies suggest that when using the arms, upper body exercise should contribute only a small percentage to the total workload. In this way, the larger muscles of the legs do most of the work. Utilizing too much arm musculature in the exercise can increase HR and blood pressure above appropriate aerobic exercise levels. To calculate the exercise workload, the rider first performs comfortable exercise using only the legs with the exercise HR in the low range of the target zone. Note the workload on the dial, add 10-20% to the work, and use the arms until this additional workload is achieved (Table 6.2). Recheck HR to be sure it is in the target zone. In general, the use of the arms should add no more than 10-15 bpm to the legs only HR.

Cycling with Arm Exerciser

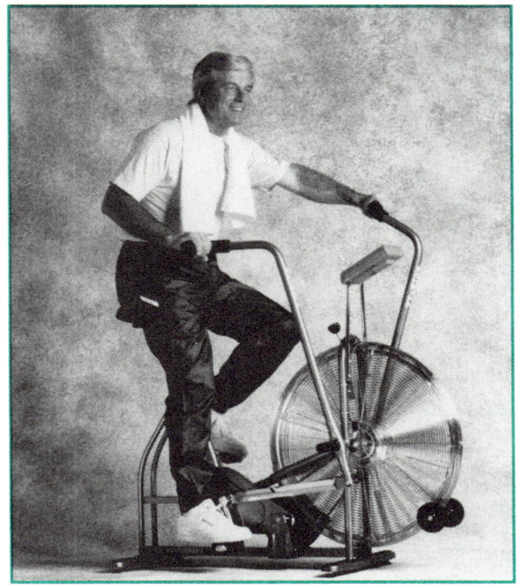

Figure 6.13. Some stationary cycles also provide arm exercise. The arms' contribution to the total energy expenditure should be only 10 to 20%. Photo was provided by Schwinn Bicycle Co.

Calculation of Workload Using an Arm and Leg Cycle Ergometer

1. Exercise at a comfortable pace using only the legs with HR in the low range of the target zone.
2. Record workload (kpm/min, watts, kcals, etc.).
3. Add 10 to 20% to the leg workload.
4. Exercise with arms and legs until calculated workload is achieved.
5. Check HR to make sure it is in the target zone.
6. If HR is too high or low, reduce or increase workload accordingly.

Example

Female: Age 44
Target HR 132 bpm
Target HR Zone 127-137 bpm

Cycles with legs at 127 bpm, workload at 300 kpm/min.

300 kpm/min x .10 (10%) = 30 kpm/min.

300 kpm/min + 30 kpm/min = 330 kpm/min.

Exercise with arms and legs at 330 kpm/min.

HR monitored at 135 bpm.

Table 6.2.

Low-Sit Cycling

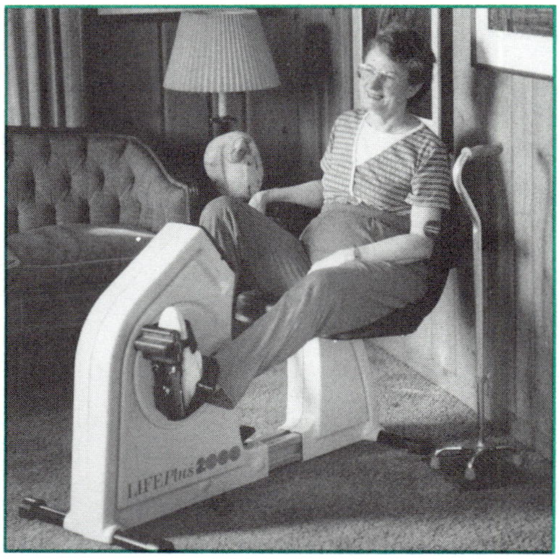

Figure 6.14. The low-sit cycle provides cycling exercise in a comfortable position. Photo was provided by LifePlus.

A new method of cycling involves the leg cycling movement from the low-sit position rather than upright (Figure 6.14). In this position, the seat and legs are parallel to the floor. The position is comfortable and allows more blood (venous return) to get back to the heart and thus increases the heart's output (stroke volume) more than the upright cycling position. For a similar oxygen consumption (or caloric expenditure), the HR is generally lower than in the traditional cycling position. Involving the arms in this exercise also increases the burning of calories and promotes upper body muscle tone.

The low-sit cycling in the semi-reclining position may be especially useful for pregnant women or individuals with high blood pressure. In the semi-reclining position, both gravity and the fetus have less effect on blood flow coming back to the mother's heart.

ROWING

Like cycling, rowing is a non-weight-bearing exercise and therefore is easier on joints and uses less calories than some other aerobic activities. Rowing stresses the use of the upper torso and arms although the legs also are utilized (Figure 6.15). The combination of upper and lower body exercise is a definite advantage. Upper body tone can be an expected benefit. The arm rowing movement primarily involves the biceps, brachioradialis, and brachialis muscles of the upper arm and the trapezius and other muscles of the upper back. On some piston type instruments, the upper body position can be reversed so that the triceps in back of the arm and pectoral muscles of the chest also can be exercised (Figure 6.16).

Types of Rowing Exercisers

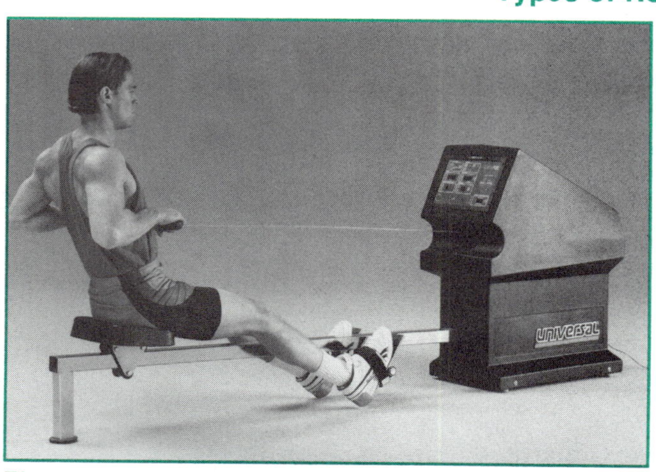

Figure 6.15. This arm and leg aerobic exerciser can fit conveniently in the home or office. Photo was provided by Universal Gym Equipment, Inc.

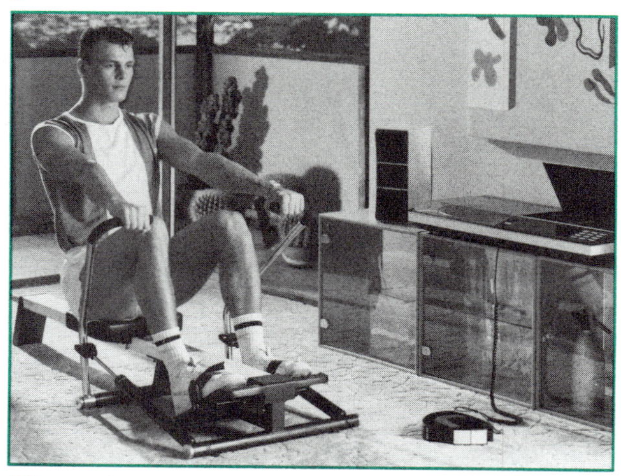

Figure 6.16. On rowers with arms, the body position can be reversed, so that additional arm and chest muscles can be strengthened.

In using the rower, the resistance on the arms should be relatively low. Remember, the upper body should contribute only 10-20% of the total work when using both arms and legs in exercise (Table 6.2). Thus, the lower body exercise should be emphasized unless specific goals include more enhanced arm development. Vigorous arm work can be especially unwise in middle-aged individuals just beginning an exercise program. Likewise, vigorous upper body exercise generally is not recommended for individuals with cardiovascular disease.

One disadvantage of most rowers is that the resistance can only be adjusted for the arms; the leg resistance cannot be altered. If the arm resistance is increased very high, then the arms will contribute beyond the acceptable 20% of the total work. The NordicRow offers a unique rower with leg as well as arm adjustable resistance (Figure 6.17). These adjustments allow the workload to be increased at the legs while remaining lower at the arms. Resistance exercises also can be performed separately on arms or legs.

Rowing with Leg Resistance

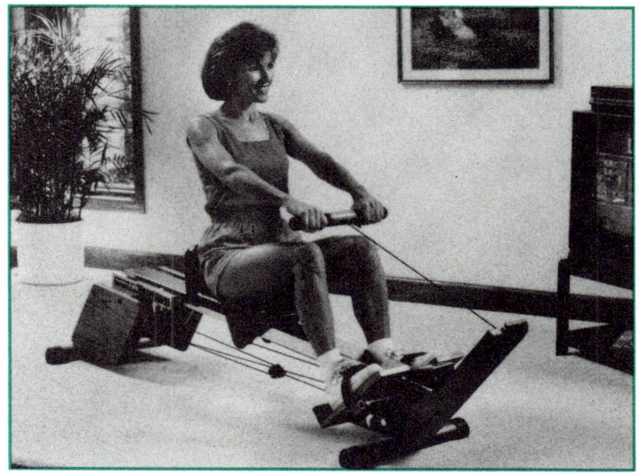

Figure 6.17. The Nordic Row combines the activities of rowing and resistance exercise with separate resistance settings for legs and arms. Photo was provided by NordicTrack.

SWIMMING

Swimming has been called the most complete form of exercise. The diverse movements in the water involve flexibility, strength, and aerobic exercises (Figure 6.18). In addition, moving in cool water is often refreshing and relaxing. Swimming is one exercise where fatness can make the exercise easier. Unlike muscle, the fat tissue is less dense than water, and it therefore floats. Since fatter individuals do not have to work as hard to prevent sinking, the work is easier to propel the body through the water. This advantage also provides a disadvantage—fatter people use less calories than lean people when swimming.

Swimming

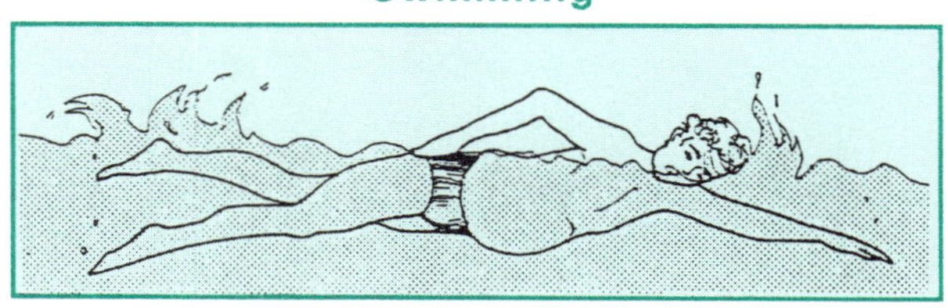

Figure 6.18. The target HR zone for swimming is lower than that for other aerobic exercises.

Since the body is supported by water, the risk of joint and muscle injury is very low in aerobic swimming. For many years, water exercises have been used by athletes and race horses as a means of continuing to exercise when injured. In addition, water activity is recommended for arthritis and cardiac patients. This mode of exercise may be the least traumatic exercise for joints and muscles of all aerobic activities.

This does not mean that swimming exercise is easy. Swimming can elicit appropriate target HR's and caloric expenditure; however, some research suggests that the exercise target HR should be 10-15 beats lower than with other aerobic exercise. The horizontal position allows more blood to return to the heart which increases stroke volume. This increased output with each heartbeat causes fewer beats to be necessary to pump blood out of the heart to the working muscles. The cool water also has a HR lowering effect. One of the ways of judging the potential benefits to the CV system of

Oxygen Pulse of Various Activities

Activity	O_2 Pulse (ml/beat)
Swimming	16.0
Jogging	15.0
Walking with Hand Weights	14.5
Ski Simulator	14.5
Walking	14.0
Low-Sit Cycling	13.0
Cycling	12.5
Rowing	12.5
Stepping	12.5
Aerobic Dance	11.5
Circuit Resistance Training	10.5
Racquetball	10.0
Weight Lifting	8.0

Table 6.3. Values are derived from exercise at the same moderate heart rate (~130 bpm).

various exercises is to compare the oxygen pulse (Table 6.3), which is the ratio of total body oxygen consumption (energy used) to HR expressed as ml of oxygen per beat.

It is beneficial for total body oxygen consumption to be high while HR is relatively low; thus, the heart is working relatively easy in providing the oxygen to support a relatively high total body workload. Swimming exercise is associated with a high oxygen pulse because of the relatively high oxygen consumption at a relatively low HR. In other words, swimming is an excellent exercise for the heart.

Exercise intensity can be varied by stroke and by speed. In general, it is best to use both arms and legs together in a swimming workout. Since the resistance of the water on the arms is relatively low, it is not likely that the arm exercise will be too strenuous for the CV system. The rate of the swimming strokes should be varied so that the target HR is maintained for at least 30 min. Lap swimming is the easiest method to ensure that the swimming is aerobic.

Water aerobics offers an excellent alternative to land aerobics. These exercises offer the intensity of land aerobics without the high impact forces on the legs. In addition, the water offers the potential for greater arm resistance than the air on land and thus provides added upper body benefit.

CIRCUIT RESISTANCE TRAINING

CRT

Many different forms of exercise can be performed at moderate intensity and maintained continuously for at least 30 min and thus be considered aerobic. One mode which is gaining increasing acceptance as an effective fitness activity is **circuit resistance training (CRT)**. This type of resistance training is described in Chapter 8 on page 118. By using relatively light resistance and greater repetitions than traditional weight training, CRT can benefit both the muscular and the CV systems. Another key to the aerobic nature of this activity is the limited rest period (15-30 sec) between exercises. With these limited rest periods and lighter loads, the HR can be maintained within the appropriate CV target zone. CRT is especially useful in maintaining CV fitness and in providing a combination of muscular strength and CV fitness aspects in a program.

While all aerobic activities benefit the CV system, the energy expenditure may be very different for various activities. Therefore, some aerobic exercises will be more effective than others if weight loss is a primary goal. Exercise and weight loss are discussed in detail in Chapter 9. In Table 6.4, a list of caloric costs of various aerobic activities is presented. A more complete listing can be found in Appendix A.

HEALTHY ACTIVITIES

Some activities may be too mild in nature to be classified as effective aerobic or CV exercise. In golf, the low intensity walking the fairways can be beneficial, but this walking is interrupted by the golf swing and the anxious process of searching for a lost ball. Or worse, an electric cart is used, and most of the benefits of this sport are lost. Walking with a push golf cart is the best way to reap the health benefits of this activity. Other games, such as bowling, are so physically mild that they do not tax the CV system enough to improve CV fitness. But they have other healthy effects.

Hunting and fishing are other activities that often are not associated with vigorous effort. The intensity of these activities varies greatly and ranges from the restful watching of the baited fishing line to the maximal effort of dragging decoys and equipment through a muddy marsh. Recent studies on deer hunting in Michigan indicate that the HR's can be very high when stalking and shooting at a deer. In addition, the risk of irregular heart beats increases due to the excitement of the hunt. Thus, hunters should participate in CV fitness exercises prior to the hunting season, and individuals with CV disease should be cautious about the type of hunting and fishing undertaken.

Even though many of these sports and games may not promote large increases in CV fitness, these and many other activities can be beneficial to the body. Even routine, daily movement can be beneficial to many of the body's systems. It is wise to take advantage of opportunities to move around rather than sit. One key to life-long good health may be the willingness to avoid being sedentary. Mild, everyday activities such as housekeeping, walking on errands, walking stairs, etc. may be all the activity that is necessary to keep one healthy if these tasks are performed very frequently.

One strategy for increasing the activity level is to "manufacture activity," that is, purposefully put yourself in situations that require you to be active. For example, get a pet so that you will be motivated to play with it or walk with it (Figure 6.6). Maintain a large lawn or mow it more frequently (Figure 6.19). Plant a flower or vegetable garden to provide motivation to get out and moving. Plant trees or bushes and maintain them (Figure 6.20). Clean the house or the car more often and at a more rapid pace (Figure 6.21). The list of "work activity" is unending. The motivation for movement may come from active hobbies or from actual work. In either case, this active life-style will promote feelings of accomplishment as well as help improve health status.

Caloric Cost of Various Aerobic Activities

Activity	Cal/hour*
Running 6 min/mi	1,100
Cross-country skiing	725
Jogging 10 min/mi	710
Rope jumping 75 skips/min	650
Stepping	650
Rowing	600
Swimming 40 yds/min	500
Aerobic dance (moderate)	480
Cycling and arm work	480
Cycling 10 mph	400
Aerobic dance (low impact)	360
Walking 17 min/mi	325

* Estimates for a 150 lb (68 kg) man or woman at a typical pace. Caloric costs are increased or decreased depending on the body weight, terrain, surface, wind, etc.

Table 6.4.

Mowing Lawn

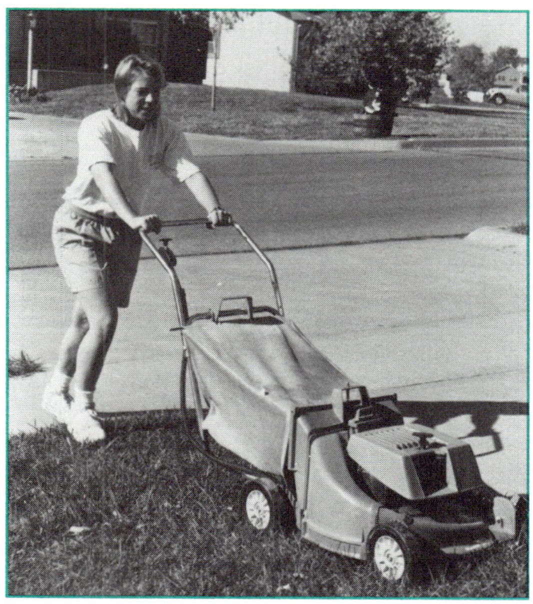

Figure 6.19. Such work-type activity accomplishes health benefit as well as home improvement.

An optimal life-style strategy might be to combine "healthy" activities with "fitness" activities. It is very beneficial to incorporate some moderate intensity CV exercise in the life-style. Thus, gardening, cleaning, or golfing can be performed four times per week, and aerobic dance or swimming performed twice per week. It may be necessary to alternate weight-bearing activity with nonweight-bearing activity to decrease the strain on the legs (Inventory # 28 on page 277).

Individuals who feel that the intensity and time commitment for any aerobic training are too great can still benefit from consistent low intensity, brief activity, especially if it is performed everyday. These benefits perhaps relate to the relaxing effect of participating in the activity as well as the physiological adaptations caused by consistently repeating the activity. Therefore, the most important criterion for selecting an activity is *enjoyment*. Find something that you like enough to do every day, or alternate two enjoyable activities. Exercise has no health value if an individual dislikes it so much that he or she "drops out." Although not all exercise will enhance aerobic capacity, almost all low intensity, nonstressful activity will enhance health and decrease the risk of disease and death.

Trimming Trees

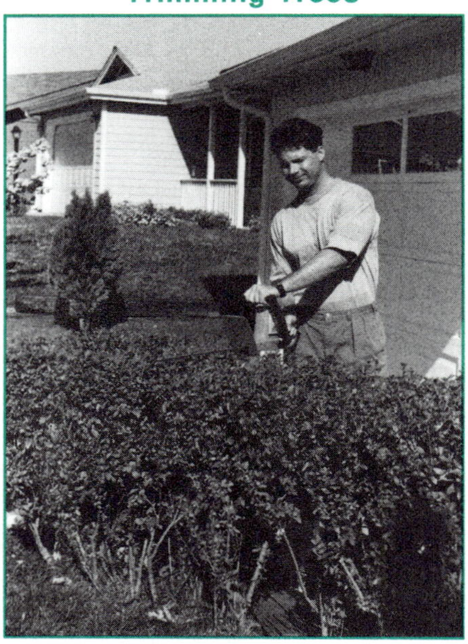

Figure 6.20. Mild activity can benefit health status and feeling of well-being.

Cleaning Windows

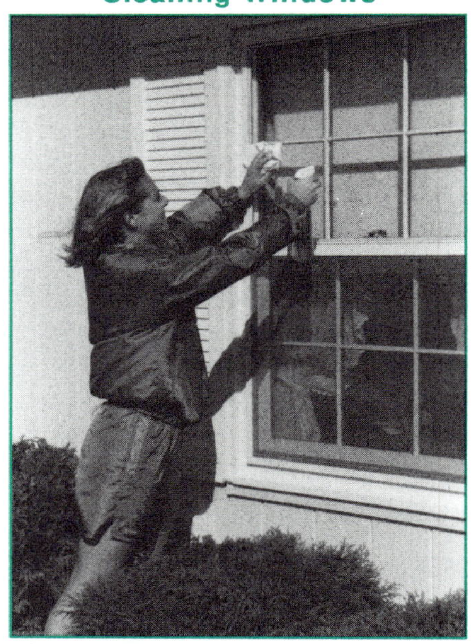

Figure 6.21. The bending and stretching associated with cleaning has excellent health benefits.

Suggested Readings

Cooper, K. *The Aerobics Way.* New York: M. Evans, 1977.

Stamford, B.A. and P. Shimer. *Fitness Without Exercise.* New York:Warner Books, 1990.

Thomas, T.R. and B.R. Londeree. Energy cost during prolonged walking vs jogging exercise. *Physician and Sportsmedicine.* 17:93-102, 1989.

This chapter is adapted from a chapter which first appeared in T.R. Thomas and C.J. Zebas. *Scientific Exercise Training.* Dubuque: Kendall/Hunt, 1987. Parts are used with permission.

CHAPTER

7

FLEXIBILITY AND STRETCHING

Carole Zebas

Learning Objectives

- Distinguish among the terms flexibility, warming-up, and stretching.
- Explain what happens physiologically when muscle temperature is elevated.
- Explain what happens biomechanically when muscle and connective tissue are stretched.
- Distinguish among ballistic, static, passive, and proprioceptive neuromuscular facilitation exercises.
- Determine when warming-up or stretching should take place in a fitness program.
- Describe the benefits of a flexibility program.
- Describe the basic fundamentals of designing a flexibility program.
- Determine which muscles should be involved in the design of a flexibility program.

Important Terms

ballistic stretching
elastic
flexibility
passive stretching
proprioceptive neuromuscular facilitation (PNF)
static stretching
stress relaxation
stretching
stretch reflex phenomenon
viscoelastic
viscous
warming-up

INTRODUCTION

Examples in everyday living point out the importance of warming-up or "loosening up" before beginning an activity. For instance, those who live in cold climates know that a car engine will function more effectively if it is allowed to warm-up first. Likewise, a balloon can be blown up to its maximum capacity if it is stretched before air is introduced into it. Handball players who warm-up before playing also are "warming-up" the ball, even though they may not be aware of it. A warm ball will bounce better than a cold one. The human body is no different. It functions more effectively if it is allowed to warm-up or stretch before it begins an activity. It is the purpose of this chapter to explore the general topic of flexibility.

Warm-Up and Stretch

Several Questions Commonly Asked When Planning a Flexibility/Stretching Program

1. What are the differences between flexibility, warming-up, and stretching?
2. What are the benefits of warming-up or stretching before an activity?
3. What physically happens to the body during the warm-up or stretching process?
4. What type of exercises are best for warming-up or stretching?
5. When should warming-up or stretching exercises be done?
6. What do I need to consider in designing my own flexibility program?

DEFINING THE TERMINOLOGY

The terms flexibility, warming-up, and stretching have all been used to describe pre-exercise activity. **Flexibility** generally is defined as the range of motion about a joint. However, it also can refer to the amount of extensibility in the muscles and connective tissues surrounding a joint. The definition which is used depends upon how the flexibility is measured. If a goniometer (i.e., an instrument designed to measure range of motion) is used, flexibility is described in terms of how many degrees of displacement a segment of the body makes about the joint. If a measurement such as the sit-and-reach test is used, flexibility is described in terms of how many inches the muscle allows a part of the body to move. (See Chapter 14 , Inventories 1-9 for examples of Flexibility Testing.)

Measuring Flexibility

Warming-up and **stretching** are processes for obtaining flexibility. Warming-up is the elevation of muscle temperature to allow for a greater range of motion or muscle extensibility. Stretching, on the other hand, is the active motion of extending the connective tissues found in and around the muscles. Confusion between the terms exists because the terms often are used interchangeably.

BENEFITS OF FLEXIBILITY TRAINING

Very few exercisers would argue against the benefits of flexibility training. Generally, there are three acknowledged reasons for warming-up or stretching to become more flexibile.

Reasons for Warming-up or Stretching

1. Preventing muscle and connective tissue injuries from occurring. The most common of these injuries is the strain which involves the overextension of the muscle or the tendon of the muscle. (See Chapter 13 on Preventing Fitness Related Injuries.)

2. Improving the range of motion about a joint so that activities requiring any great amount of segment displacement can be done to the fullest.

3. Preventing muscle soreness due to a training error. One such training error is trying to do too much too quickly when first beginning a fitness program.

PHYSIOLOGICAL AND BIOMECHANICAL CHANGES

Physically speaking, there are two major changes occuring within the muscle and connective tissue during flexibility training. One is a physiological change in the temperature of the muscle and two is the biomechanical change in the elasticity of the muscle.

PHYSIOLOGY OF MUSCLE TEMPERATURE ELEVATION

Warm-Up the Muscles

Muscle tissue temperature may be elevated by activities such as light jogging, walking, taking a hot shower, or sitting in a sauna. On the other hand, temperature may be raised by performing an activity at a submaximal level. For instance, hitting serves in tennis at less than maximum speed would assist in elevating the temperature of the muscle. It generally is thought that a warmed muscle is less likely to become injured because it would take a greater force and length of stretch to "tear" the muscle.

Several benefits accrue from the elevation of muscle tissue temperature. Circulation is increased making oxygen more available to the muscle cells. This results in more energy being made available for muscle contraction. The increase in muscle temperature also speeds up the metabolic processes to produce more forceful contractions. Additionally, the elevated temperature reduces muscle stiffness, making the muscle more extensible. This, in turn, makes the muscle contraction smoother. Finally, the elevated muscle tissue temperature helps to relax the muscle and make it perform more efficiently.

BIOMECHANICS OF MUSCLE ELASTICITY

Connective tissues are found in and around the muscles. They are the tendons, muscle sheath, ligaments, and joint capsules. These are the structures which can enhance movement or can inhibit it.

These important connective tissues have **viscoelastic** properties which are responsible for length increases. One of these properties is termed **viscous** and is characterized by the ability of a tissue to remain permanently deformed once it has been subjected to stretch. This same effect can be seen in pulling taffy. Once the taffy has been stretched, it does not return to its original shape. The second property, which is called **elastic,** has just the opposite effect. Once it has been subjected to a stretch, it returns back to its original shape. This is much like the effect of removing a rubber band from around a package. Once it has been removed, it returns to its original shape.

Viscous and Elastic Properties

Both viscous and elastic properties are found in connective tissue, thus the term viscoelastic. The property which acts to a greater degree is dependent upon the type of stretching, the temperature to which it has been subjected, and the rate at which the stretch has been applied. The domination of the viscous property is desirable for increased range of motion or extensibility of the muscle. The stretching exercises which enhance this property are the ones which are of a long, slow stretch variety. An example of this type of exercise is the static stretch. As the temperature rises, the viscous property dominates. This lends support to the idea that the muscle tissue temperature should be elevated before stretching begins.

TYPES OF STRETCHING EXERCISES

The types of stretching exercises commonly used to improve flexibility are categorized as ballistic, static, passive, and proprioceptive neuromuscular facilitation (PNF). The decision on which type of stretching exercise to use depends to a great extent on the nature of the fitness activity and the safety involved in performing the exercise.

BALLISTIC STRETCHING EXERCISES

Ballistic stretching exercises are characterized by bouncing movements. An example might be a side bending exercise in which one hand is placed on the hip and the other hand is raised overhead. The trunk is bent sideways in a direction toward the hand which is on the hip. The quick sideward movement causes arebounding action of the trunk back to the standing position. This action is repeated several times in succession to give an appearance of "bouncing."

Bouncing: Good or Bad

The ballistic type of exercise generally is considered to be be less effective and less beneficial than the other types. It is less effective because of the **stretch reflex phenomenon**. When a muscle is stretched, a sensory structure within the muscle becomes active. This nerve and muscle complex is the "muscle spindle." It is a modified muscle fiber contained within a capsule and has a sensory nerve spiraled around its center. The muscle spindle is sensitive to any stretch placed on the muscle and serves as a protective device to prevent overstretching. When the muscle is stretched, the muscle spindle and, more specifically the sensory nerve is activated. An impulse is sent to the central nervous system which, in turn, sends impulses via the motor nerves to cause contraction of the muscle fibers. The bouncing action of the ballistic type exercise causes the reflexive action which inhibits the stretch.

An added disadvantage to the ballistic type exercise is the potential for injury and muscle soreness. There is some speculation that the rapid lengthening and shortening of the muscle and connective tissue may result in small tears. This may eventually develop into a more serious injury problem.

STATIC STRETCHING EXERCISES

Static stretching exercises are characterized by a long, slow stretch through a range of motion with the ending position being held for 10-60 seconds. The length of time the stretch is held depends on when the program was begun. If the stretching is occurring during the earlier stages of the program, the 10-second time period would be appropriate. As the muscles become accustomed to the stretches, more time can be added. An example of this exercise might be one for stretching the muscles of the lower leg. The person performing the exercise leans forward against a solid object (e.g., a wall) with the leg which is not being exercised in the forward position. The body is lowered forward toward the solid object or wall as the extended leg, with its knee in an extended position, is being stretched. (Figure 7.1.)

A Static Stretch Exercise

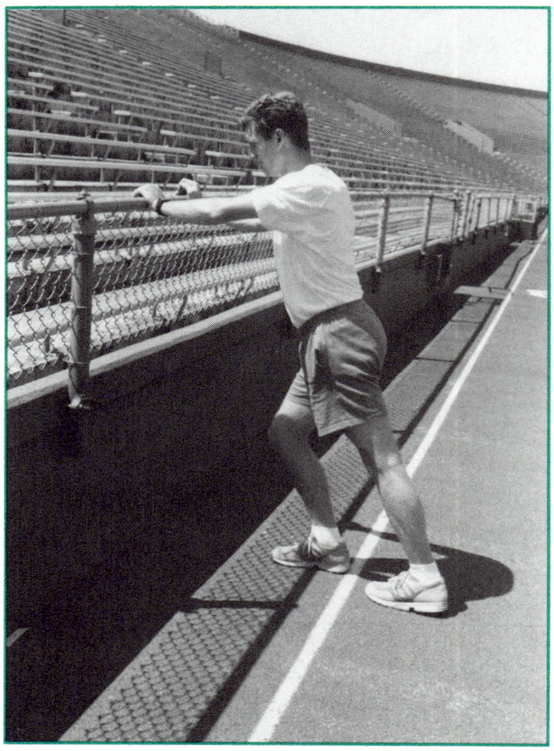

Figure 7.1. The muscle is placed on stretch and held for 10 to 30 seconds.

The static stretching exercises are the most popular of all the exercises for improving flexibility. They also are the least likely to cause the microtears associated with the ballistic type motion and the most likely to promote greater extensibility of the muscle and connective tissue. One of the reasons for this advantage is the delayed activation of the stretch reflex. Another reason is a phenomenon known as **stress relaxation**. The viscoelastic properties mentioned earlier respond to stretching by creating and reducing tension. The elastic property reacts to stretching by creating tension in the muscle or connective tissue. The viscous property reacts to the rate and duration of the stretch. The slower rate and the longer duration of the stretch results in a reduced tension in the tissues and allows for stress relaxation. This is desirable because it allows the performer to increase the range of motion of the stretch.

PASSIVE STRETCHING EXERCISES

Passive stretching exercises involve two people, one who actively moves another person's limbs through a range of motion and the other whose limbs are passively being moved. Generally, these exercises are of the static stretch variety; however, they may be ballistic also. An example might be an exercise designed to stretch the hamstrings. The person performing the exercise sits on the floor with the legs extended. A partner reaches over the exerciser's shoulder and grasps one of the legs just above the ankle. The partner then draws the leg up toward the chest of the exerciser. The exerciser, in this case, does no active moving of the leg. (Figure 7.2.) The major disadvantage of this exercise is the potential overstretching of a muscle.

A Passive Stretch Exercise

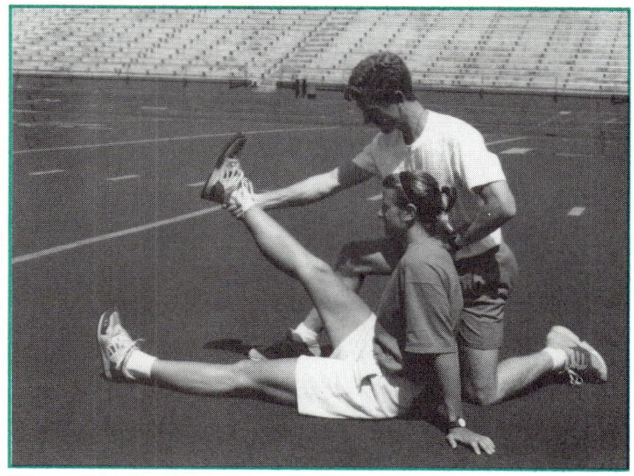

Figure 7.2. The exerciser plays a passive role as her partner moves the limb actively through a range of motion.

PROPRIOCEPTIVE NEUROMUSCULAR FACILITATION EXERCISES

Proprioceptive neuromuscular facilitation (PNF) exercises were first designed to rehabilitate patients with paralysis. They were based, in part, on the concepts of reflex activation and inhibition. Modified versions of the PNF exercises were adopted by such people as athletes and fitness participants. One modified version, involving two people, incorporates a slow stretch with an isometric contraction. An example might be an exercise in which the hamstrings are stretched. The person performing the exercise is in a back-lying position with both legs extended. One leg is then bent at the hip and brought upward toward the head as far as possible. When the leg has reached the limit of its range of motion, an attempt is made to return it to its original position. However, a partner provides resistance to this motion by prohibiting any forward movement from occurring. This is the isometric contraction. After approximately 10 seconds, the resistance is removed and the exerciser attempts to move the leg in the original motion toward the head. Some exercise specialists encourage the partner to assist in the last stretch, thus making it a passive motion on the part of the exerciser. (Figures 7.3.-7.5)

The PNF exercises do not activate the stretch reflex as quickly as the ballistic type exercises. Also because of the slow and long movements, stress relaxation is promoted. Thus, the muscle can be stretched further and range of motion can be increased. See Table 7.1 for a summary of the protective effect of all flexibility exercise types.

A PNF Stretch Exercise - First Phase

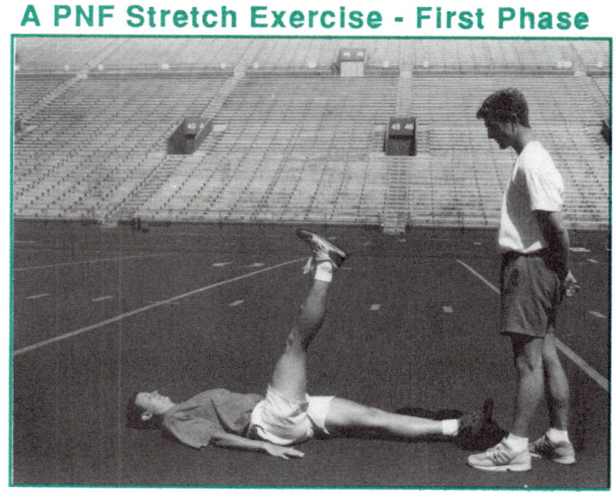

Figure 7.3. The exerciser moves the leg through a range of motion by pulling it toward the head as far as possible.

A PNF Stretch Exercise - Second Phase

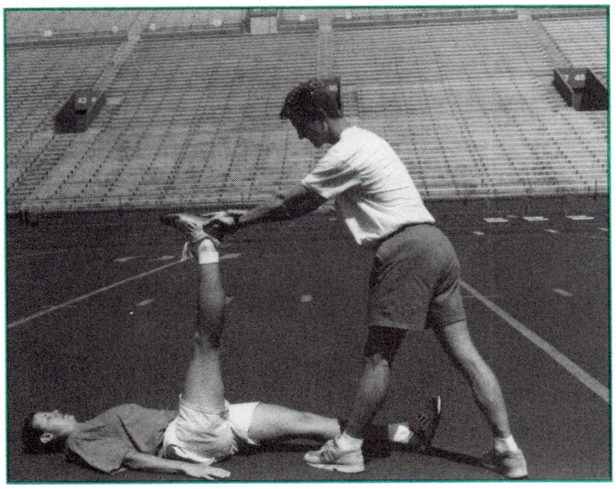

Figure 7.4. The partner provides resistance as the exerciser attempts to move the leg back toward the ground. This causes an isometric contraction of the hamstrings and gluteals.

A PNF Stretch Exercise - Third Phase

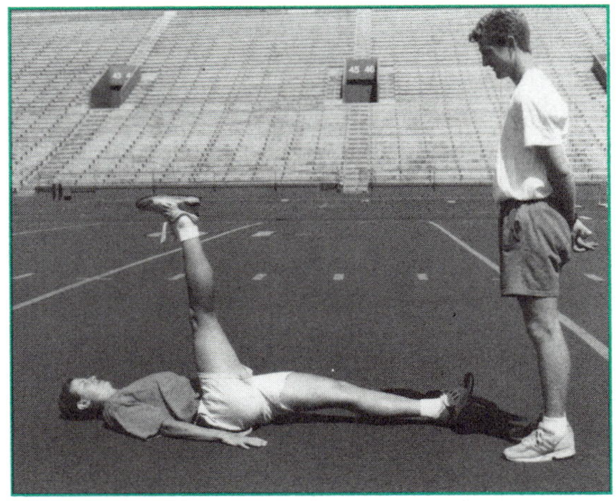

Figure 7.5. The exerciser attempts to move the leg toward the head.

Protective Effect of Stretching Exercises

Type	Physiological Response	Protective Effect
1. Ballistic	Causes rapid lengthening and shortening of muscle and connective tissue	Greater muscle tension Greater reflex action Less stress relaxation
2. Static	Causes delayed activation of stretch reflex Greater stress relaxation	Less muscle tension Less reflex action
3. Passive	Depends upon whether action is static or ballistic	Depends upon whether action is static or ballistic
4. PNF	Causes delayed activation of stretch reflex Greater stress relaxation	Less muscle tension Less reflex action

Table 7.1.

WHEN TO STRETCH

There has been considerable discussion as to when exercises to improve flexibility should be performed. Tradition tells us that stretching exercises should be performed prior to a fitness activity such as running or cycling. However, the consensus now among exercise specialists is that some fitness activities are not rigorous enough to warrant stretching beforehand, and the risk of injury is minimal. On the other hand, if the exercise involves quick movements or large ranges of motion, stretching prior to the activity may be desirable. The key seems to lie in the muscle temperature at the time of the activity. This can be summed up in this way:

Stretching Guidelines

Activity Not Vigorous	If the fitness activity is not a vigorous one, the activity itself may serve as the vehicle for elevating muscle temperature. In this case, begin with submaximal effort until muscles have been warmed. Then stretch after the activity.
Activity Vigorous	If the fitness activity is a vigorous one, elevate muscle temperature by doing a submaximal activity or light jogging or walking. Then perform stretching exercises. Stretch after the fitness activity also.

DESIGNING A FLEXIBILITY PROGRAM

A flexibility program should be designed to fit your primary fitness activity goals. When that has been determined, consider the following general suggestions for a safe and effective program:

Important Considerations

1. Stretch after muscle temperature has been elevated. Warm-up activities such as jogging, walking briskly, or submaximal efforts of an activity can be used to elevate the muscle temperature.
2. Wear comfortable and loose fitting clothing.
3. Stretch the major muscles involved in the fitness activity.
4. Stretch both the agonist and antagonist muscles (e.g., quadriceps and hamstrings).
5. Exercise both sides of the body equally.
6. Stretch slowly to the point of discomfort, but not to the point of pain.
7. Concentrate on being relaxed throughout the movement, and continue smooth and rhythmic breathing.
8. Hold each stretch for 10 to 60 seconds.
9. Repeat each stretching exercise 2-4 times before moving on to the next exercise.
10. Avoid stretching areas of the body which are "overflexible".

SAMPLE STRETCHING EXERCISES

The most fundamental flexibility program includes several basic muscle groups. Table 7.2 and Figure 7.6 have been developed to assist you in identifying the general location of the muscle and its primary movement responsibility.

Muscles and Their Movements

Muscle	Location	Primary Movement
Quadriceps	Front of thigh	Extends the knee
Hamstrings	Back of thigh	Bends the knee
Gastrocnemius/soleus	Back of lower leg	Extends the ankle
Anterior tibialis	Front of lower leg	Bends the ankle
Iliopsoas	Front of hip	Bends the hip
Adductors	Inside of thigh	Draws leg inward
Erector spinae*	Back side of trunk	Straightens the trunk
Gluteus maximus	Back of hip	Extends the hip
Gluteus medius	Side of hip	Extends leg sideward
Abdominals*	Front side of trunk	Bends the trunk
Pectoralis	Upper chest	Bends the shoulder Draws arm inward
Deltoid	Shoulder	Draws the arm sideward and upward
Biceps	Front of upper arm	Bends the elbow
Triceps	Back of upper arm	Extends the elbow
Latissimus dorsi	Upper back	Extends the shoulder Extends arm sideward

* *These muscles rotate the trunk also*

Table 7.2. Examples of exercises which stretch the muscles listed in Table 7.2 may be found in Figures 7.7-7.23.

Muscles of the Body

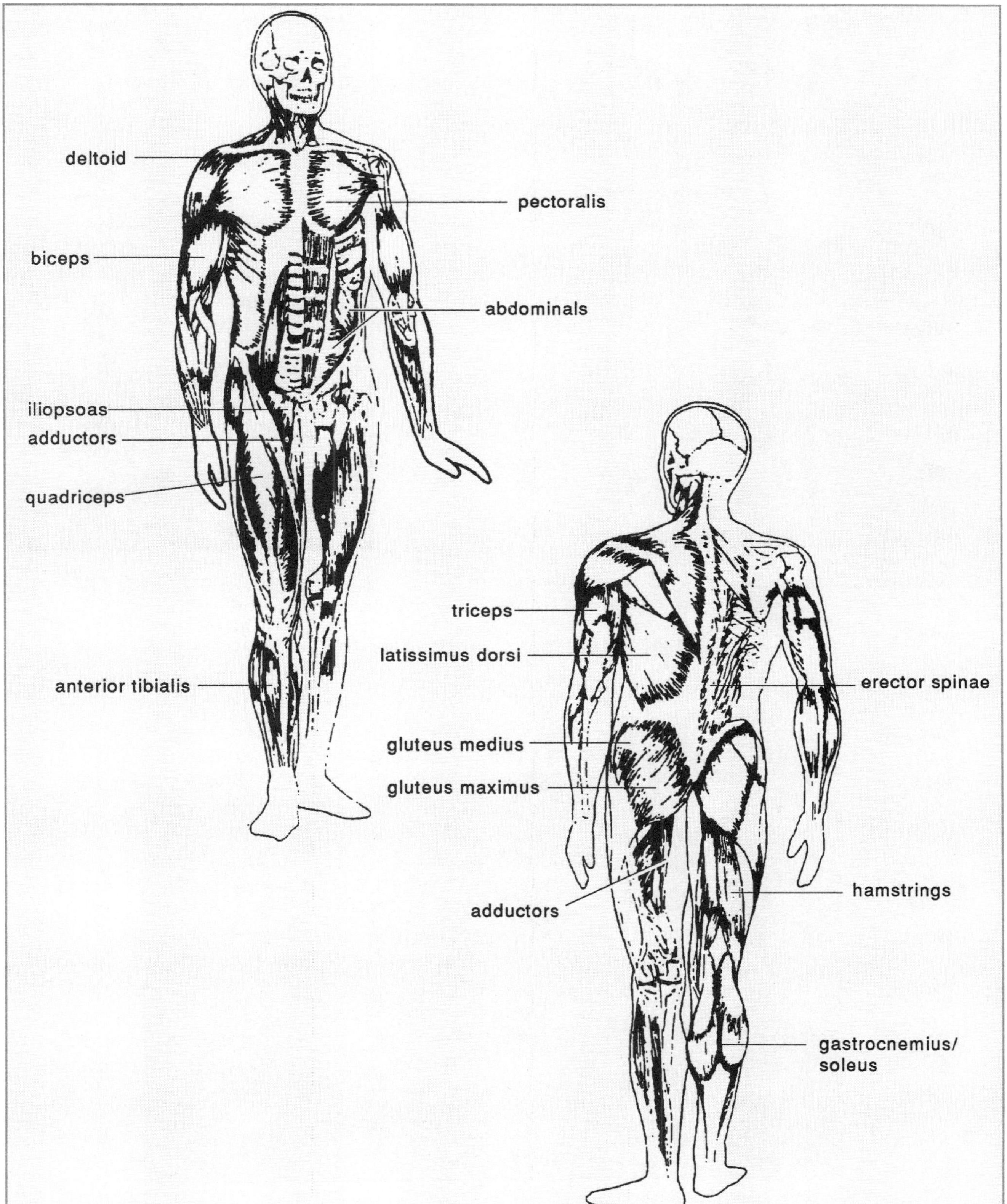

Figure 7.6. *Reproduced with permission of Cramer Products, Inc., Gardner, KS.*

Quadriceps (upper front leg) Stretch

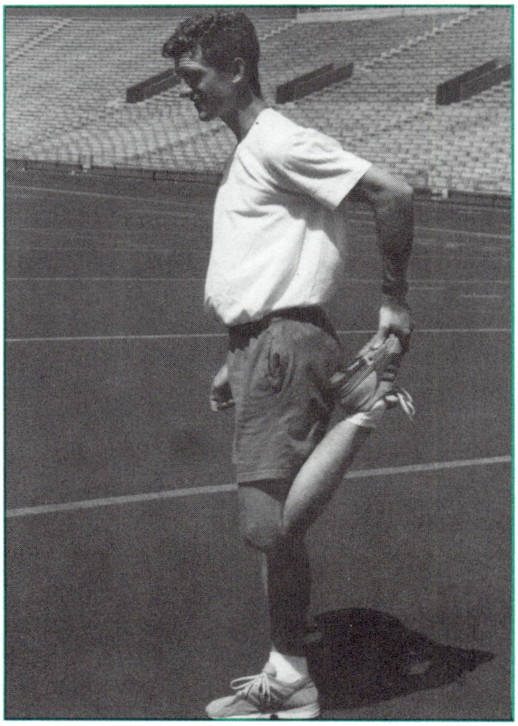

Figure 7.7. Grasp one leg at the foot and draw the heel toward the buttocks until a stretch is felt. For better stability, face and lean against a wall or chair for support.

Quadriceps and Hip Flexor (front of hip) Stretch

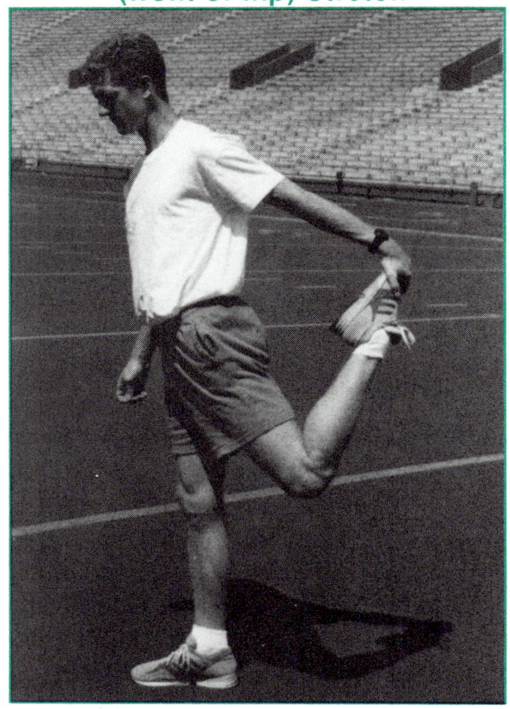

Figure 7.8. By extending the leg at the hip, the hip flexors can be stretched as well as the quadriceps.

Hamstrings (upper back leg) and Hip Extensor (buttocks) Stretch

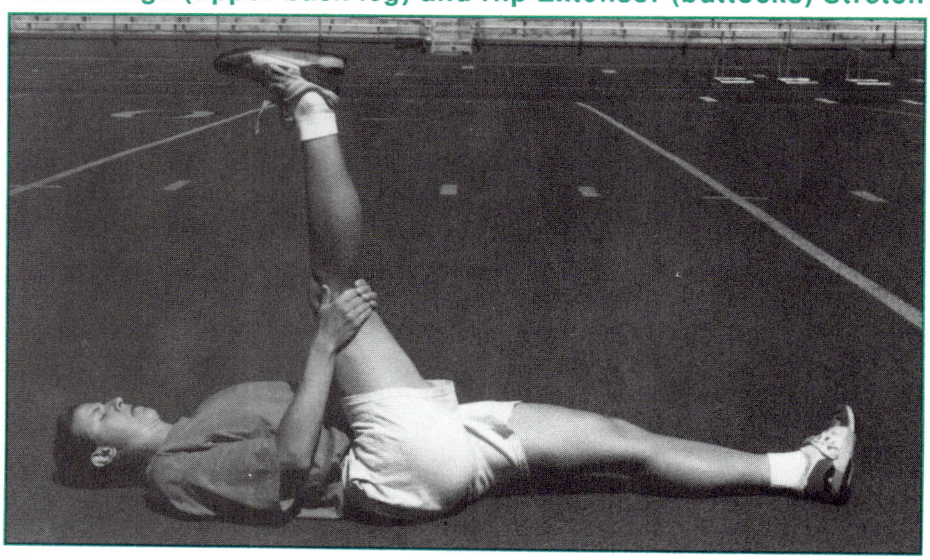

Figure 7.9. Lie on the back with one leg extended on the ground. Grasp the other leg behind the knee and draw toward the chest until a stretch is felt in the back of the leg and buttocks.

Gastrocnemius/Soleus (lower back leg) Stretch

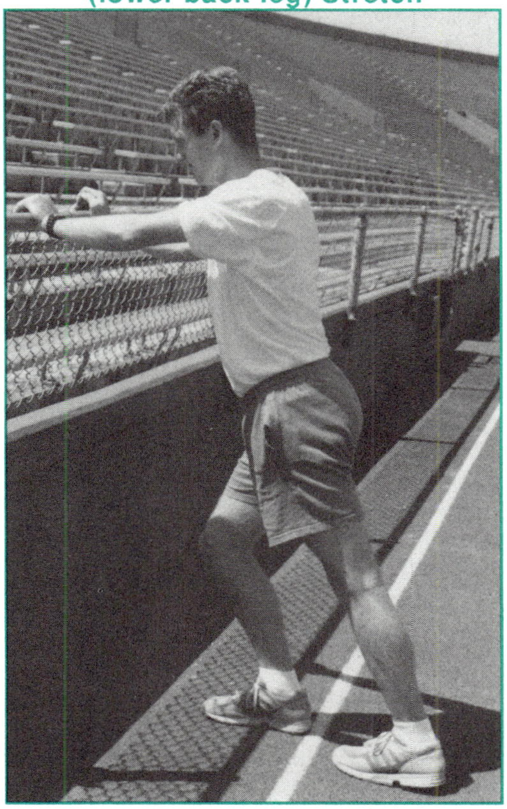

Figure 7.10. Lean against a wall or other solid object. Place one leg forward with the other leg extended backward. Keeping the heel on the ground, lean forward and downward at the ankle so that a stretch is felt in the lower leg.

Anterior Tibialis (lower front leg) Stretch

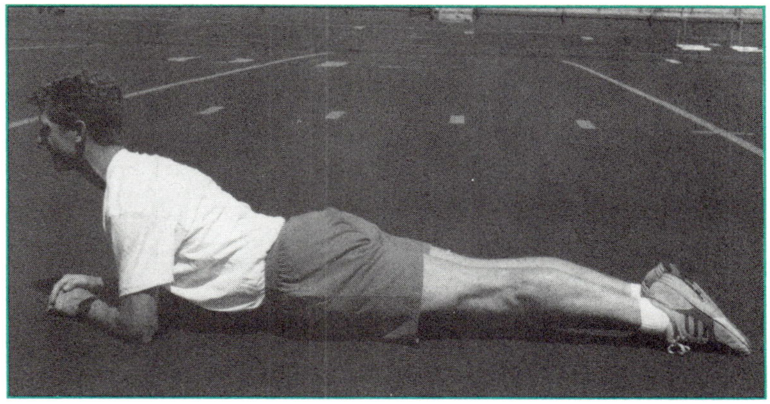

Figure 7.11. Extend the body while being supported by the lower arms and the toes. Lower the body toward the floor until a stretch is felt on along the front portion of the lower leg.

Hip Adductor (groin) Stretch

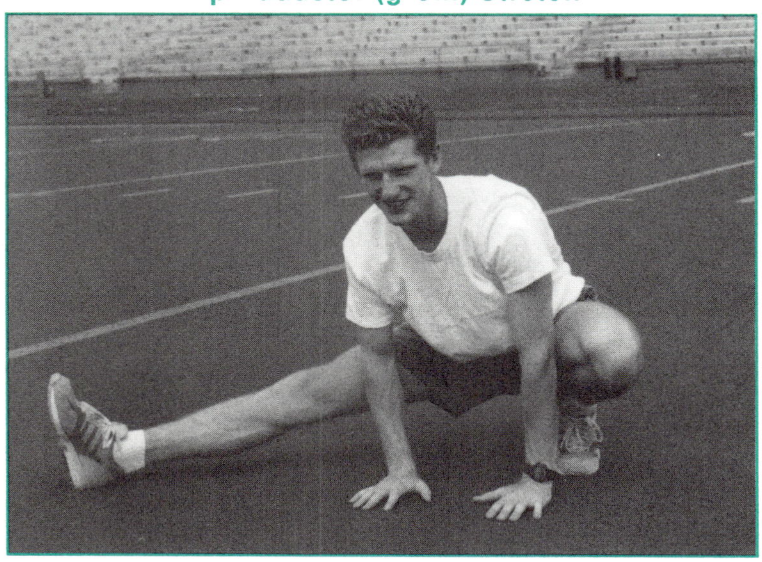

Figure 7.12. Assume a squat position with one leg bent at the knee and the other leg extended to the side with toes pointing upward. Move the body toward the ground until a stretch is felt. This exercise also may be started with the body in a standing position with one legextended to the side and the other slightly bent at the knee. Move toward the ground until the position in the photo is reached.

Hip Abductor (outside of hip) Stretch

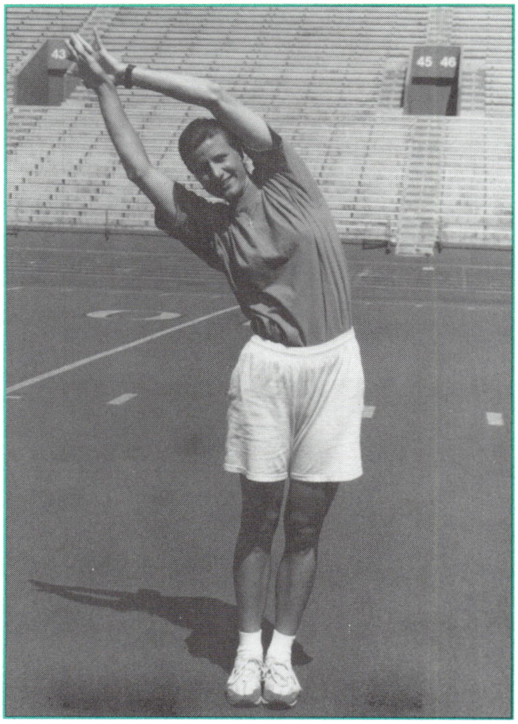

Figure 7.13. Assume a standing position with arms overhead. Lean to one side so that a stretch is felt along side of the body. Be sure there is no bending forward at the waist.

Hip Adbuctor Alternate Stretch

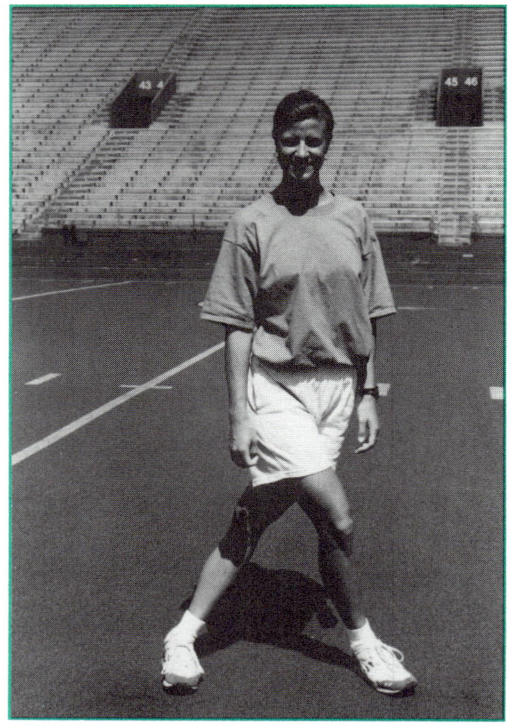

Figure 7.14. In an upright standing position, cross one leg over the other. The stretch should be felt on the back leg. For a greater stretch, take a longer side step.

Hip and Trunk Stretch

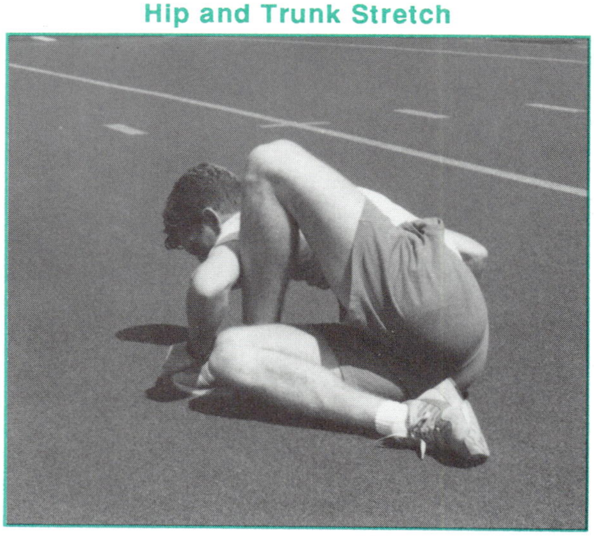

Figure 7.15. In a seated position, tuck the right leg under the left leg. Bring the left leg over the right leg and twist the body to the right until a stretch is felt along the buttocks and trunk. The hands may be placed to the outside of the left leg or the inside of the left leg depending upon the amount of flexibility.

Lower Back and Gluteals (buttocks) Stretch

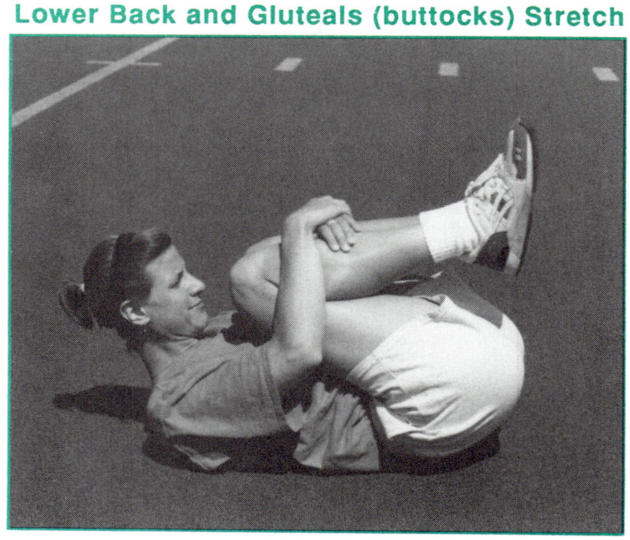

Figure 7.16. Lie on the ground and bend both legs and grasp around the knees. Pull the knees toward the chest and at the same time lift the shoulders off the ground. The stretch should be felt in the lower back and buttocks.

Abdominal Stretch

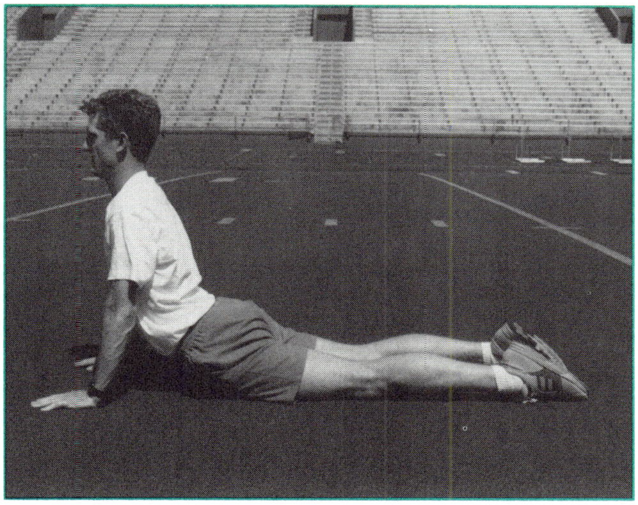

Figure 7.17. Lie on the ground and support the upper body with the arms. Arch the back until the stretch is felt in the abdominal muscles.

Chest and Abdominal Alternative Stretch

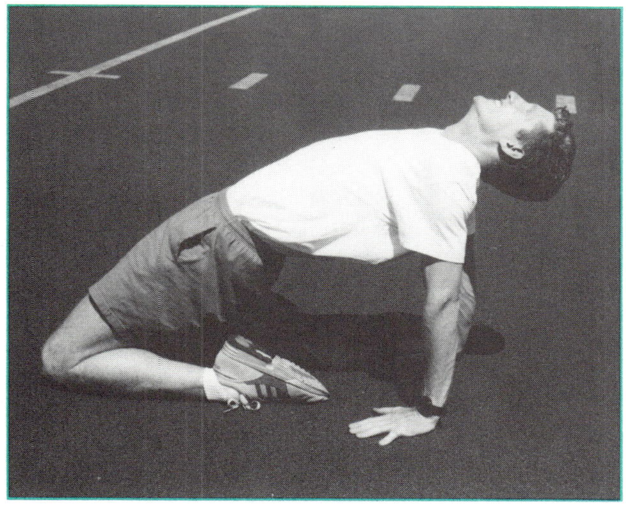

Figure 7.18. Kneel down and lean back so that the hands are resting on the floor near the small of the back. Lower the body toward the floor until a stretch is felt in the chest and abdominal region.

Pectoralis, Deltoid, and Biceps (upper arm and chest) Stretch

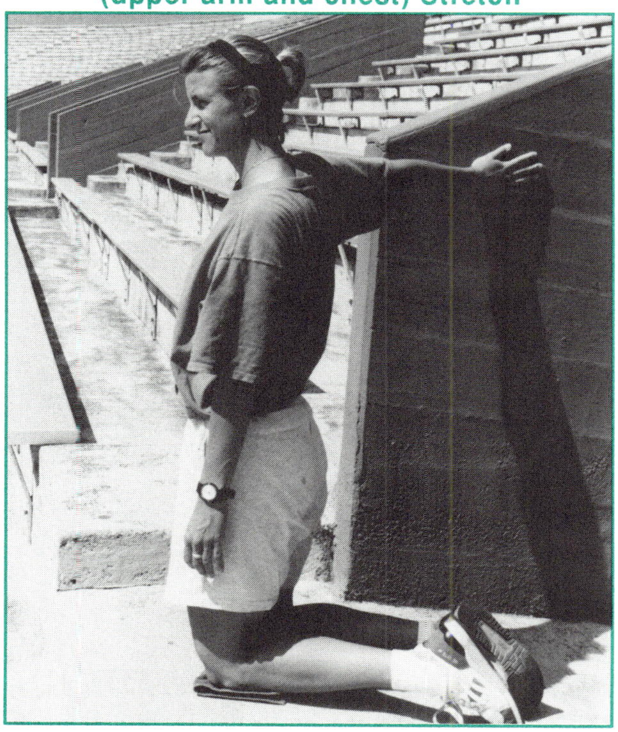

Figure 7.19. Stand with the body sideways to a wall or solid object. Extend the arm closest to the wall in a backward direction. Step sideways toward the wall until a stretch is felt in the upper arm and chest.

Pectoralis and Deltoid (chest and shoulder) Stretch

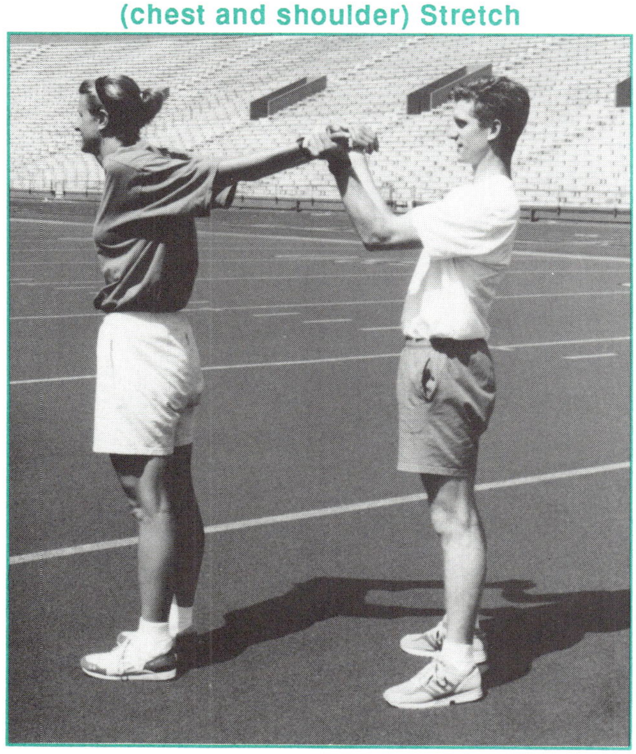

Figure 7.20. This is a partner- assisted stretch. A partner stands in back of the exerciser. The exerciser reaches back with both arms. The partner grasps the wrists and gently draws the arms together in back until a stretch is felt in the chest and shoulder.

Biceps (upper front arm) Stretch

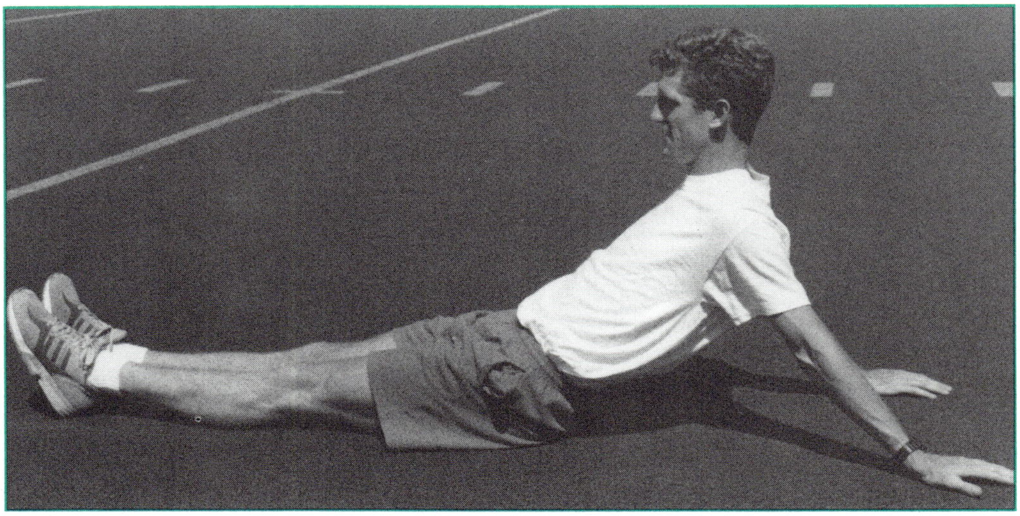

Figure 7.21. Sit on the ground and extend the arms in back of the body. Lower the body by moving the extended arms away slowly until a stretch is felt in the upper front arm.

Triceps (upper back arm) Stretch

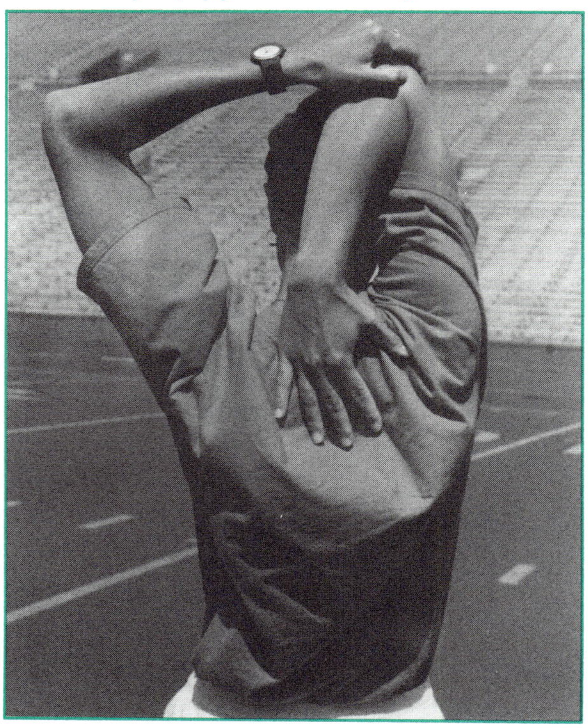

Figure 7.22. Reach in back of the head with one arm. Push the downward at the elbow with the opposite hand until a stretch is felt in the upper back arm.

Ankle Stretch

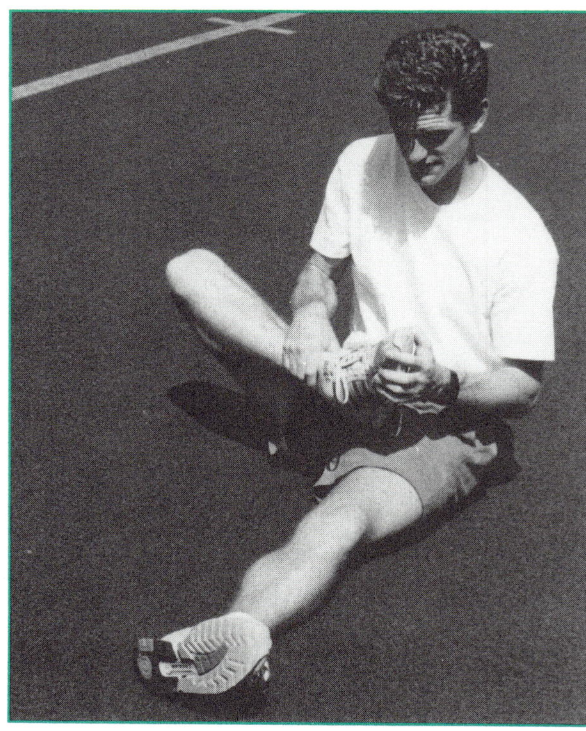

Figure 7.23. Grasp the foot and rotate it in all directions.

Suggested Readings

Anderson, B. *Stretching.* St. Bolinas, CA: Shelter Publications, Inc., 1980.

Beaulieu, J. E. *Stretching for All Sports.* Pasadena, CA: The Athletic Press, 1980.

Borms, J. Importance of flexibility in overall physical fitness. *International Journal of Physical Education.* 21:15, 1984.

Croce, P. *Stretching for Athletics.* New York: Leisure Press, 1984.

Roundtable Discussion: Flexibility. *National Strength and Conditioning Association Journal.* 6(4): 10-22, 71-73, 1984.

Safran, M. R. et al. The role of warm-up in muscular injury prevention. *American Journal of Sports Medicine.* 16(2): 123-128, 1988.

Safran, M. R. et al. Warm-up and muscular injury prevention: an update. *Sports Medicine.* 8(4): 239-249, 1989.

Sapega, A. A. et al. Biophysical factors in range-of-motion exercise. *The Physician and sportsmedicine.* 9(12): 57-65, 1981.

Taylor, D. C. et al. Viscoelastic properties of muscle-tendon units: the biomechanical effects of stretching. *American Journal of Sports Medicine.* 18(3): 300-309, 1990.

Zebas, C. J. & M. Chapman. *Prevention of Sports Injuries: A Biomechanical Approach.* Dubuque, IA: eddie bowers publishing, inc., 1990.

This chapter is adapted from a chapter which first appeared in T. R. Thomas. *Muscular Fitness Through Resistance Training.* Dubuque, IA: eddie bowers publishing, inc., 1991.

CHAPTER

8

MUSCULAR FITNESS

Tom Thomas

Learning Objectives

- Understand the role of resistance training in gaining muscular strength.
- Understand the role of resistance training in improving health status and gaining cardiovascular fitness.
- Describe the types of muscular contractions.
- Comprehend the methods of providing resistance to muscles.
- Understand the strength curve and the resistance techniques used to match it.
- Realize the specificity of resistance training to improve various physical skills.
- Know the terminology associated with resistance training.
- Understand strategies to maximize strength and power gains.
- Be able to develop a resistance training program.
- Contrast resistance training for strength, fitness, and muscle tone.

Important Terms

circuit resistance training (CRT)

concentric contraction

constant resistance

eccentric contraction

isokinetic contraction

muscular balance

overload

periodization

power training

resistance training

spot reduction

static resistance

strength training

supercompensation

tone

variable resistance

INTRODUCTION

The term "total fitness" has a variety of definitions and interpretations. Most people would consider muscular strength and tone a part of total fitness. Exercise scientists agree that aerobic training is the most important component of a fitness program since the health of the heart, lungs, and blood vessels are so critical to total health. But aerobic training alone may not produce adequate muscular function to efficiently perform many daily activities. Movements such as opening a stuck window or opening a garage door can cause injury to muscles not used to exerting such force. While aerobic training will improve the function of the muscle groups used in the exercise, it generally does not affect other muscles. Since most aerobic activities rely on the leg muscles, these exercises may not stimulate adequate gains in upper body strength. Therefore muscular resistance training must be used to supplement the aerobic program, especially relative to the upper body.

Total Fitness

TYPES OF MUSCULAR CONTRACTION

Skeletal muscle can be stimulated to contract in a variety of different ways. Basically muscular contractions can be divided into two types.

1. Static or isometric in which the internal muscular tension is equal to the external resistance and no movement occurs
2. Dynamic in which muscular tension produces movement

Dynamic contractions in which the internal muscular tension is greater than the external resistance is called **concentric**. In this type of contraction, the muscle shortens and the associated bones move toward each other. In **eccentric contractions**, the internal muscular tension is less than the external resistance, and the bones move apart. The muscle is "stronger" when contracting eccentrically, and it can handle more weight in this "negative" movement than in the "positive" concentric contraction.

The understanding of concentric and eccentric contractions is very important in prescribing exercises for specific muscles. For example, in the push-up, the same muscle groups are involved in both the up-phase and the down-phase of the exercise (Figure 8.1). This exercise would be prescribed only if the goal was to strengthen the triceps or the chest muscles. It would not be a good exercise for developing the biceps or back muscles.

Another type of dynamic contraction is **isokinetic** in which the muscle moves at a specific controlled speed. This type of contraction requires an external device to alter resistance so that the speed of contraction is the same throughout the range of movement. This type of contraction may be important in exercising the muscle at high speeds, which approximate those used during physical activity and sports performance.

Concentric and Eccentric Contractions

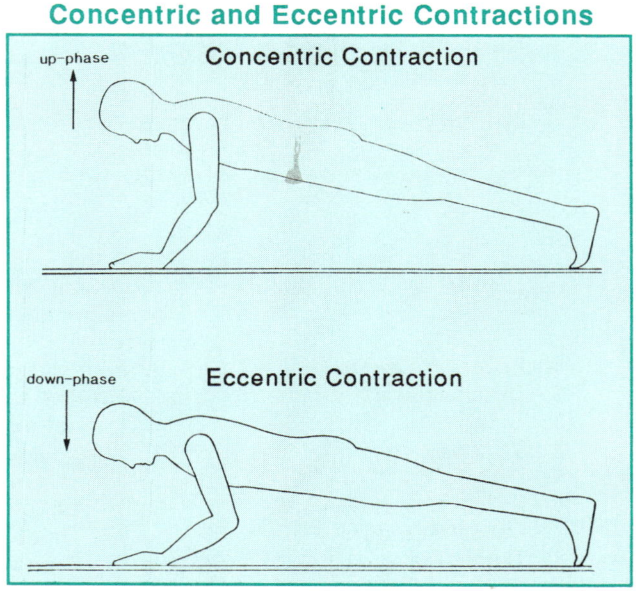

Figure 8.1. The same muscle groups (pectorals and triceps) control the movement in both the up and down phases of the push-up.

Major Muscles of the Body

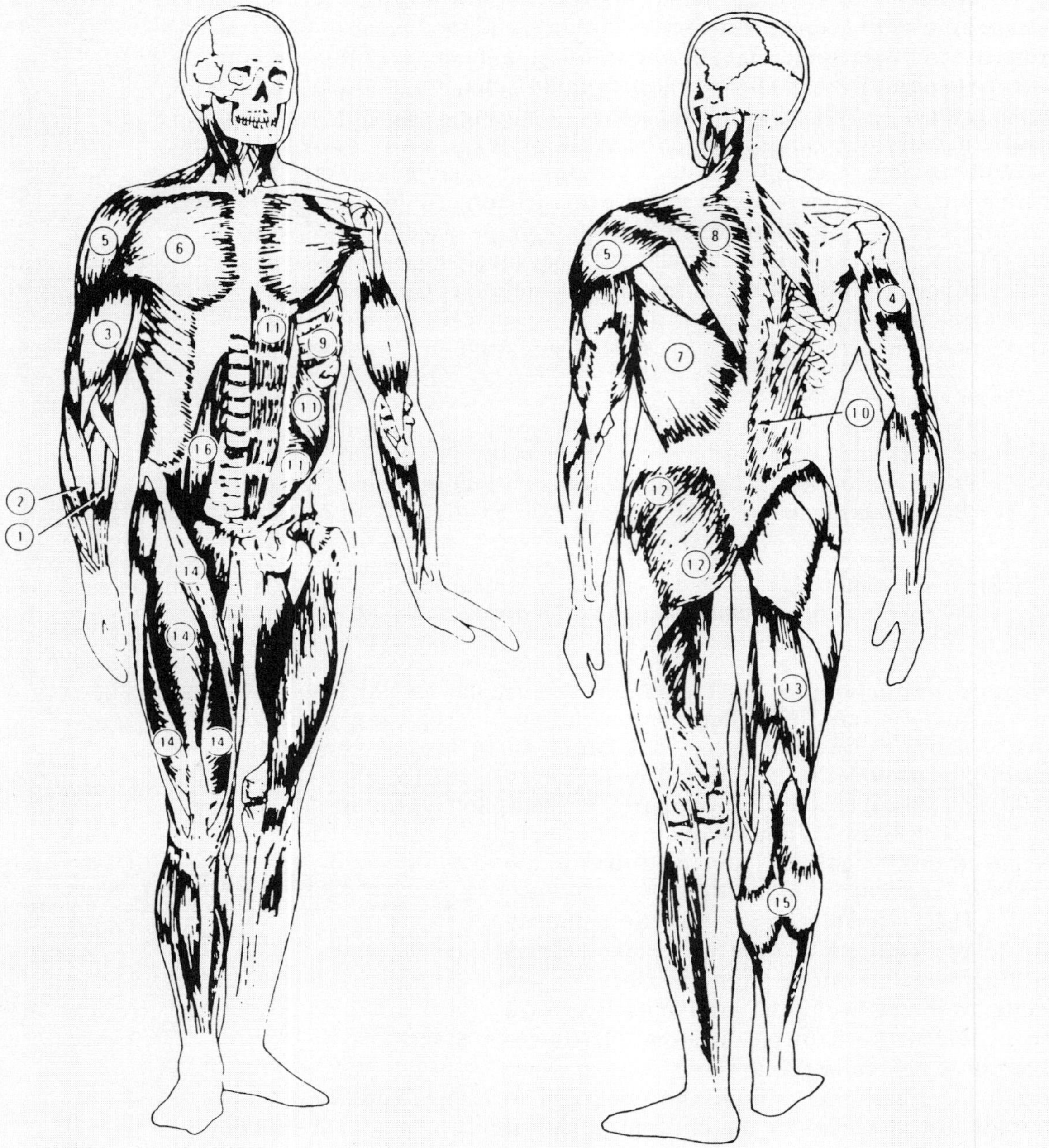

1. Forearm flexors
2. Brachioradialis
3. Biceps
4. Triceps
5. Deltoid
6. Pectoral muscles
7. Latissimus dorsi
8. Trapezius
9. Serratus anterior
10. Erector spinae (spinal extensors)
11. Abdominal muscles
    a. Internal and external obliques
    b. Rectus abdominis
    c. Transversalis
12. Gluteal muscles
13. Hamstrings
14. Quadriceps muscles
15. Gastrocnemius, soleus muscles
16. Iliopsoas (under abdominal muscles)

Reproduced with permission of Cramer Products, Inc., Gardner, KS.

METHODS OF PROVIDING RESISTANCE

Nearly any type of muscular activity may be beneficial in developing or maintaining the fitness of muscle. Simply raising the arms over the head can provide a beneficial effect to the muscles involved in the movement. In raising the arms over the head, the weight of the hand and arm provide the resistance for the muscles. Improvement in muscular strength and performance, however, generally requires a method of providing a greater overload resistance to stimulate the muscle to produce greater forces.

Muscle Fitness

Just as there are many kinds of muscular contractions, there are a variety of ways of providing external resistance for muscular exercise. Currently the study of resistance devices is one of the most dynamic aspects of the fitness boom era. Major equipment manufacturers are spending millions of dollars in developing new resistance machines. The goal of this investment is to make instruments which provide the most appropriate type of resistance for the muscle. Unfortunately, the type of resistance that is actually best for training muscle is unknown. This is an area which is being vigorously researched by exercise physiologists in the U.S. and other countries.

STATIC RESISTANCE

When resistance is immovable by the muscular force, it is termed static or isometric. These terms indicate that the load is so heavy, the muscle cannot move it, and thus the muscle length remains the same during the contraction. Because **static resistance** provides the muscle with stress only at a specific point in the range of motion, strength gains are "angle specific." That is, the strength gained occurs in a very limited area of the working range. For example, if an individual attempted to lift a heavy desk by flexing the biceps muscle, the strength gain would be limited to the arm angle at which the contraction was performed. Of course, the elbow angle could be changed several times which would allow the muscle to be worked through the range. This requires a very long workout period for each muscle and generally is not feasible. Regardless, such exercises would have little relevance to the way the muscle is actually used during activity. Very few activities utilize static muscular contraction.

Static Problems

Another disadvantage of using static resistance is the relatively large increase in blood pressure during the exercise. In addition, the pressure in the chest, called intrathoracic pressure, can be elevated. Both of these effects diminish the heart's ability to pump blood to the working muscles and to other organs such as the brain. These effects can be especially dangerous in the older individual. Static or isometric resistance training programs are not recommended for most people. Many better ways exist for providing resistance to the muscle.

Static exercise can be used for brief time periods by young adults when other resistance exercises are not available (e.g., vacation). In addition, isometric instruments can be used for testing muscular strength. The cable tensiometer and hand grip and back dynamometers are examples of such testing instruments.

Universal Free Weights

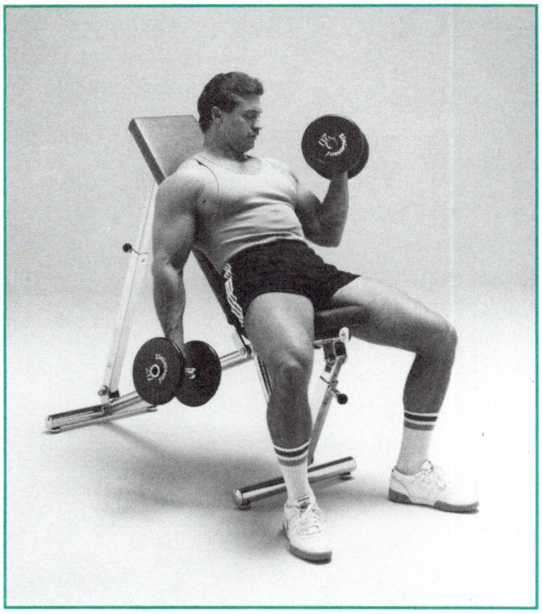

Figure 8.2. The dumbbell resistance remains constant throughout the range of motion. Photo was provided by Universal Gym Equipment, Inc.

Universal Lat Pulldown and Biceps Curl

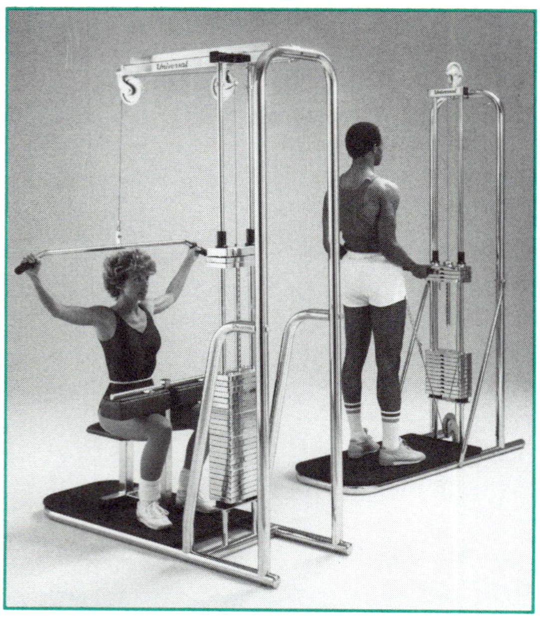

Figure 8.3. The lever system of the machine does not change and the resistance remains constant throughout the range of motion. Photo was provided by Universal Gym Equipment, Inc.

ISOTONIC RESISTANCE

Isotonic methods are the traditional types of weight lifting. These include the standard free-weight barbell and dumbbell (Figure 8.2) as well as some weight lifting machines (Figure 8.3). Isotonic resistance provides a "constant load" on the muscle throughout the entire range of motion. The muscle must contract with both concentric and eccentric dynamic contractions to raise and lower the weight, respectively. If the isotonic exercise is performed correctly, the muscle is stressed throughout its complete contraction range. Since the muscle is "stronger" when contracting eccentrically, it is less overloaded during this phase of the exercise. In addition, **constant resistance** exercises do not tax each joint angle equally. The skeletal lever system causes the muscle to be stronger at certain angles. Therefore, at points where the muscle is strongest, the weight will tax it less than at points where the muscle is weakest. For example, in the biceps curl, a 100 lb barbell might cause the muscle to develop maximal tension at 180° and 45° joint angles (beginning and end of the lift). But at 100° joint angle (middle of the lift), the muscle is not taxed as much. This constant resistance technique may cause some points in the range of motion to develop greater strength gains than others. This selective improvement may be beneficial in that the weaker points might catch up to the stronger points in the contraction range. On the other hand, constant resistance training may be a disadvantage since the strongest points in the range may not develop to their full capacity.

Momentum or inertia of the weight also is altered from the start of the lift to the end, and this changes the load which the muscle feels through the range of motion. This is one reason why free-weight exercise is traditionally performed at slow speeds in an attempt to lessen the effect of momentum. Some of the variable resistance and isokinetic machines which do not use weight stacks, have eliminated the effect of inertia on the resistance.

Barbell free-weights require both the dominant and non-dominant limbs to share the load equally. Thus, muscular balance between the two sides of the body is better maintained. In addition, free-weight lifting requires balancing the bar in many directions and not just the direction of the lift. This may require additional beneficial muscular activity during the exercise. These potential advantages of free-weights are countered by the greater skill required to perform free-weight exercises than machine exercises. Increased danger of losing control and even dropping the weights are risks for the novice. A partner also is required for spotting on some lifts. Because of these potential problems, use of free-weight, constant-resistance exercises require appropriate training and supervision. Heavy free-weight lifting is recommended only for experienced weight lifters and power athletes with the primary goals of maximizing muscular bulk and muscular strength balance.

VARIABLE RESISTANCE

The newest and commercially most competitive area of resistance equipment is the development of **variable resistance** machines. With this equipment, the resistance is altered throughout the range of motion in an attempt to match the changing capabilities of muscle at different joint angles. Many techniques have been devised to alter resistance during the range of motion. One of the first methods was developed by Nautilus, which used a "nautilus shell" shaped cam to alter the load. In this system, as the pulley cord is moved around the cam, the resistance arm distance is altered and thus the resistance felt by the muscle is changed throughout its range of motion (Figure 8.4). Such a cam potentially allows the resistance to be increased at the strongest points in the movement range and decreased at the weakest points, thus a "compound resistance" change.

Another novel system, developed by Universal, mechanically alters the load by physically moving the weights to change the resistance arm length (Figure 8.5). Such a system causes the resistance to continually increase throughout the concentric phase of the range of motion, and decrease during the eccentric phase. These are "linear resistance" changes. In the example of the shoulder press, the resistance somewhat matches the muscular strength curve because the lever system for the triceps muscle causes increased strength through the concentric range of motion. For other lifts, such as the biceps curl, the resistance overshoots the muscle capabilities late in the concentric phase of the lift. Momentum allows the lift to be completed.

Other examples of innovative mechanisms which produce variable resistance include the Soloflex resistance bands or weight straps. As these straps are stretched through the concentric range of motion, the resistance is increased (Figure 8.6). In Keiser strength equipment, muscular movement causes an engine-like piston to compress air in a pneumatic cylinder, thus increasing the resistance through the range-of-motion. A built-in system of linkages attached to the machine

Nautilus Shoulder Press

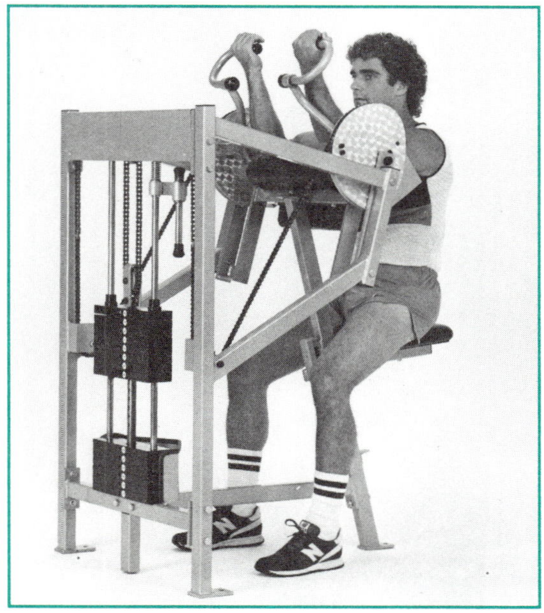

Figure 8.4. The variable resistance cams are shown at the shoulders of the exerciser. Photo was provided by Nautilus Sports/Medical Industries, Inc.

Universal Centurion Shoulder Press

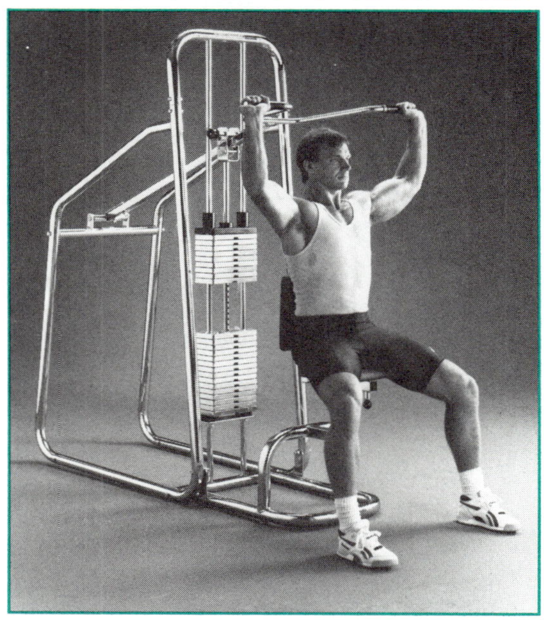

Figure 8.5. The resistance arm changes throughout each phase of the lift. The resistance increases through the concentric phase range of motion and decreases through the eccentric phase. Photo was provided by Universal Gym Equipment, Inc.

Soloflex Shoulder Press

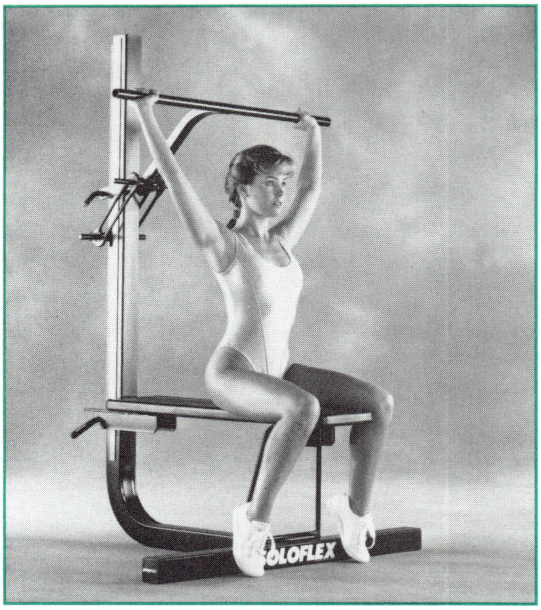

Figure 8.6. Stretched weight straps are shown on the vertical stand. Photo was provided by Soloflex, Inc.

Keiser Leg Extension

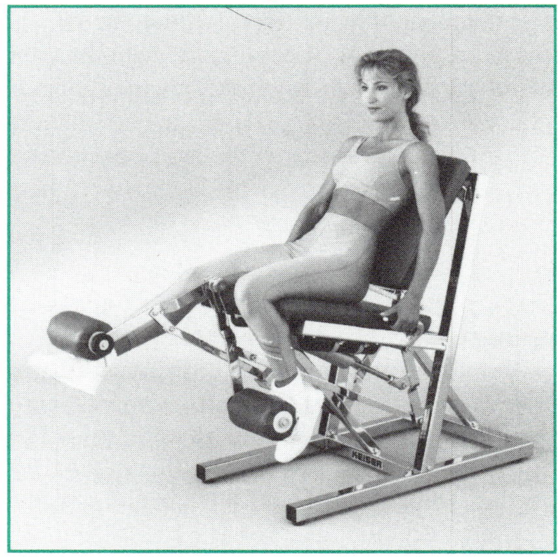

Figure 8.7. Air cylinder is shown under the seat. Photo was provided by Keiser Sports Health Equipment.

Hydra-Fitness Shoulder Press/Lat Pull

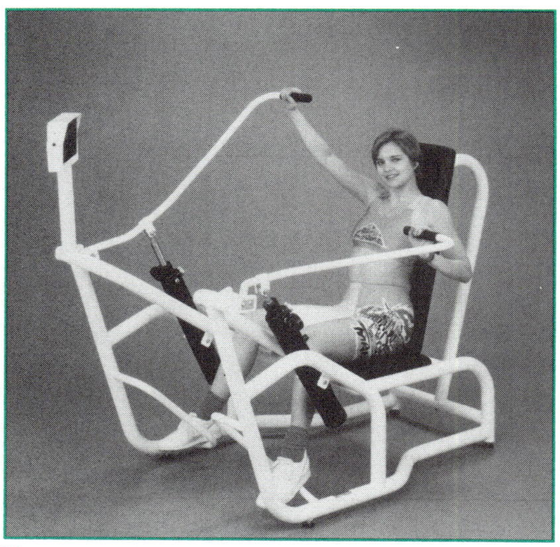

Figure 8.8. Hydraulic cylinders are shown at the knees of the exerciser. Photo was provided by Hydra-Fitness Industries.

also adjusts the resistance (Figure 8.7). The Hydra-Fitness exercise machines alter resistance with hydraulic cylinders in which hydraulic fluid provides the resistance for concentric contractions (Figure 8.8). These machines are called "double positive" because the initial movement works one muscle concentrically and the return movement works the opposite muscle concentrically.

Additional variable resistance systems are being developed at a rapid pace. Each has a different mechanism attempting to match resistance with muscular function. The success of these strategies may depend on how well an individual's strength curve of a given muscle matches the specific resistance curve of the machine.

Although certain systems seem to have theoretical advantage, very little research has examined the muscular strength - resistance match-ups of the various types of strength equipment. Current scientific findings do not support the use of any one type of variable resistance mechanism. Rather, all systems seem to improve muscular strength. The development of various training devices seems beneficial since nearly anyone interested in muscular training can find equipment which suits him/her. The selection of one variable resistance system over another then may relate to the specific goals of an individual. For example, some machines are easier to work at higher speeds than others. Machines which do not utilize actual weights, e.g., hydraulic machines, are especially useful for high speed lifting.

ISOKINETIC RESISTANCE

Another kind of muscular training which uses a form of variable resistance is isokinetic exercises. In this "same speed" technique, the movement speed is set on a dial. This speed setting is the key distinguishing characteristic of true isokinetic equipment. Speed of the instrument is selected and not the amount of resistance. The machine allows the movement to proceed no faster than the set speed no matter how much tension is produced in the contracting muscle. By this mechanism, an exact resistance can be matched to the force capabilities of the muscle. If a maximal effort is attempted at all joint angles, the machine resistance is maximal at all joint angles. The advantage of such a machine is to tax the muscle maximally throughout the range of motion. Isokinetic resistance training involves no eccentric contraction, only concentric. This may be an advantage since eccentric movements have been associated with muscular soreness. However, the lack of eccentric training also may be a disadvantage since most sports activities require eccentric contractions. For example, the rapid bending of the knees to lower the torso in making a tennis stroke or gathering for a jump shot or spike, all require eccentric contractions of the quadriceps muscles.

Dial the Speed

Cybex by Lumex, a noteworthy isokinetic testing instrument, has a recording of the performance which is valuable in muscular function testing (Figure 8.9). The major advantage of isokinetic exercise is the ability to train at high speeds and thus develop the force and speed aspects of power. Most individuals lift weights at 60-100 degrees/sec. Many power events (e.g., jumping and sprinting) are performed at speeds two to three times greater than this. Previous research indicates the "performance power" is improved only when muscle is trained at speeds equal to or greater than the performance speed. If this principle is true, the use of traditional weight training lifting speeds may not maximally improve muscular function at speeds necessary for elite power performance.

A major disadvantage of isokinetic muscular training is that the resistance of the machine is solely dependent upon the user's motivation. The effort can be minimal, maximal, or somewhere in-between. The instrument controls only the speed of movement. Because of the potential for "cheating," isokinetic exercise, in the present form, may not achieve all of its theoretical capabilities as a training tool. Some coaches and athletic trainers have questioned the appropriateness of isokinetic training since the muscle seldom performs isokinetically during sport activities. In addition, the device provides resistance only when the speed of the lift equals the set machine speed. During the initial phases of the exercise, as the muscle accelerates to the set speed, no resistance is encountered. Therefore, the resistance is not maximal through the initial range of motion, especially at fast movement settings.

Cybex 350

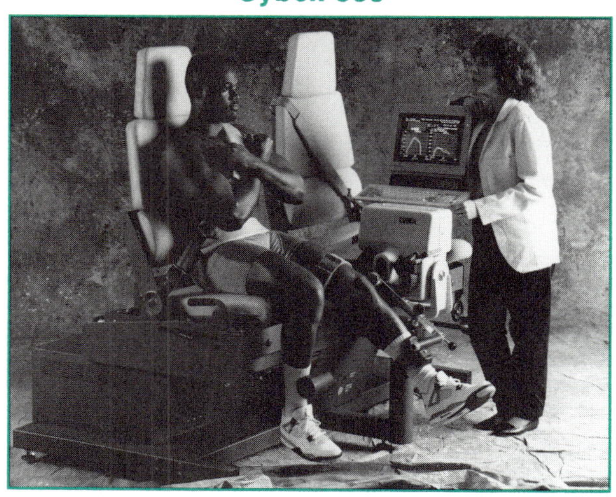

Figure 8.9. An isokinetic testing instrument. Photo was provided by Cybex.

Studies comparing isotonic, variable resistance, and isokinetic muscular training methods have not been conclusive. However, some studies have suggested greater gains can be obtained with isokinetic training in highly motivated individuals. All types of muscular training have been shown to produce strength gains if the workload is heavy. Whether all methods will improve muscular power and sports performance is unknown.

BODY WEIGHT RESISTANCE EXERCISES

Many techniques can be utilized to develop skeletal muscle fitness without the use of weight equipment. Most of these methods rely on part or all of the body weight to provide the resistance during the exercise (Figure 8.10). While these techniques may not be as effective as machine training in developing maximal muscular strength and bulk, they are very adequate in improving general muscular fitness.

Body Weight Exercise

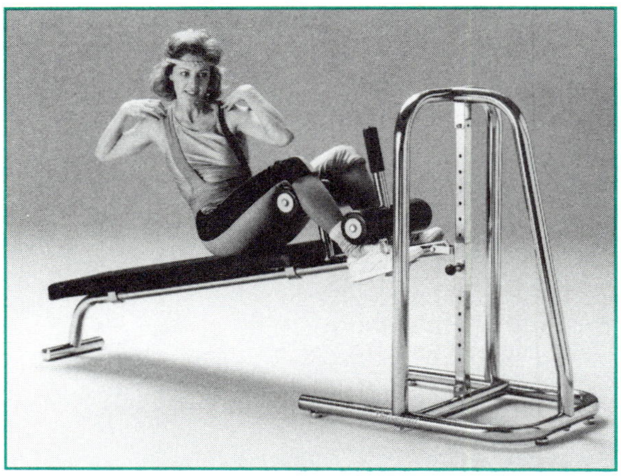

Figure 8.10. The upper torso provides the resistance for the abdominal muscles during the sit-up. Photo was provided by Universal Gym Equipment, Inc.

Many common exercises require the muscles to lift the body weight off the floor. These activities require dynamic muscular contractions, both concentric and eccentric. The sit-up, push-up, and pull-up are examples of these activities. Running or jumping also are body weight lifting exercises which stress specific muscles and can be used to improve muscular fitness. One limitation to such activities can be the difficulty in exercising opposite muscle groups to maintain muscular balance (e.g., quadriceps and hamstrings).

Body weight activities generally are sufficient to maintain muscular strength and improve muscular tone. With the addition of weights to the body or by increasing the resistance with a partner, substantial strength improvements may be observed.

RESISTANCE TRAINING PROGRAMS

Some general principles are important regardless of the goals of the **resistance training**. However, some strategies used in the resistance training sessions vary according to the specific goal of the individual. Strength Assessments can be found in Inventory #27 on page 273.

WORKOUT TERMS

In traditional weight training terms, a "repetition" is moving the resistance through one complete range of motion and returning to the starting position (Table 8.1). The amount of resistance or weight which requires a single maximal contraction is called a one repetition maximum (1 RM). This feat indicates the maximal strength of a specific muscle or group of muscles. The amount of resistance which can be lifted only twice is called a 2 RM, and so on. A training "set" is a single series of multiple repetitions. For example, an individual may perform a 6 RM exercise in each of two sets for a total of 12 repetitions.

Resistance Training Workout Terminology

Term	Definition
Repetition	Moving a resistance through one complete range of motion and Returning
One Repetition Maximum (1 RM)	The amount of resistance which can be moved only one time through the range of motion and returned.
Set	A single series of repetitions.
Rest Period	The time between sets.
Work Period	The time during which the repetitions are performed.

Table 8.1.

STRENGTH TRAINING

Strength is best increased by exerting near maximal forces a few times each workout, i.e., high resistance, low repetition exercises. Typically the resistance is 70-85% of 1 RM with four to eight repetitions to failure (4-8 RM). Early research using untrained men and traditional free-weight training indicated that three sets of six RM on alternative days produced the greatest increments in dynamic strength. Some research evidence suggests that three sets are optimal and five sets produce no greater increase in strength. Regardless of the method, the key goal is to provide the muscle with an **overload** or a greater workload than it is accustomed. **Supercompensation**, the muscular rebuilding process, probably requires 24-48 hours. This process is longer after more intense, heavy exercise than after light lifting. In addition, supercompensation may take less time in well-trained individuals. The time necessary for muscular rebuilding, therefore, dictates that alternate day workouts using the same muscle group are likely to be more effective than working the same muscle group each day. Since most research dealing with dynamic **strength training** has utilized untrained men, it is unknown if the repetitions, sets, and frequency principles apply to well-trained individuals. Athletes and coaches have sometimes questioned the results of research which used non-athletes. Indeed, strength training research has not always produced results observed by ardent weight lifters. Athletes and other experienced lifters use a variety of heavy resistance programs apparently with good success. This supports the concept that maximal motor unit recruitment, regardless of the techniques, is a key to muscular strength gains.

Allow Time to Rebuild

Lifting speed does not seem to be important in the development of muscular strength. When using weights, fast speeds should not be attempted due to the risk of injury and the increased use of momentum in the exercise, which tends to reduce the tension required by the muscle. Likewise, the time between sets does not appear critical to the amount of strength gains. Usually trial and error is used by experienced lifters to determine the rest period. Rests of one to three minutes have been suggested for heavy resistance training.

Lighten Up

Heavy resistance training is not appropriate for most individuals with fitness goals. Adequate strength gains can be achieved with lighter loads and greater repetitions. Even if the goal is to improve performance in recreational sports, a lighter load strength program will be effective. An individual interested in general muscular fitness, sports performance, or muscular tone should use a "scaled down" strength program of 3 sets of 12 repetitions using a 15 RM load (about 65% of 1 RM) (Table 8.2). In other words use 12 reps of a resistance which could be handled for 15 reps. This strategy illustrates a key principle for most people: Do not lift to failure. Other principles related to strength resistance training are listed in Table 8.3.

Resistance Training Programs

Resistance Training Goal	Strength	Muscular Tone	CV Fitness
Load (% of 1 RM)	60-70	50-60	40-60
Repetitions (number)	10-12	12-20	12-15
Sets (number/exercise)	3	6-10	1-2
Exercises or Stations (number/workout)	10-12	10-12	6-8
Rest periods (seconds)	120-180	60-90	10-20
Frequency (days/week/muscle group)	2-3	2-3	3-4

Table 8.2.

General Principles for Effective Resistance Training

1. Move the resistance through the full range of motion.
2. Breathe during each phase of the lift to prevent large increases of intrathoracic pressure.
3. Know the muscle(s) affected by the exercise.
4. Exercise antagonistic muscles to avoid imbalance. For example, quadriceps exercises should be accompanied by hamstrings exercises and pectoralis exercises accompanied by exercises using the upper back muscles such as the infraspinatus, posterior deltoid, and teres minor.
5. Stretch the active muscle and joints before and after exercise to prevent loss of flexibility.
6. Warm-up with calisthenics and light lifting before the workout. Cool-down with similar light exercises after the workout.
7. Do not exercise just after eating.
8. Do not use the same muscle in sequential exercises. For example, do not perform the shoulder press and bench press in sequence because both use the triceps extensively.
9. Heavy lifting (75-100% of maximum) is reserved for competitive athletes and weight lifters.
10. After their competitive careers, athletes need to reduce resistance training loads and intensity.

Table 8.3.

Training Phases

In general, heavy loads and few repetitions are utilized to build strength. Also part of this system is "pyramiding" in which loads are progressively increased during the exercise session. Loads also are progressively increased or "pyramided" over a given time period in the program. The training regimen uses cycling or **periodization** in which the exercise intensity is varied workout to workout and over set time periods to avoid staleness and training plateaus. Each major muscle group is exercised two times per week, once heavy and once medium. At least two days rest is taken between sessions using the same muscle groups. The chest and legs are exercised on Monday (heavy) and Thursday (medium), and the back, shoulders, and arms on Tuesday (heavy) and Friday (medium).

Time to Fine Tune

A simpler program can be performed by young athletes or athletes participating in sports which do not necessarily require maximal strength efforts. In this simpler system three sets of six repetitions (6 RM) are used for each muscle group and all body parts three times per week (alternate days). It is important that the muscles associated with the sport be emphasized and muscular balance maintained. This program is very effective in producing strength and hypertrophy gains in previously untrained young adults.

A program similar in intensity to the Epley system can be used for any sport in which maximal muscular strength and power are required. Such intense training generally is reserved for high-level competitive athletics and is especially effective in power sports such as football, basketball, volleyball, and track and field. This high intensity program is not necessary nor recommended for the recreational athlete.

The Periodization "Phases" Progress from Light to Maximum Intensity

Phase 1	Phase 2	Phase 3	Phase 4	Phase 5
10 reps 3 sets 1st set 65% of 1 RM 2nd set 70% 3rd set 75% 1-2 minutes between exercises 1-2 week duration	8 reps 4 sets 1st set 65% 2nd set 70% 3rd set 75% 4th set 75% 2 minutes between exercises 1-2 week duration Reduce loads by 5% on medium days e.g., 1st set = 60% of 1 RM	6 reps 4 sets 1st set 65% 2nd set 75% 3rd set 75% 4th set 80% 2 minutes rest between exercises 1 week duration Reduce loads by 5% on medium days	10, 8, 4, 3 reps 4 sets 10 reps at 50% 8 reps at 60% 4 reps at 80% 3 reps at 85% 2 minutes rest between exercises 1 week duration Reduce loads by 5% on medium days	Rest (Actvity but no resistance training) 1-2 week duration **Start again at Phase 1.**

Power Training

High Speeds

Power training can be incorporated into this strength regimen by using power drills on non-lifting days (Wednesday and weekends) or before the strength routine on leg days (Monday and Thursday). Power drills might include high knees, ankle flips, stair runs, hopping, jumping, and plyometrics.

Power resistance training also can be performed on a fifth workout day in which lighter loads and faster contractions are used. Loads of about 40-60% can be used with lifts made as rapidly as possible. Such a program is feasible only when non-weight resistance equipment is available. Momentum caused by rapidly lifting free-weights and weight stacks can reduce the resistance on the muscle and increase the risk of injury. Some form of power training should be incorporated into the resistance program whether in-season or off-season.

Maintenance

Once strength and power are gained, they are fairly easy to retain. Maintenance training during the season can include using the medium day only, each muscular group used one day per week. As an alternative, one exercise can be performed for each muscle group twice a week (heavy and medium) at intensities equivalent to phase 3 of the cycle.

Training Exercises

Keep a Log

Example exercises are listed below. Alternatives which affect similar muscular groups can be used. Illustrations at the end of the chapter provide descriptions of the exercises and the muscles involved. Additional exercises can be selected if the sport demands greater training of specific muscle groups. The sequence of exercises are arranged so that the same muscle group is not used in successive exercises. The complete cycle is performed and then repeated for the second and third sets. If equipment is limited, the second set for a given lift can immediately follow the first set using a three minute rest period. Inventory #29 on page 279 contains workout records for logging daily resistance training workouts.

Exercise Examples

Monday (heavy) and Thursday (medium)	Tuesday (heavy) and Friday (medium)	Monday-Friday (4 times/week)
Chest and Legs 1. Bench Press 2. Squat 3. Incline Press or Chest Butterfly 4. Leg Curl 5. Heel Raise 6. Leg Extension or Leg Press 7. Ankle Flexion 8. Hip Extension and Flexion	**Arms, Shoulders, Back** 1. Arm Curl 2. Shoulder Press 3. Lat Pull 4. Arm Extension 5. Upright Row 6. Incline Shoulder Press 7. Bent-over Row 8. Shoulder Shrug	**Abdominal-Trunk** **One set of 25 each** 1. Incline Sit-Up or Roman-Chair Sit-Up 2. Abdominal Curl on machine 3. Knee Raise or Knee Lift

MUSCULAR ENDURANCE

Muscular endurance is best improved by moving a submaximal resistance as many times as possible. That is, low resistance (25 to 50% of maximum) is used with many repetitions. The use of traditional resistance training as a means of obtaining endurance generally is not very effective. Not only are such workouts very time consuming, but other forms of activity such as distance running, swimming, and cycling produce superior results. Most of the popular "endurance" programs (e.g., 2-3 sets of 12-20 RM) are actually providing better muscular strength training than endurance. These programs do increase strength and when performed in a circuit can even produce small increases in aerobic capacity. On the other hand, high speed, 30 sec isokinetic workbouts may enhance "anaerobic endurance." Such improvement may be valuable in longer anaerobic events such as wrestling and middle distance running.

Repeat
Repeat
Repeat

MUSCULAR BALANCE

Research studies in sports medicine suggest that **muscular balance** is very important in preventing muscular injury as well as in enhancing success in certain athletic events. Most of the information regarding muscular balance has been obtained by testing the leg muscles. It has been suggested that the hamstrings in the back of the leg should be at least 60% as strong as the quadriceps in the front of the same leg when tested at slow speeds, 60 to 120 degree per second (°/sec).

Front to Back
Side to Side

$$\frac{\text{hamstrings strength}}{\text{quadriceps strength}} \times 100 > 60\%$$

When tested at faster speeds of 180°/sec or greater, the hamstrings strength becomes closer in magnitude to the quadriceps and at 300°/sec approaches 85-90%. Thus, when the legs are tested at speeds which more closely correspond to sports performance rates, the strength between the two muscle groups approaches equality.

$$\frac{\text{hamstring strength}}{\text{quadriceps strength}} \text{ (at > 180°/sec)} \times 100 > 80\%$$

The two hamstring muscles (right and left) should be nearly equal or exhibit no more than 10% difference in strength or power at any testing speed. The same is true for the two quadriceps muscle groups.

$$\frac{\text{weak hamstrings}}{\text{strong hamstrings}} \times 100 > 90\%$$

$$\frac{\text{weak quadriceps}}{\text{strong quadriceps}} \times 100 > 90\%$$

Tests of muscular balance are most accurately performed isokinetically on devices such as the Cybex. If the leg muscles are not in balance, the susceptibility to leg injury is higher. In addition, successful performance is less likely, especially in competitive sprinting and jumping.

Antagonists

It is not known whether muscular balances in other parts of the body are as important as leg balance. However, an effort should be made to work antagonistic or opposite muscle groups in the training program. For example, triceps exercises should be combined with biceps exercises. Chest exercises should be performed with exercises for the back muscles. It may be tempting to concentrate solely on triceps strength exercises to help improve skills such as the volleyball spike and the basketball shot since this is the primary arm muscle involved. But complete neglect of the biceps can cause muscular imbalance to develop which may detrimentally affect the skill and increase the risk of injury. Some research indicates that antagonistic muscles are active during movements of the agonist and thus gain some benefit. For example, during the biceps curl, the triceps are active as a stabilizer and therefore benefit from the exercise. These findings imply that it may not be necessary to spend equal amounts of time on agonist and antagonist muscles. Rather, the primary moves of the activity or sport should be emphasized.

In the general fitness program it is important to lift with opposing muscle groups. Isolating specific muscles may not be as important as in athletic weight training. Simply spending equal time using muscles in the front and back of each limb and front and back of the torso should be sufficient.

It is important to make the weaker side work as hard or harder during the exercise as the stronger side. If a double limb machine is used for the training, concentration is necessary to ensure the weak limb is working adequately. Single limb exercises may be necessary to increase the performance of the weaker side or weaker muscle group.

MUSCULAR TONE

The majority of fitness conscious Americans use muscular training for aesthetic purposes. That is, they desire to develop a leaner, stronger appearance.

Muscular Tone Requires Two Processes

1. The strengthening and hypertrophying of muscle
2. The loss of subcutaneous body fat.

The use of strength exercises to **tone** a specific area of the body is called **spot reduction**. Nearly all types of strength training exercises will strengthen muscle and cause it to increase in size. Moderate changes in strength and lean body weight can occur with resistance as light as 40-50% of maximum using 10-15 repetitions. Although greater hypertrophy occurs with the use of heavier weights, the lighter loads are recommended for muscular toning in the general fitness program (Table 8.2).

Whether resistance exercises will cause the loss of superficial (under the skin) body fat is controversial. Some scientific evidence supports the theory that resistance exercises such as sit-ups and circuit weight training will decrease fat cells in the exercised area and reduce total body percent fat. If fat loss does occur in muscular training, it will be minimal. Greater body fat losses can be expected from vigorous, routine aerobic exercises. Weight-bearing activities (walking, jogging, rope jumping) are especially effective. Prolonged aerobic exercise (>20 min) promotes the mobilization of fat from body depots and the utilization of fat by muscle.

Fat is Mobilized from at Least Three Areas*

1. Stomach (abdomen)	2. Seat (gluteal)	3. Thigh (femoral)

* Listed numerically from easiest to hardest.

The mobilization seems to occur in this particular order. That is, theoretically, it will be most difficult to lose fat from the thigh region and easiest to lose fat from the abdominal region. Regardless, a substantial period of time is required to lose fat in a given area. (See Chapter 9 for more details.)

In summary, a degree of muscular tone can be achieved with resistance exercises. Optimal means of achieving total body tone is the combination of resistance training with aerobic conditioning.

Mobilze the Fat

CARDIOVASCULAR FITNESS

Utilizing resistance training as a means of conditioning the cardiovascular system generally is ineffective. Traditional forms of heavy resistance training produce virtually no improvement in cardiovascular efficiency. In some types of circuit resistance training, small cardiovascular benefits can be obtained. However, circuit training itself is not an adequate program for development of optimal cardiorespiratory fitness.

Resistance training causes the heart to work very hard. One reason for this extra strain is the constriction of blood vessels in the muscle caused by the vigorous muscle contraction around the vessels. This narrowing of the vessels increases the resistance to blood flow, and the heart pumps more forcefully in an attempt to push the blood into the muscle (Figure 8.11).

Heavy Resistance Exercise Elevates Blood Pressure

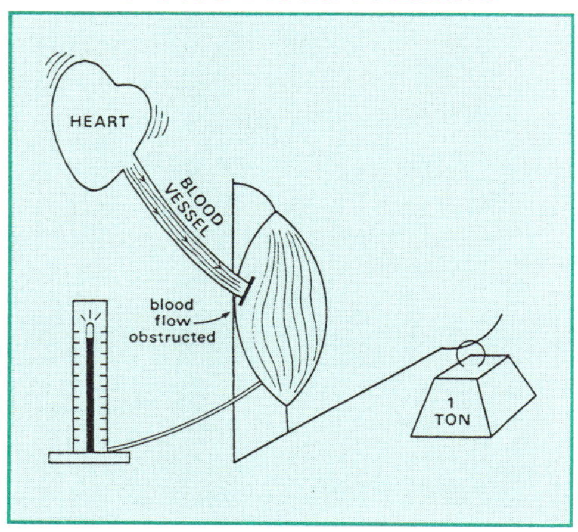

Figure 8.11. Intense muscular contractions increase the resistance of the blood vessels and the heart must contract more forcefully.

Another cause for this increased strain on the heart is the pressure in the chest cavity around the heart. One of the most important principles related to safe resistance training is breathing during each phase of the lift. Breathing keeps the air passages open which prevents the dramatic pressure buildup that can occur in the chest during straining exercise. Closing the air passages during a lift induces a reflex called the Valsalva maneuver in which the blood flow into the heart is reduced and the heart must pump against a greater resistance and blood pressure is increased (Figure 8.12). The idea of holding the breath during the lift to maintain torso stability may be correct mechanically, but this practice simply puts too much strain on the heart and vascular system.

Breath-Holding During Resistance Exercise

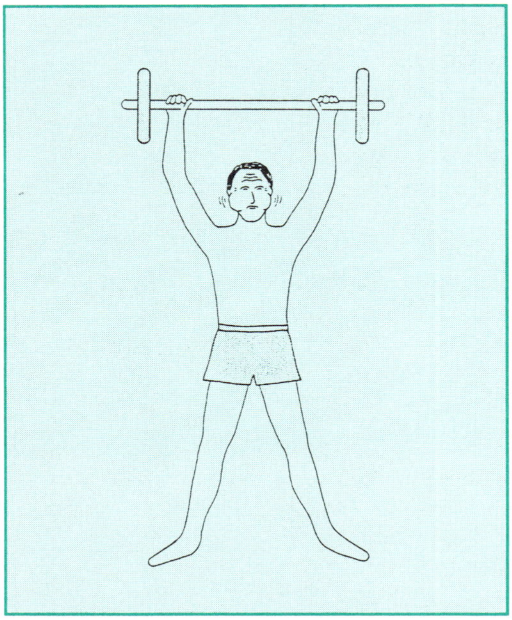

Figure 8.12. Holding the breath will increase the resistance in the chest cavity surrounding the heart.

tems to consider: breathing muscles and the heart. Inhalation is an active muscular process requiring more chest muscle activity than exhalation. Since the exercising muscle is strongest in the eccentric (lowering) phase, this easier phase of contraction for the lifting muscles should be associated with the hardest phase of breathing for the respiratory muscles-inhalation. On the other hand, chest (intrathoracic) pressure increases during exhalation which increases the force of the heart necessary to eject blood. Using this heart physiological process as a guide, the eccentric muscular contraction of the lift should be associated with the hardest phase for the heart-exhalation. Unfortunately, chest muscle and heart activities suggest opposite sequences for breathing. Therefore, physiologically the exhalation-inhalation sequence probably is not critical, and comfort or desires can be used as a guide for breathing. Most experienced heavy lifters inhale during the eccentric phase and exhale during the concentric phase. But more important is simply the act of exchanging air during each phase of the lift. In the general muscular fitness program, coupling the eccentric phase with exhalation and the concentric phase with inhalation is probably better for the heart.

Breathing also must be stressed outside the weight room. Resistance exercises such as sit-ups and push-ups as well as shoveling dirt or chopping wood require the exchange of air during the maneuver. Once again, breathholding should be avoided. This will require some practice at first since most individuals habitually hold the breath during these types of exercises. Other safety guidelines for heart health are listed as follows (Table 8.4.).

Guidelines for Resistance Training Based on CV Health

1. Resistance training using loads greater than 50% of maximum should not be performed by individuals with known cardiovascular disease or high blood pressure.
2. Resistance training with loads greater than 50% of maximum should not be performed without medical clearance by individuals with cardiovascular disease risk factors such as smoking, obesity, or elevated blood fats.
3. Individuals over 45 years of age usually should not perform resistance exercises using loads greater than 60% of maximum (~20 RM).
4. Persons interested in general muscular fitness should use loads of 40 to 60% of maximum.
5. Persons interested in general muscular fitness should not lift to complete failure.
6. Breathing should be continuous and rhythmic throughout the lifts. The Valsalva maneuver should be avoided.
7. Heavy resistance training using loads greater than 75% of maximum should be reserved for competitive athletes.
8. After their competitive playing days, athletes should decrease the loads of resistance training workouts.

Table 8.4.

Circuit Resistance Training (CRT)

Resistance training for general fitness is somewhat different in intensity than a program designed to maximize strength and power (Table 8.2). Cardiovascular fitness is not developed using heavy resistances. Rather, lighter loads are used and the number of repetitions increased. In addition, the time between exercises is reduced to 15 seconds and a sequence of exercises is performed in close succession. The goal of such a routine is to maintain heart rate and oxygen consumption within a target zone necessary to elicit cardiovascular or aerobic training. The exercise intensity should be maintained continuously for 30-45 minutes.

Bulk Down with CRT

A **circuit resistance training (CRT)** program is the best type of resistance exercise system for producing a desirable aerobic effect. Such a routine will not produce maximal strength and bulk gains. But strength gains can be significant and the continuous, moderate exercise promotes beneficial changes in body composition and cardiovascular fitness. Likewise, improvements in aerobic capacity will not be maximal. But adequate gains can be expected and maintenance of aerobic fitness is possible with the CRT routines. Multistation resistance systems are ideal for CRT programs (Figure 8.13).

This type of program is recommended for individuals interested in aerobic fitness. It is also beneficial for the recreational athlete who seeks general fitness and wishes to improve tennis, racquetball, basketball, jogging, etc. performance. Individuals interested in optimal cardiovascular fitness must use other aerobic activities as the primary exercise. However, CRT can supplement and serve as a short-term substitute for the regular aerobic program. Aerobic exercisers may find the CRT routine a welcome diversion from the normal exercise routine.

Centurion Multi-Station Machine

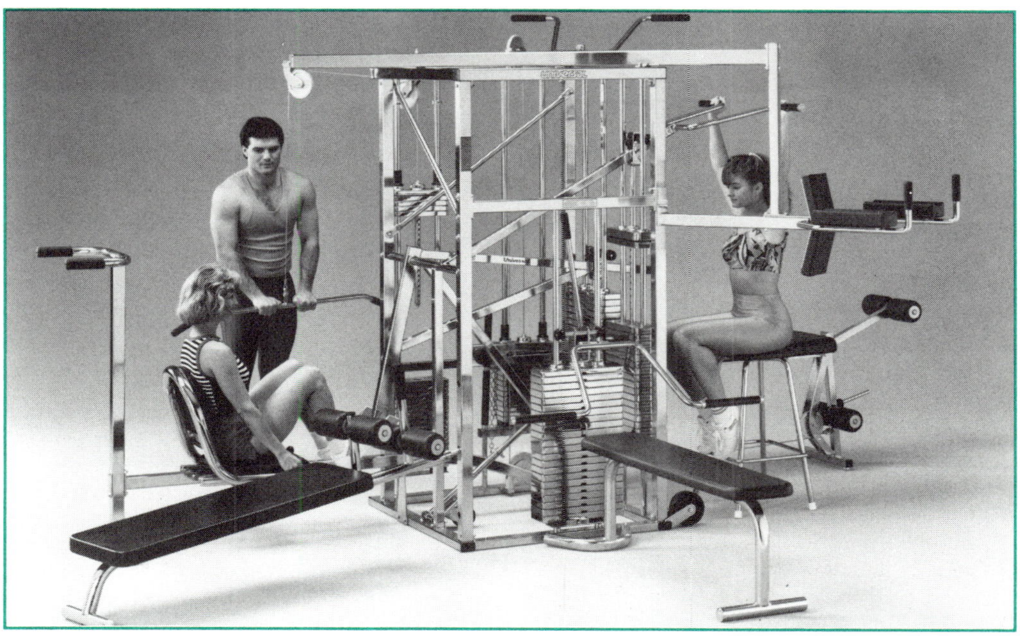

Figure 8.13. Machines which allow rapid movement from station to station are excellent for circuit resistance training. Photo provided by Universal Gym Equipment, Inc.

Alternate with CRT

Like strength resistance training, CRT can be performed on alternate days. A Monday, Wednesday, Friday program is outlined below, but a better strategy is a two day per week CRT program alternated with a three day per week aerobic program, and the total conditioning program is five times per week. For example, jogging or aerobics is performed on Monday, Wednesday, and Friday and the CRT workout on Tuesday and Thursday.

Inserting an aerobic vehicle in the CRT routine can enhance the cardiovascular component of the workout and provide diversity. Aerobic "ergometers" are instruments which provide a means of performing aerobic exercise (Chapter 6). Some are relatively inexpensive and can provide a warm-up and cool down exercise as well as be included in the CRT routine. Such exercise should be performed for 3-5 minutes at a CRT station to allow the cardiovascular system to adapt to the exercise.

CRT Exercises

Generally, free-weights are not appropriate for CRT. Machines which allow rapid changes in the loads are best because delays between exercises can lessen the potential cardiovascular effect.

Lighter But More

The program described below is for three times per week using lighter weights and more repetitions than the heavy resistance program designed for athletes. For each exercise, 12-15 repetitions are performed using loads of 40 to 50% of 1 RM. It is not necessary or desirable to lift to failure in this type of training. To determine the 40-50% resistance, simply use a load which causes near fatigue after 18-20 repetitions. If no aerobic mode is used, a 15 second rest is taken between each resistance exercise. After completion of the total sequence (1-13), the routine is repeated omitting #1 and #2. After two cycles, the session is ended with cool down (#15) and stretching (#16). The total routine is designed to be completed in 45-50 minutes (Table 8.5).

Sample CRT Program

Monday, Wednesday, Friday *or* **Tuesday, Thursday, Saturday**

1. stretching exercises - 6 minutes - no rest period
2. warm-up on cycle - 4 minutes
3. chest press or shoulder press
4. lat pull or pull-up - no rest period
5. ski ergometer - 3 minutes
6. incline sit-ups or abdominal curl
7. leg press or squat - no rest period
8. treadmill walk - 3 minutes
9. trunk extension
10. leg curl
11. knee raise or knee lift
12. heel raise - no rest period
13. rowing ergometer - 3 minutes
14. repeat stations 3 through 13
15. cool down on cycle - 5 minutes
16. stretching exercises - 6 minutes

Table 8.5.

Other resistance exercises and other modes of aerobic ergometers can be used in the CRT routine. A single aerobic ergometer can be used in each three minute aerobic session during the routine, but a variety may help keep the routine more enjoyable. It is important to utilize all muscle groups. More upper body resistance exercises can be substituted for the lower body exercises if jogging, aerobics, skiing, or other leg activities are the primary exercise modes in the aerobic program. Appendix A contains workout records for logging CRT training bouts.

Variety is the Key

As an alternative to the described CRT program, the ergometers can be used during the "rest period" itself. Following each resistance exercise, the aerobic ergometer is used for a 30 to 60 second recovery period. In this way, the heart rate remains continuously elevated, and no real rest is taken during the exercise session. This method is often called "super circuit resistance training."

Suggested Readings

Fleck, S.J. and W.J. Kraemer. *Designing Resistance Training Programs*. Champaign, IL: Human Kinetics, 1987.

Gettman, L.R. and M.L. Pollock. Circuit weight training: A critical review of its physiological benefits. *The Physician and Sportsmedicine*. 9:44-60, January, 1981.

Hurley, B.F. and P.F. Kokkinos. Effects of weight training on risk factors for coronary artery disease. *Sports Medicine*. 4:231-238, 1987.

Kraemer, W.J. and S.J. Fleck. Resistance training. (Parts 1-4). *Physician and Sportsmedicine*. 16:March-June, 1988.

Powers, S.K. and E.T. Howley. *Exercise Physiology: Theory and Application to Fitness and Performance*. Dubuque: Wm. C. Brown, Chapters 8 and 21, 1990.

Riley, D.P. *Maximum Muscular Fitness: Strength Training Without Equipment*. West Point: Leisure Press, 1982.

Thomas, T.R. *Muscular Fitness through Resistance Training*. Dubuque: eddie bowers publishing, inc., 1991.

CHAPTER 9

WEIGHT MANAGEMENT STRATEGIES

Jerry Mayhew

Learning Objectives

- List the useful purpose of storage fat and the harmful effects of excess storage fat.
- Describe the major techniques for measuring body composition.
- Describe the effects of calorie restricted diets on body composition and health.
- List the essential nutrients.
- Discuss the body's need for protein and differentiate between complete and incomplete proteins.
- Illustrate how the long-haul concept of weight control works
- List some of the ways to reduce the fat content of the diet.
- Discuss the relationship among exercise, oxygen consumption, caloric expenditure, and weight control.
- Discuss the role of exercise in a weight-gaining program.
- Discuss the different effects of aerobic and anaerobic exercise on body composition.

Important Terms

amino acids
bioelectrical impedance
body composition
carbohydrates
complete proteins
complex carbohydrates
creeping obesity
density
diet
elevated post-exercise oxygen consumption (EPOC)
essential fat
fat mass (FM)
fat-free mass (FFM)
fat-soluble vitamins
hydrostatic weighing
hypoglycemia
incomplete proteins
infrared reactance
insulin
insulin overshoot
lean body mass (LBM)
long-haul concept
major minerals
malnourished
minerals
obese
saturated fats
set-point
simple sugars
skinfold
skinfold caliper
storage fat
trace minerals
undermuscled
undernourished
underweight
unsaturated fats
water soluble vitamins
yo-yo dieting

BODY COMPOSITION

A topic of great interest to most individuals engaged in a fitness program is their body composition. Many people begin exercise programs because they feel they are "overweight". Actually the term "overweight" is a misnomer and instead of denoting someone who has an excessive amount of fat, it simply refers to an individual who is above the average weight for a given height. Therefore, it is a classic mistake to evaluate ourself simply by what the bathroom scales say without regard for how that weight is distributed between lean tissue and fat.

Overweight vs. Overfat

The term **body composition** refers to the components that makeup the body's weight. The body weight (or more correctly the body mass) recorded by the scales is composed of main parts or components. For determining body composition, the two major components of the body mass are the **fat-free mass (FFM)** and the **fat mass (FM)**. The relationship between these components can be denoted by the simple mathematical expression:

Body Mass (kg) = **Fat-Free Mass** (kg) + **Fat Mass** (kg)

While height does not dictate one's weight, average body weights have been developed based on heights. The range for body weights based on height is quite wide and should be taken only as a crude guideline. Thus, the term "overweight" refers to people who have a large fat-free mass for their height such as football players or weight lifters. To the contrary, the term "overfat" is more appropriate to use for those who have a larger fat mass than appropriate for their body weight.

The fat-free mass is the functional, active tissues of the body. Of course, the largest contributor to the fat-free mass comes from skeletal muscle. The average person has about 40% of the body mass composed of muscle. However other active tissues such as bones, organs, glands, etc. are also grouped together in the FFM.

40% is Muscle

Some authorities refer to the fat-free mass as the **lean body mass (LBM)**, although there is a technical difference between the two. The FFM, as its name implies, contains no fat, while the LBM contains a small amount of essential fat. Although the terms often are used interchangeably, there is sufficient difference to warrant mentioning.

The fat mass is the non-active, storage tissues of the body. The total fat mass is divided into essential fat and storage fat. The **essential fat** is required for normal body functions, such as the covering around some nerve tissues and part of the cell wall. Storage fat, as you might guess, is that which is placed in reserve and is the fat which most people watch so closely. The storage fat is most easily seen as it accumulates around the waist, on the hips, and over the thighs.

Too Much Storage Fat

While most people might wish to have no fat, it is a physiological impossibility. **Storage fat** serves such useful purpose as a reservoir for energy when food is not readily available, an insulator to hold in body heat, and a padding to cushion vital areas from trauma. The problem for most people in modern society is that they may have too big a reservoir, are too well insulated, and have too much padding.

Despite the usefulness of a certain amount of fat, an excess of storage fat may have several negative effects on a person.

Negative Side Effects of Excess Storage Fat

1. Causes extra work for the heart.
2. Increases chances of high blood pressure.
3. Is a greater risk during surgery.
4. Increases the chances of developing diabetes.
5. May increase the chances of getting cancer by trapping dangerous chemicals in the body.

Creeping Obesity

The excess storage fat may not be a problem now, but it can become a major threat to health as you get older. An extra 200 calories eaten each day beyond the amount needed by the body can result in a gain of 20 lbs. a year. By the time the average college student is 45 years old, he or she could have easily lost 25 lbs. of muscle mass and gained 35-40 lbs. of fat. When this person steps on the scales he or she sees a gain of only about 10-15 lbs., but the distribution of that gain is what is important. This slow, almost unnoticed process of fat gain is sometimes referred to as **creeping obesity**.

REFERENCE STANDARDS

13% or 23%

The two-component model of body composition allows you to assess the relative contribution of each component to the total body mass. This is the proportion of the total body mass which is fat. In the average college male who weighs 75 kg (165 lbs.), the fat mass is equal to be about 96 kg (22 lbs.),or 13% of his total body mass. The average college female weighs about 61 kg (135 lbs.) and has a fat mass equal to about 13.8 kg (31 lbs.), or 23% of her total body mass. Recall that the proportion of the total body mass which is lean tissue may be represented by 100 - %fat. Therefore, a male who is 13% fat would be 87% lean and have about 65 kg (143 lbs) of fat-free mass. The average female who is 23% fat would be 77% lean and have about 47 kg (104) of fat-free mass.

Body Fat Calculation

$$\% \text{ Fat} = \frac{\text{Fat Mass (kg)}}{\text{Total Body Mass (kg)}} \times 100$$

The greatest interest to most people is their relative amount of body fat (% fat)

The difference in body composition between men and women is mostly genetic. Recall that essential fat is that which the body must maintain in order to function normally. in men this is approximately 3% of their body mass, while in women it is about 13%. The greater essential fat in women is a function of their potential to bare children. The storage fat in men and women is about the same and amounts to about 10% of the body mass.

MEASUREMENT TECHNIQUES

Underwater Weighing

The most widely accepted technique for measuring body composition is underwater or **hydrostatic weighing**, also known as densitometry. This method is based on the Archemedian principle that an object displaces an amount of water equal to its volume. By placing a person in water, the body volume can be calculated from the weight lost during submersion. The ratio of a body's weight to its volume is its **density**. Previous research has shown that fat tissue has a density of 0.900 g/ml and thus has a tendency to float, while muscle tissue with a density of 1.100 g/ml has a tendency to sink. In simplest terms, the degree to which a person floats or sinks determines the body's density. The more an individual sinks, the higher the density, and the less fat in the body. The more a person floats, the less dense the body and the more fat it will contain.

Sink or Float

To perform the underwater weighing procedure, the individual is suspended from a very accurate scale and then submerged under water. As the person submerges, all the air possible is blown out of the lungs, although a small residual volume will always remain. This residual volume can be estimated using several different procedures and mathematically removed for the weight registered on the scale while the individual is submerged. Although the density of the body can exist between the extremes of all fat and all muscle, the values are more likely to lie between 1.000 and 1.088 g/ml.

Siri Equation

$$\% \text{ fat} = \frac{495}{\text{Density}} - 450$$

The body density can be converted to an estimate of % fat using the Siri equation.

Therefore, if a male weighed 85 kg (187 lbs.) and had a density of 1.069 g/ml, he would be 13.0% fat. If another male had a body weight of 100 kg (220 lbs.) but had a density of 1.069 g/ml, he too would be 13.0% fat. Despite having the same %fat, the second male would have 87 kg of fat-free weight compared to the first male's 74 kg. Most college men will have %fat values between 5% and 35%, and most college women will be between 15% and 45%. Most authorities agree that when men exceed 20% fat and women exceed 30% fat, they are considered **obese**.

Ouch- 20% plus or 30% plus

Bioelectric Impedance

A recent development in the field of body composition measurement is the ability to measure the amount of fat-free mass from an estimate of the body's capacity to conduct a small electrical current. Called **bioelectrical impedance**, the method used two pair of electrode placed on the back of one hand and the top of one foot. A very small electrical current is passed from one electrode to the other. Since more of the current conducted through water and because most of the water lies in the fat-free mass, the current will

Bioelectrical Impedance

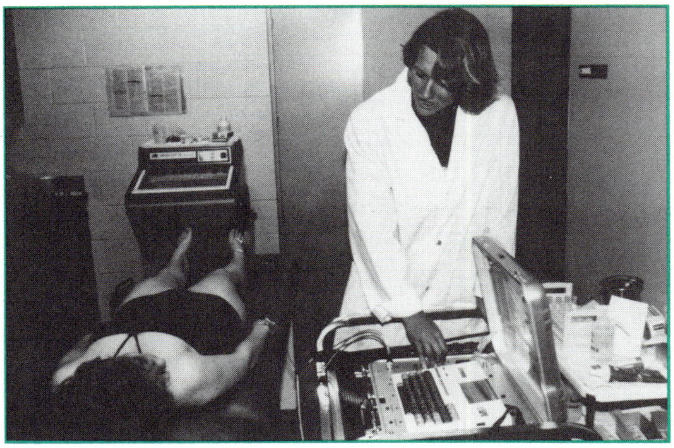

Figure 9.1. The conducting electrodes are located on the subjects right hand and foot.

travel better through a person with more fat-free mass and less fat mass.

Research comparisons of bioelectrical impedance with the more widely accepted underwater weighing procedure have produced mixed results. Bioelectrical impedance is accurate for individuals in the middle of the body composition range, that is 12-16% for men and 20-26% for women. Outside these ranges the bioelectrical impedance techniques may over estimate the relative fat content of lean people and underestimate the relative fat content of fat people. This technique should be used with caution for estimating ideal weight since already lean people might attempt to lose more weight, while those with too much fat might be satisfied with the excess (Figure 9.1).

Infrared Reactance

Fat Layering

An even simpler technique than bioelectric impedance is the **infrared reactance** method. This approach uses the speed with which infrared waves pass through body tissues of different densities to estimate fat layering. An insulating rubber cover is placed over the biceps muscle and a reading taken from the infrared sensor. The microprocessor attached to the sensor calculates the degree of fatness and projects it to a total body fat estimate.

The infrared reactance method suffers from the same shortcomings as the bioelectric impedance technique. That is, it tends to overestimate the fat content of lean individuals and underestimate that of fat individuals. Increasing the number of sites measures with infrared reactance improves prediction somewhat but still leaves it less proficient than underwater weighing or skinfold measurements.

Skinfold Thicknesses

Are You Thick-Skinned

Perhaps the most widely used method for evaluating body composition is the **skinfold** thickness technique. Since approximately 50% of an individual's body fat lies just under the skin, it is possible to pinch double folds of fat in certain locations about the body and estimate the total amount of fat present. Such areas as the back of the arm (triceps), on the back (subscapular), above the waist (suprailiac), on the abdomen (abdominal), and over the front of the thigh (thigh) are excellent places for determining skinfold thickness values. While it is relatively easy for a person to tell if there is too much fat in a given area simply by pinching with the fingers, more accurate measurements require the use of a **skinfold caliper**. This instrument gives a reasonably accurate measurement of the thickness of a double fold of fat on the surface of the body. Skinfolds values for six commonly measured sites are shown in Table 9.1. Body composition analysis can be found in Inventory 19and 20 on pages 253 and 257.

Skinfold Values for College Men and Women*

Skinfold Sites	Men Percentile			Women Percentile		
	20	50	80	20	50	80
Triceps (mm)	6.7	10.4	14.1	13.6	18.6	23.5
Subscapular (mm)	7.5	12.0	16.5	9.2	15.4	21.6
Abdomen (mm)	9.1	16.0	22.9	12.1	18.7	25.3
Suprailiac (mm)	9.2	16.2	23.2	11.4	18.1	24.8
Thigh (mm)	8.0	12.5	17.0	19.5	26.2	32.9
Calf (mm)	6.0	9.5	13.0	13.5	18.8	24.1
Sum of 6 (mm)	**46.5**	**76.6**	**106.6**	**79.3**	**115.8**	**152.2**

* Data from randomly selected students (n = 600) enrolled in a Wellness class at Northeast Missouri State University.

Table 9.1.

Over 100 equations have been developed to allow the prediction of body composition from skinfold measurements. Because there are so many prediction equations, the questions often arises, "Is the skinfold technique as accurate as other methods of determining body composition?" Since the equations used to predict body density from skinfold measurements are based on a standard measure such as underwater weighing, the former cannot be more accurate than the latter. No matter how good the criterion measurement of body composition is, there is always some error associated with it. For example, the measurement error associated with the underwater weighing technique is about 2%. Therefore, if we calculate the error associated with a given criterion measurement techniques and add that to the error associated with skinfold measurements, the margin of error for estimating %fat from skinfold thickness is about 3-5%. This means that if an individual is predicted to have 13% fat, their actual value is likely to lie between 10% and 16%.

Plus or Minus 3-5%

Despite the potential error associated with skinfold measurements, they are nevertheless a valuable technique for providing a quick and ready reference for body composition determination. It usually takes less than five minutes to measure several skinfolds and calculate the estimate of an individual's %fat. The more skilled the examiner at skinfold measurement, the smaller the error that will be made and the more accurate the prediction of body composition will be.

Although skinfold measurements are quick and convenient and provide a reasonably accurate measurement of an individual's body composition, they may not be appropriate to track the temporal changes in body composition resulting from diet or exercise programs. Recent research has indicated that an exercise program may cause changes in the body composition that are not detected by the less sensitive skinfold measurements. Thus students who exercise for a week and request to have their skinfolds remeasured may be disappointed to find hardly any changes in body composition. The errors associated with the method are greater than the potential changes that the person can invoke in just one week of exercise. Over several months of exercise, however the skinfold technique might provide a rough gauge of the success of the program in reducing the body's fat layer.

Fat: Where it's At

The reader should not forget the other alternative consequence of an exercise program: gaining fat-free mass. Although the exerciser may not have reduced the skinfold measurements and hence is predicted to have the same %fat, perhaps the muscles have developed in size and strength. For these reasons, it may be best if skinfold prediction techniques produce a range within which the person's %fat might lie. This might help avoid the disappointment that can accompany the failure to decrease the skinfold thickness after a month of hard aerobic exercise.

Recent research has noted a difference in the skinfold fat patterning of various individuals. For example, men have a different fat patterning than women. Men tend to store most of their excess fat around the waist, producing that "spare tire" or "pot-bellied" look. Women tend to place their fat around the hips and over the thighs, giving that "saddle bag" appearance. In obese men, more fat is deposited in the lower abdominal region, giving them a "pear-shaped" appearance. In obese women, more of the excess fat is deposited in the upper trunk. Recent research has noted that the pear-shaped person who deposited most of the body fat in the abdominal and upper trunk regions is at greater risk of developing heart disease than those whose major fat deposits are located on the thighs and hips. Waist/Hip ration analysis can be found in Inventory 20 on page 257.

NUTRIENTS RELATED TO EXERCISE

The Everday Struggle

Perhaps no more mystery or myth surrounds our daily lives than that related to our diet. For centuries people have been looking for that magic food, the one that will make us young, keep us thin, or increase our physical performance. But, alas, no one has found any such food despite the barrage of advertisements that claim to have the perfect food.

Because of the fixation most people have with the food they eat, the word "diet" has become synonymous with what you do not eat rather that what you do eat. In its correct usage, **diet** is the sum total of those foods which we eat. If your diet is not adequate to meet the caloric demands for a day, you are said to be **undernourished**. If your diet is lacking in essential elements to keep you healthy, you may be **malnourished**.

Each Day a Person Needs Six Basic or Essential Nutrients to Maintain an Adequate Diet

1. carbohydrates
2. fats
3. proteins
4. vitamins
5. minerals
6. water

We have been taught since elementary school that the way to get the 6 essential nutrients is from the Four Basic Food Groups (Table 9.2). Recently these four food groups have been reorganized into a pyramid as a guide to food selection (Figure 9.2). Diet Analysis experiments can be found in Inventories 22 and 23 and Appendix B.

Basic Food Groups

4 Food Group	Servings per day
1) Dairy	2
2) Protein	2
3) Fruits and Vegetables	4
4) Grains and Cereals	4

Table 9.2.

Pyramid Food Guide

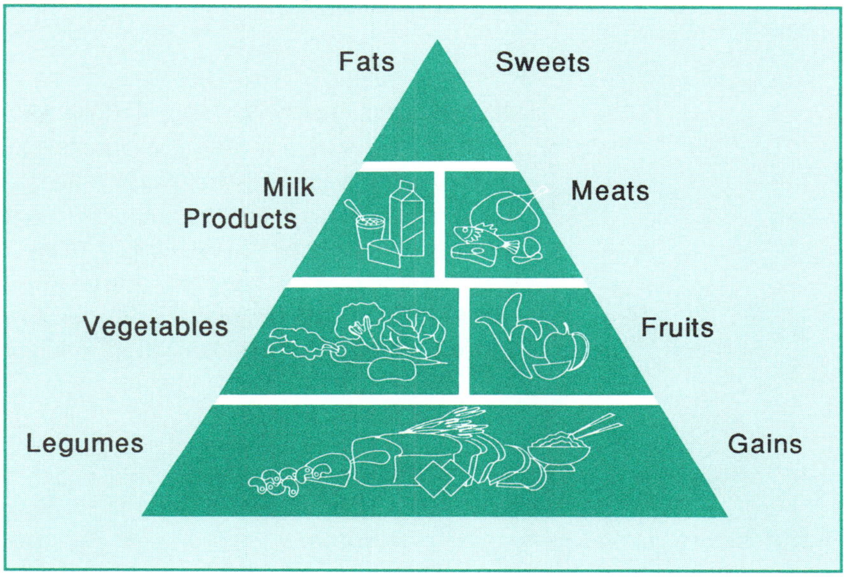

Figure 9.2.

CARBOHYDRATES

Carbohydrates are the mainstay of an individual's diet. These are the nutrients that provide the primary fuel for running the body. **Carbohydrates** may be divided into two categories: simple sugars and complex starches.

Fuel the Body

Simple sugars are easy enough to identify. These are the things that many of us have grown to love all too well. Cookies, candy, and soda are but a few examples of simple sugars. While they taste great, simple sugars may not be all that good for us. Beyond the damage they might do to teeth, simple sugars cause a sudden upward surge in blood sugar as they are absorbed quickly from the intestines. To counter this phenomenon, the body produces a huge outpouring of **insulin**, a hormone that assists in transporting sugar across the cell membranes in the body. Once the sugar in the blood stream is rushed into the cells, you might experience an unusually low blood sugar level and feel rather tired, rundown, and droopy,

The sugar surge and purge is exactly what happens in the typical "coffee break". Feeling a bit wary, you eat a candy bar and have a soda, which sends your blood sugar soaring. The **insulin overshoot** begins to load that blood sugar into cells and for a while you feel revived. But the excess insulin production causes more blood sugar to be delivered into cells than you want, and you begin to come crashing down from the "sugar high". If it is going to be some time before you eat again, you might wind up feeling worse than you did before you ate your candy bar.

Take a Potato Break

To rescue yourself from the hazards of simple sugars, try eating **complex carbohydrates.** These are the foods rich in starches that take longer to break down in the intestines, thus releasing their sugars into the blood stream more slowly. While the "potato break" is not likely to replace the coffee break, such complex carbohydrates as pasta, breads, rice, and potatoes will moderate the blood sugar levels and keep you going longer.

Increased Need During Exercise

The average college student eats about 45% of the total diet as carbohydrates. For individuals who increase their activity level by means of an exercise program, the need for carbohydrates is increased to approximately 8 grams per kilogram of body mass. The increased energy output required for an exercise program should be met by increasing the carbohydrate intake to about 60% of the daily total. Because of the life-style of most college students, this can be difficult to achieve.

Percent of Nutrients from Different Sources

Nutrient	Curent Levels	Recommended Levels
Carbohydrates	45%	60%
Fats	43%	28%
Proteins	12%	12%

Table 9.3. Note the intake level of proteins remains constant so this points out that the change needs to be in fat consumption

FATS

One of the things that makes it difficult to get sufficient carbohydrate intake is the large amount of fat in the average diet. A college student consumes about 43% of the daily total as fats. This is comparable to the national average and well above the maximal 30% level recommended for good health. The higher level of fat may contribute to heart disease, cancer, and strokes. Table 9.2 gives the current nutrient intakes and those recommended for good health.

Saturated versus Unsaturated Fats

Solid or Liquid

Like carbohydrates, fats come in two broad categories. One category is **saturated fats** in which every atomic bond on the long-chain carbon backbone of the molecule is occupied (Figure 9.3). Many of these fats are solids at room temperature and are derived mostly from animal sources, such as butter, margarine, cheese, and mayonnaise.

The other category is the **unsaturated fats**, which do not have all their carbon bonds occupied and are liquids at room temperature. The exceptions to the latter rule are palm and coconut oils, which are highly saturated but also liquids at room temperature. This draws attention to avoiding "tropical" oils in the foods we consume. These are the fats that tend to increase the level of cholesterol in the blood and contribute to heart disease.

Saturated and Unsaturated Fats

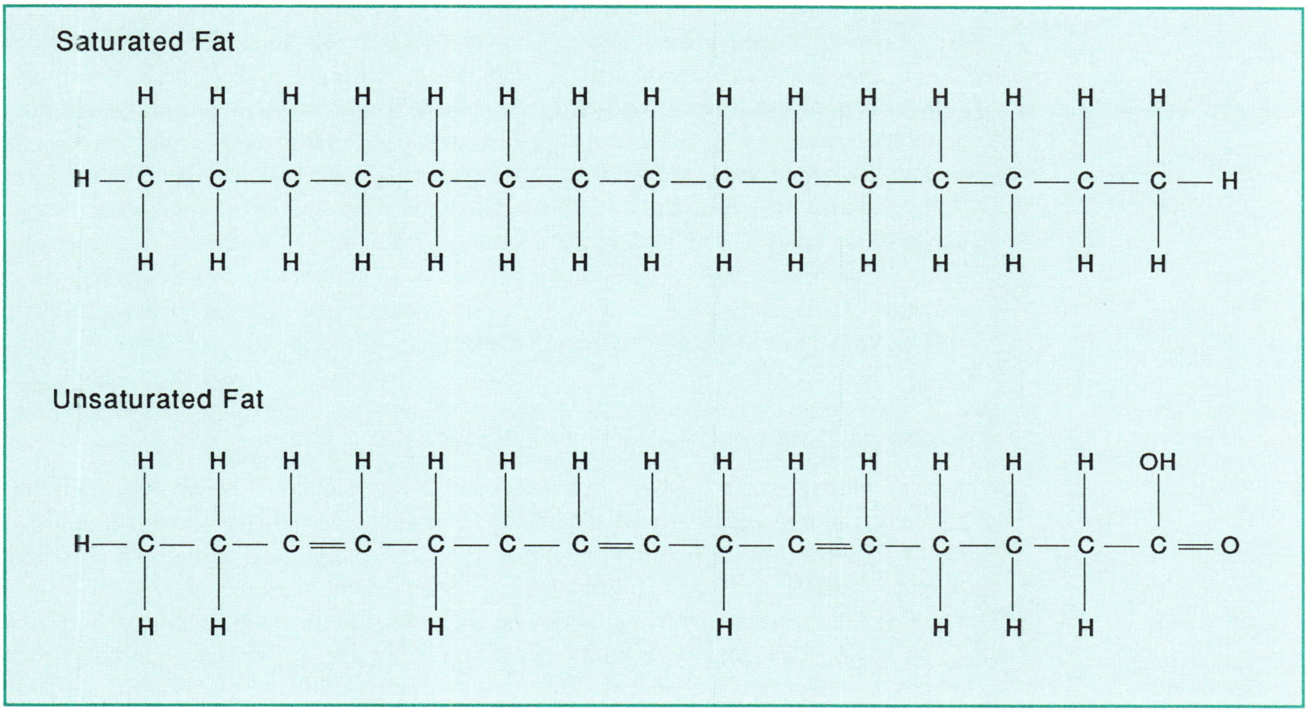

Figure 9.3.

Reducing Fats in the Diet

It is not simply enough to say that you are going to cut down on the fat intake in your diet. Many of the fats you consume are hidden, and while you think you are eating little fat, you are, in fact, consuming too much. Such foods as whole milk, cheese, ice cream, eggs, red meat, nuts, French fries, fried chicken, mayonnaise, and salad dressing contain far more fat than we require. It is often the fat in these foods that gives them their desirable taste and keeps us returning for more. In order to cut back on the amount of fat in your diet, you may have to make a strong effort to control your intake of certain foods.

Fat and More Fat

This may require you to learn new behaviors and acquire new tastes. Select low-fat dairy products such as ice milk, skim milk, and low-fat cheeses. Switch from red meats to low-fat white meats such as chicken and fish. In fact, red meat could well become a side dish in the modern diet and not the main focus of each meal with no loss of protein intake.

If you find it hard to know which of the foods you eat contain hidden fats, you might do well to switch your diet to more fresh fruits, vegetables, and whole grain products. In order to appeal to our taste buds and speed the cooking process, many dormitory foods are high in fats. Likewise, the fast-food business prepares many of the foods by deep-fat frying or grilling. Lately, however, the continued emphasis on reducing the fat intake in the diet has prompted many of these establishments to offer new, low-fat foods. The well-known fast-food restaurants now have light menus with reduced calorie and fat contents. More salads and fresh vegetables are being offered.

But before you switch totally to the salad bar and await your weight to begin dropping, consider the results of a recent study at Southern University. Researchers positioned themselves at the exits from the hot-lunch line and the salad bar line and asked students if they would sell the lunches they had just selected. Returning to the laboratory with the lunches they had purchased, the investigators analyzed the meals for their content of calories, carbohydrates, fats, and proteins, as well as other nutrients. Surprisingly, the salads, topped with rich dressings, cheeses, nuts, and other fatty foods, had about the same calorie and fat content as the meat-and-potatoes lunches. Just eating at the salad bar may not be cutting your calories and fat intake. To lower the fat in your diet will take a very deliberate, conscious effort on your part.

Beware of Salad Bars

PROTEINS

Perhaps the biggest myth surrounding diet and exercise is the idea that anyone engaged in a fitness program needs extra protein. Some people think this extra protein is used for energy during exercise, while others think that the additional protein goes for repair of cells damaged during exercise. Both of these ideas are not supported by research findings. Proteins are not good sources of energy for exercise since it requires so much to break them down into a form that is usable by the working cells. No more than about five percent of the daily energy needs come from protein, and this is only after it has gone through a lengthy digestive and chemical conversion process. As for the damaged cells after exercise, there is sufficient protein in the average diet to supply all the rebuilding materials the body needs for repair of cells. There is some recent evidence that during the first two weeks of a strenuous exercise program the body may require slightly more protein than usual, but his phenomenon soon subsides, and the body functions very well on the 12% protein intake of the normal diet.

Too Much Protein

How much protein in the diet is enough? As mentioned earlier, the average protein intake should be about 12% of the total caloric consumption. Another way of viewing it is to say that the average college male should get more than enough protein to supply all the needs resulting from an exercise program. Some research shows that highly trained athletes may require slightly more protein than the average exerciser. Protein intake levels of 1.2-1.5 g/kg may be necessary for individuals engaged in competitive athletics.

Supplements

Another myth about the exercising person is that a protein supplement will increase the benefit derived from a conditioning program. These supplements take many forms from powders to shakes to bars. As we have seen from looking at the average student's diet, this additional protein is not necessary, and indeed may be harmful to the vigorous exerciser. The large molecules of protein consumed in the diet are composed of smaller building blocks called **amino acids**. These amino acids differ in their composition from carbohydrates and fats only in the configuration of the molecules and in the fact that they contain nitrogen. Unlike plants, the body does not use nitrogen and therefore must get rid of it. The nitrogen by-products of amino acid breakdown are converted to urea and carried to the kidneys and flushed out. In order to rid the body of this urea, water must be mixed with it to produce urine. This water may be drawn from the body during times of heavy exercise when it is vitally needed. Thus, an individual who consumes a protein supplement might be at some risk of suffering from dehydration during times of heavy sweating. In addition, if the individual is using the protein supplement in lieu of dietary protein they may be missing vital nutrients that accompany the intake of dietary protein.

Complete versus Incomplete

Proteins can generally be considered in two class: Complete or incomplete. **Complete proteins** are those that contain all the essential amino acids required by the body since the body cannot store these basic building blocks. The foods containing complete proteins are meat, milk, cheese, eggs. **Incomplete proteins** are those which are lacking one or more of the essential amino acids needed for proper function in the body. Examples of these are breads, nuts, legumes, and seeds. Individuals who wish to reduce their fat intake by decreasing their intake of meats, eggs, and cheese may not get an adequate daily supply of complete protein. This can be remedied by combining a small amount of a complete protein like milk with several incomplete proteins like cereals, grains, and legumes.

Amino Acids are a Must

VITAMINS

Vitamins are organic substances required in small amounts to maintain normal physiological function in the body. They cannot be stored by the body and must be ingested on a regular basis. Because several vitamins have been identified as elements in enzymes that aid in the digestion and utilization of food by the body, many people feel they have some magical power or supply additional energy beyond that provided in food alone. Millions of dollars are spent each year on vitamin supplements in the hope that they will make up for inadequate diet. As with most nutrients, there is a correct amount of each vitamin required to maintain optimal body function. Unfortunately, some people still think that the more vitamins they take, the better they will perform. To compound the problem, many of these people take the vitamin pills in lieu of nutritious meal which renders the vitamin pill ineffective since the intestinal tract will be rather quiescent without food to stimulate the digestive process. Therefore, few of the vitamins are actually absorbed and most of them pass through the system to be eliminated.

Save Your Money

Water-Soluble

Vitamins come in two categories, those soluble in water and those soluble in fat. The **water soluble vitamins** include vitamin C and B-complex group. Vitamin C serves many purposes in the body and is found in foods such as citrus fruits, strawberries, tomatoes, broccoli, potatoes, and cabbage. The B vitamins are involved in the production of many enzymes regulating metabolism and can be found in green vegetables, meats, whole-grain foods, and milk. Excess intake of the water-soluble vitamins may be

Food Sources for Vitamins and Minerals

Vitamins	Food Sources	Minerals	Food Sources
Fat Soluble		Calcium (Ca)	milk, cheese, green vegetables
Vitamin A (retinol)	liver, animal products, green vegetables, carrots, sweet potatoes, fish liver oils	Phosphorus (P)	milk, lean meats, cheese, grains
Vitamin D (cholecalciferol)	milk, fish liver oils, eggs	Magnesium (Mg)	whole grains, nuts, milk, green vegetables
Vitamin E (alpha tocopherol)	vegetable oils, salmon, seeds, whole grains, margarine	Potassium (K)	whole grains, meats, fruits, potatoes
Vitamin K (phylloquinone)	intestinal bacteria, green vegetables, whole grains	Sodium (Na)	salt, milk, meat
		Chlorine (Cl)	salt
Water Soluble		Iodine (I)	iodized salt, sea food, milk
Vitamins B Thiamin (B_1)	whole grains, nuts, pork	Iron (Fe)	liver, meats, dried apricots, beans, wines, oysters
Riboflavin (B_2)	liver, milk, dairy products	Copper (Cu)	liver, meat, drinking water
Niacin (nicotinic acid)	meats, whole grains, legumes, peanuts	Fluorine (Fl)	water, seafood
Pyridoxine (B_6)	meats, whole grains, bananas, eggs	Sulfur (S)	meats, eggs, cheese, milk, (sulfur amino acids)
Folicin (folic acid)	beans, green vegetables (spinach), whole wheat, liver	Chromium (Cr)	meats, yeast, vegetable oils
Cyancobalamin (B_{12})	meat and animal products (not present in plants)	Cobalt (Co)	animal products - vitamin B_{12}
Panthothenic Acid	liver, meats, eggs, whole grains	Selenium (Se)	meats, seafood, whole grains
Biotin	peas, beans, meats	Molybdenum (Mo)	organ meats, whole grains, legumes
Choline	egg yolk, liver, grains	Zinc (Zn)	liver, meats, seafood, whole grains, cocoa
Vitamin C (ascorbic acid)	citrus fruits, tomatoes, green peppers, brussel sprouts	Manganese (Mn)	whole grains, soybeans, tea, coffee, bananas

Table 9.4. Reprinted from T.R. Thomas and C.J. Zebas. *Scientific Exercise Training.* Copyright © by Kendall/Hunt Publishing Co.

eliminated by the kidneys. Individuals who consume large doses of these vitamins may notice their urine will be a bright yellow or deep gold color. In some cases, however, the body is not able to rid itself of all the excess water-soluble vitamins, and toxic side effects may result. For example, one of the minor side effects of excess vitamin C intake is diarrhea.

Fat-Soluble

The **fat-soluble vitamins** are A, D, E, and K. Their functions include bone formation and growth, tooth development, cell membrane maintenance, and blood clotting formation. Because they dissolve in the fats of the body, they are much more difficult to remove when there are excesses. Prolonged excessive intake of fat-soluble vitamins may have toxic side effects, such as damage to the liver, kidneys, and bones. As long as the diet is adequate, selected from among the Four Basic Food Groups, and of a wide variety, vitamin supplementation should not be necessary. Table 9.4 provides suggested food sources for vitamins and minerals.

No to Vitamins and Mineral Supplements

MINERALS

Minerals are inorganic substances which serve a wide variety of uses in the body. Minerals can be classified by their need in the body: major minerals and trace minerals. **Major minerals** such as calcium, phosphorous, sodium, potassium, and magnesium are required in larger amounts for normal bodily function. **Trace minerals** such as iron, zinc, copper, iodine, and chromium are required in much smaller amounts to maintain normal body function. As with vitamins, there is almost no need to take a mineral supplement provided you eat an adequate diet. Indeed, the ingestion of excess minerals in the form of supplements may have a toxic effect. See Table 9.4 for suggested food sources rich in minerals.

WATER

Perhaps the most overlooked nutrient in our daily diet is water. While you may live for quite sometime with deficiencies of the other nutrients, you can live for only several days without water. Among its major functions are the maintenance of body temperature, the assistance in food digestion, and the regulation of blood volume. You might think that just because you do not drink a lot of water that your body gets by just fine without it. A great many of the foods you consume are largely water and provide the body with much of its requirement each day. However, it is vital that you get an adequate amount of water each day, especially if you are active and lose fluids through heavy breathing and sweating. The old adage of drinking eight glasses of water a day has merit for those involved in a rigorous exercise program.

"8" Glasses Per Day

DIETING TO CHANGE BODY COMPOSITION

LOSING WEIGHT

Calorie Restricted Diets

Diet and Lose Muscle

Almost everyone has been on some form of caloric restriction at one time or another in an attempt to lose body weight. The main objective when "going on a diet" is to preferentially reduce body fat content. In order to achieve this goal, the person must produce a negative caloric balance in which the number of calories expended by the body is greater than the number of calories taken in. Far too often the pattern for these caloric-restrictive diets is to eat substantially less than required for normal daily activity and hope for quick reductions in body weight. This approach may seem feasible during the first few days when five to 10 lbs. may be lost. However, this is mostly water loss as the body draws on its supply of stored sugar (glycogen) to maintain itself. After the first few days the weight loss slows as the body protects itself from further water loss. Some fat is withdrawn from storage deposits during this time, but the protective mechanism of the body begins to search for an alternative source of fuel. The amino acids stored as muscle protein is the next best source, and the body actually begins to break down muscles tissue in an effort to meet the energy demand. As much as one-half of all weight lost on a "diet" can be due to muscle tissues loss.

The loss of muscle tissue becomes self-defeating as the calorie-restricted diet continues. Because active tissue is lost by the degradation of muscle, the body's metabolic rate slows. Now, the few calories the person was eating on the calorie-restricted diet is able to meet the new energy demand, and there is no longer a negative calorie balance. In time, the body actually becomes accustomed to the new lower level of calorie intake and no longer requires as much to operate. Weight loss slows, and it becomes difficult to reduce further without again decreasing the caloric intake. Some authorities note that if individuals plan to maintain an ideal body weight by caloric restriction alone, they will be mildly hungry every day for the rest of their lives.

Yo-Yo Dieting

Watch Out for the Crash

Beyond the fact that most of the weight lost in "crash" diets is water and disregarding the loss of muscle tissue, a person can undergo some severe psychological changes with such extreme dieting. Moods change, tempers shorten, and lethargy sets in. The person feels less like doing anything and so begins to rest more, which reduces the caloric expenditure, making the dieting procedure even less effective. Satisfied with a modest weight loss or frustrated when the weight reduction stops, the person goes "off the diet" and may even reward himself with an eating binge that replaces nearly all the weight lost in the past several weeks. This describes the classic pattern of **yo-yo dieting.**

Recent research on "yo-yo" dieting has shown that while individuals may lose 10 lbs. while dieting, they are likely to gain back 12 lbs when not dieting. In addition, more of the regained weight goes on as fat than as muscle as the body attempts to avoid experiencing the famine condition it just endured. Therefore, several years of this cyclic pattern could leave the person with a weight that is 10, 15, or 20 lbs. greater than when the dieting started, and most of the gain is in the form of fat.

Diet and Gain Fat

Set-Point Theory

It has been hypothesized that a person's weight returns to a predetermined level after dieting because of a weight-governing mechanism in the brain. The weight-regulator, called the **set-point,** alerts the body to conserve energy when someone goes on a severe calorie-restricted diet. Once the person goes off the diet, the body weight attempts to regulate itself to return to its previous level.

The set point can be altered, but it is slow process. While we all may have seen people who lost 30, 40, or 50 lbs on diets, failure to maintain the new weight is often seen in 70-80% of these cases. If the weight loss is slow, there is a much greater chance for success in maintaining the new body weight.

BODY COMPOSITION CHANGES WITH DIETING

Long-Haul Concept

Individuals interested in losing weight should not become frustrated if the desired weight is not lost quickly. The excess weight was not gained in two weeks or even a month, why should you think that it will all come off in that short period of time? A comforting fact seems to be that the slower one loses the weight, the greater the likelihood the new body weight can be maintained. Whether this phenomenon is due to a downward adjustment in the set-point is not known, but this could be reasonable speculation. The safe rate of weight loss is recommended to be about 1-2 lbs. per week. While that may not seem like much, a person could be 50-100 lbs. lighter in a year's time and have a much better chance of maintaining whatever new weight that is achieved. This **long-haul concept** of weight loss is the safest, most practical, and easiest for most people.

Lose Weight Slowly

Exercise

The decision of whether exercise is a useful means of reducing or controlling one's weight is still hotly debated. Those against the procedure say that a person cannot burn enough calories during an exercise session to have a meaningful impact on the caloric balance. Since an individual must burn 3,500 calories to get rid of a pound of fat, the task of losing this in a single workout seems insurmountable. Indeed it is impractical to shed one pound of fat in a day since the average person would have to either jog for 3.8 hours, swim for 5.7 hours, or walk for 9.1 hours. Applying the long-haul concept, however, the same person can lose a pound of fat a week by either jogging for 32 minutes a day, swimming for 49 minutes a day, or walking for 78 minutes a day.

Jog

Caloric Cost

As anyone who has attempted to exercise knows, the increased effort requires energy. Just how much energy a particular exercise requires may be calculated from the amount of oxygen the body needs to consume during the activity. Since every liter of oxygen consumed burns about five kilocalories, it is relatively easy to determine the caloric cost of a wide variety of exercises. The following table shows the oxygen cost for a number of activities for the average college student.

To determine the number of calories you burn during an activity, simply multiple the length of time for your participation by the value shown in Table 9.5 or Appendix A. For example, if a female plays racquetball for 60 minutes, she would burn 660 kilocalories. If nothing in her diet changes she would be able to lose one pound of fat in about four days.

Caloric Cost of Various Exercises (Kcal/min)

Exercise	Male - 165 lbs.	Female - 135 lbs.
Cross-country skiing	17.6	14.5
Jogging	13.5	11.2
Racquetabll	13.4	11.0
Cycling	12.7	10.4
Basketball	10.4	8.5
Aerobic dance	10.1	8.3
Swimming	9.6	7.9
Tennis	8.2	6.7
Skiing (leisurely)	7.9	6.5
Circuit weight training	6.9	5.7
Golf	6.4	5.3
Walking	6.0	4.9
Volleyball (recreational)	3.8	3.1

Table 9.5.

Metabolic Rate and Oxygen Consumption

The caloric cost of exercises shown in Table 9.5 may not be the only benefit derived from participation. There is some evidence that the increased oxygen consumption noted during the activity will remain elevated for some time after the person stops. This **elevated post-exercise oxygen consumption (EPOC)** means that you are burning additional calories after you complete the vigorous part of the activity. The better conditioned you become, the sooner this post-exercise elevated oxygen consumption (EPOC) returns to normal, and the fewer total calories you may burn. However, the better your fitness becomes, the better able you may be to exercise at a higher intensity and/or for a longer period of time. The higher intensity means that you will be burning calories at a higher rate than shown in Table 9.5, while the longer duration adds substantially to the total amount of calories burned.

Stop and Burn Calories

Appetite Suppression

Beyond the calories consumed during the activity and the extra ones burned after you stop, exercise may lower your caloric intake by suppressing your appetite. Contrary to popular opinion, exercise does not cause a person to eat more. If someone eats more after exercising, it is due most probably to a psychological factor rather than a physiological demand. Research with animals and humans has shown that mild to vigorous exercise reduces the appetite. The mechanism is probably related to the elevated temperature of the blood passing through the appetite control center in the brain. Because the eating pattern of most college students results in them consuming the major part of the calories for the day during the evening meal, it might be beneficial for most people to exercise in the late afternoon.

Psychological vs. Physiological

Gaining Weight

While most Americans have the problem of wanting to lose weight or body fat, some individuals desire to gain body weight. Those wishing to gain probably fall into two categories: **underweight** and **undermuscled.** While the underweight and undermuscled conditions may be separate, they could occur simultaneously. The opposite of overweight, an underweight individual is one who is significantly below the recommended weight for a given height. Although height is not the best criterion to use for determining a desirable weight, it can be used as a rough indicator. Those individuals who are more than 20% below the designated weight for a given height are considered underweight and might contemplate gaining weight. If these underweight individuals also have very low skinfold measurements (below the 20th percentile in Table 9.1), some of the weight gain can easily be fat without being a problem. It is generally not advocated for people to gain fat and most of them will not need to do so, but for those very thin people, a reserve of fat might be beneficial.

Build the Fat Reserve

The other category of those wishing to gain weight contains individuals who have an underdeveloped muscle mass. As previously discussed, simply eating more food, especially protein, will not guarantee gains in muscle mass. The only way to insure that the weight gain will be in the form of muscle is to engage in a program of resistance training.

Caloric Demand

In order for an individual to gain 1-2 lbs. of muscle mass per week, it will require intake of an additional 1,000-1,500 kilocalories per day above the normal diet. This additional caloric intake should be supplied by healthy, carbohydrate-rich foods and not by simple sugars. The best approach to achieving the high-caloric intake may be to eat five or six smaller meals spread throughout the day instead of the traditional three large ones. Fruits and fruit juices can provide substantial calories, carbohydrates, and fiber without adding a lot of bulk and fat to the diet.

Exercise Requirement for Muscle Gain

In order to insure that the majority of the weight gain is in the form of muscle, a heavy-resistance weight training program should accompany the high-caloric diet. A "bodybuilding" routine may enhance the amount of muscle added during the time of training. This type of lifting routine concentrates on large muscle exercises performed in sets of 10-15 repetitions with relatively short rest periods between sets. (See Chapter 8 for more information.)

Muscle Tone Exercises

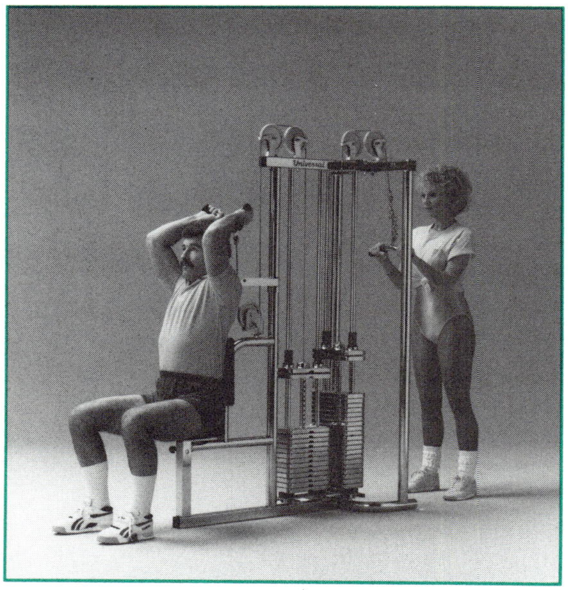

Figure 9.4. Men and women can improve muscular tone with resistance training. Photo was provided by Universal Gym Equipment, Inc.

Women versus Men

Some individuals attempting to gain weight will have more success than others. Beyond the body's efficient use of the additional calories, the levels of androgenic hormones present may influence the growth rate of muscle tissue. Those with more androgenic hormone (i.e., testosterone) will gain muscle faster than those with lower levels of the male hormone. Therefore, owing to the small amount of testosterone present, it may be quite difficult for the average female to build a great deal of muscle size despite an extensive weight training program. However, either gender can improve muscle tone with a resistance training program (Figure 9.4).

EXERCISE IN WEIGHT MANAGEMENT

While only about one-fourth of Americans are actually obese, more than three-fourths think they are overweight and would like to lose pounds. Anyone attempting to properly control body weight must seriously consider a personalized exercise program as a part of their life-style. Just as a serious commitment to maintaining an ideal body weight will require an alteration in the traditional dietary intake, so too will it demand a sound, well-designed exercise program. In addition to burning unwanted calories, the exercise program will maintain a greater fat-free weight, thus boosting the metabolic rate to allow greater food intake to assure adequate nutrition. In short, if a college student wishes to achieve and maintain a desirable body weight throughout life, a combination of nutritional control and exercise is a must.

AEROBIC VERSUS ANAEROBIC

Activities can be divided on the basis of intensity and duration. Higher intensity, shorter duration exercises can be accomplished without requiring oxygen to be delivered to the muscles. These activities are termed anaerobic and can be tolerated for only short periods of time before fatigue causes the participant to rest. All of the energy to perform anaerobic activities is supplied from carbohydrates stored in the body; therefore, anaerobic exercises are not good methods of controlling or reducing body fat. Lower intensity, longer duration exercises require a supply of oxygen to the muscles in order to avoid fatigue. The longer an individual exercises at a lower intensity, the more likely that person is to use fats as the fuel. These fats are drawn from the storage deposits in the body and help control and reduce body weight.

More is Better

USING FAT STORES

There is some evidence that aerobic exercise must last at least 20 minute before the shift to fat utilization is sufficient to be of meaningful consequence. It takes about that long for chemical reactions that withdraw fat from storage to become fully operational. Therefore, in order to concentrate the majority of your exercise on fat utilization, you need to perform moderately intense exercise for about 20-30 minutes. Longer exercise sessions will increase the amount of fat burned. Recent research has shown that exercise in the morning, despite consuming a light breakfast, may burn more fat than exercise in the late afternoon. While individuals who exercise before breakfast will have little carbohydrates to use and will use more fat to supply their energy needs, some may suffer from dizziness and fatigue because of low blood sugar (**hypoglycemia**). However, it appears that most individuals will burn significantly more fat if they can exercise before lunch than if they exercise after the noontime meal.

Take a Morning Exercise Break

COMBINATION PROGRAMS FOR CONTROLLING WEIGHT

The thoughts of sweating through tedious exercise programs for hours each day as a means of controlling their weight does not appeal to most people. Also the idea of existing on near-starvation diets for the rest of their lives is equally unappealing. But before you give up hope, consider the best benefits of both approaches. A carefully planned exercise program can require as little as an hour which includes changing into workout gear and returning to the daily routine. Couple this with a well-balance diet that provides you with nutrients, energy, and great satisfaction without giving up all of the foods you enjoy.

Plan Carefully

As examples of combining both moderate dietary alterations and exercise, consider the following. If you cut out one soda a day (150 kcal) and jog two miles (230 kcal), you create a calorie deficit of 380 kcal per day, or enough to lose a pound of fat every nine days. The two-mile jog should take you no longer than 20 minutes. If you have more time after jogging, you can spend 20 minutes lifting weights and burn an additional 138 kcal. Investing less than one hour of your day, you have created a caloric deficit of 518 kcal. If you do not change your diet, you should lose a pound of fat about every seven days.

It is hard for most of us to give up the "extras" we like to eat: chocolate bars, ice cream sundaes, or jelly-filled donuts. Psychologists indicate that sometimes the guilt that accompanies the consumption of such foods when we feel we should not be eating them is too much to bear, and we lose all hope of achieving an ideal weight. Combining exercise with moderate control of such "extras" can allow you to splurge once and a while. Go ahead, have a donut! You can burn that 390 kcal off with your jogging-weight training program and still maintain your weight.

A Life-Long Process

But be careful about falling into the rationalizing trap—"I exercised today so I can have a soda, two chocolate-chip cookies, and a bag of M & M." You just ate 1,002 kcal, or almost three times what you burned up during the exercise. While you do not want to be a slave to the bathroom scales, you should weigh periodically to determine if you are remaining stable. In addition, it would be wise to have your body composition measured every few months to assess the proportions of your weight. If you notice an increase in the fat weight in conjunction with a rise in body weight, you can make the proper adjustments by exercising more or eating less.

Weight management is a life-long process, but it need not be a ball-and-chain keeping you from enjoying yourself. A well-designed exercise program can be fun. A sensible diet can be nutritious, delicious, and rewarding. It's all a matter of life-style, and you are the master of yours.

Exercise Should be Enjoyable

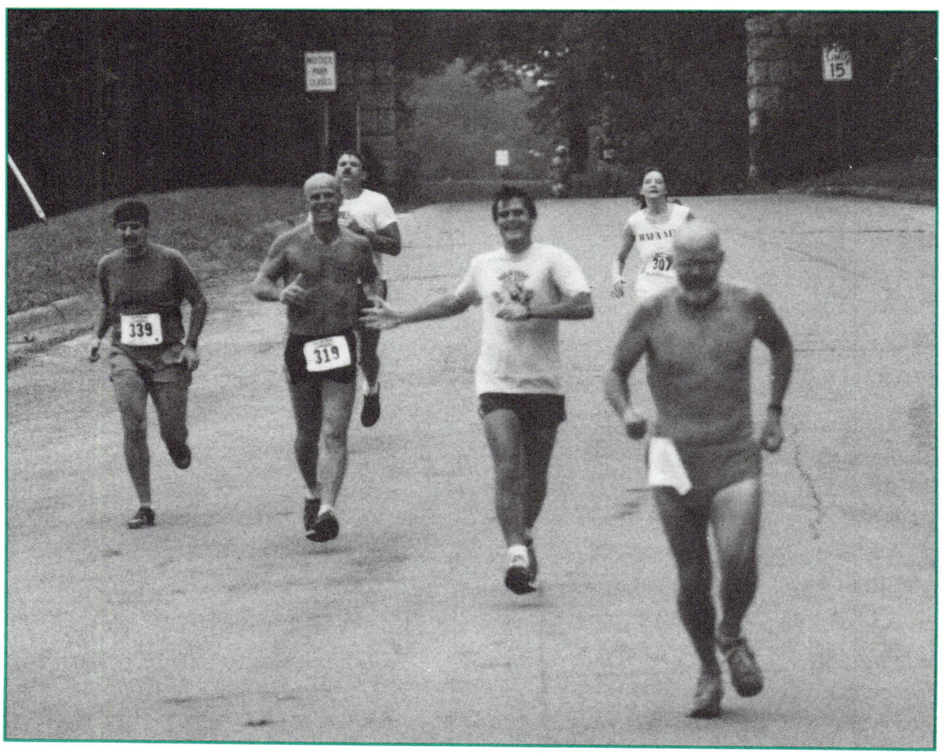

Suggested Readings

Coleman, Ellen. *Eating for Endurance.* Palo Alto, CA: Bull Publishing, 1988.

Griffin, G.C. and W.P. Castelli, *Good Fat Bad Fat: How to Lower Your Cholesterol and Beat the Odds of a Heart Attack..* Fisher, 1989

Hales, Diane. *An Invitation to Health.* (4th ed) Benjamin Cummings Publishing, 1989.

Hoeger, Werner W.K., and Sharon A. Hoeger, *Lifetime Physical Fitness and Wellness.* (3rd ed) Englewood, CO: Morton Publishing, 1992.

Ornish, D. *Dr. Dean Ornish's Program for Reversing Heart Disease.* New York: Random House, 1990.

Prentice, William E. *Fitness for College and Life.* (3rd ed) St. Louis, MO: Mosbey Year Book, 1991.

Reed, Rosalind and Thomas A. Lang, *Health Behaviors.* (2nd ed) St. Paul, MN: West Publishing, 1987.

Roberts, Scott W. *Health Wellness: An Introductory Approach.* Dubuque, IA eddie bowers publishing inc., 1989.

Thomas,Tom R. *Muscular Fitness Through Resistance Training.* (2nd ed) Dubuque, IA: eddie bowers publishing, inc., 1991.

CHAPTER 10

FEMALE HEALTH AND FITNESS

Debra Bemben

Learning Objectives

- Describe the effects of weight training on lean body mass and muscular strength in women.
- Identify potential menstrual cycle problems associated with intense endurance training.
- Discuss the benefits and risks of exercise during pregnancy for the fetus and the mother.
- Describe the relationship between menopause and bone loss in women.
- Identify ways in which women can reduce their risk for osteoporosis.
- Identify the RDA and food sources for iron in adult women.
- Differentiate between eating disorders, anorexia nervosa and bulimia.

Important Terms

amenorrhea
anorexia nervosa
athletic amenorrhea
bulimia
calcium carbonate
climacteric
cortical bone
eating disorders
estrogen
ferritin
follicular phase
iron deficiency anemia
iron depletion
luteal phase
maximal oxygen uptake (VO_2 max)
menopause
menstrual cycle
muscle hypertrophy
neural adaptations
oligomenorrhea
oral contraceptives (OC)
osteoporosis
oxygen uptake
pregnancy
progesterone
stress fractures
stroke volume
testosterone
trabecular bone

INTRODUCTION

The increased participation in exercise by women of all ages has brought attention to concerns and issues which specifically relate to the physiological function of the exercising female. The purpose of this chapter is to review the relationships between exercise training and the health of the adult female. Special health issues such as **athletic amenorrhea, eating disorders**, exercise during pregnancy, and **osteoporosis** are addressed. Finally, exercise and nutrition recommendations are given based on the current state of knowledge for each topic.

Exercise and the Female

TRAINING RESPONSES

WEIGHT TRAINING

Sex differences in strength and muscle mass are evident with men generally being stronger than women. In women, the upper body strength is about 50-60% that of men, and the lower body strength is about 70-80% that of men. Strength is affected by neural factors, i.e., the number of motor units activated during a task, and by muscle size, as force production is directly related to muscle cross-sectional area. The greater absolute strength in men has been attributed to the greater amounts of muscle mass they possess compared to women, rather than the function of the muscle itself. In fact, male and female muscle tissue is functionally similar, in that force output per kilogram of muscle tissue does not differ between the sexes.

Another sex difference relates to the potential for **muscle hypertrophy**, which is the increase in muscle size in response to weight training. Based on weight training studies, it seems that women experience less increase in muscle size compared to men, therefore, their improvements in strength are a result of **neural adaptations** to training rather than muscle hypertrophy. It has been widely accepted that women will not build muscle mass during a weight training program to the same extent as men due to their lower levels of the male sex hormone, **testosterone**. Recently, the role of testosterone in muscle hypertrophy and strength development has been questioned. When men and women were placed on the same weight training routines, women were able to achieve similar percentages in strength gains and in muscle size increases as men (Figure 10.1). These results indicate that muscle tissue of males and females has the same training potential for strength and muscle hypertrophy relative to their pre-weight training levels. The tendency for males to have greater muscle mass before training accounts for sex differences in the absolute levels of strength and muscle mass gains in response to weight training. It is evident that women desiring improvements in strength should follow the same weight training principles as men (Chapter 8). As with all exercise training, the programs should be suited to the needs and goals of the individual.

Female Strength Training

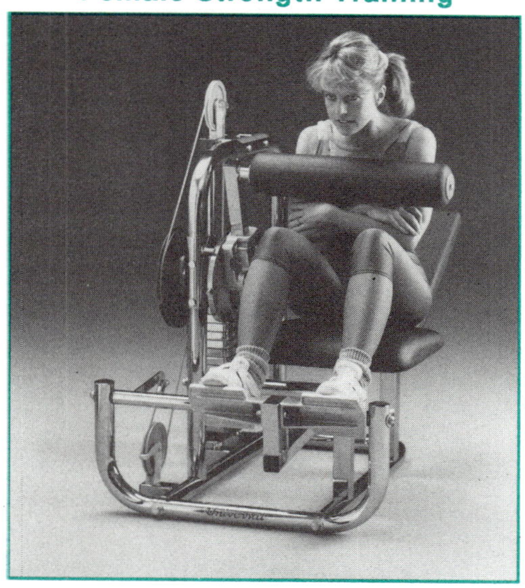

Figure 10.1. Research studies show that women can make similar strength gains as men when placed on the same resistance training programs. Photo was provided by Universal Gym Equipment, Inc.

ENDURANCE TRAINING

Sex differences exist in cardiorespiratory function, as women have approximately 28% lower maximal aerobic power, as measured by **maximal oxygen uptake (VO_2 max)** as compared to men. Several physiological factors account for this sex difference. Women have lower hemoglobin levels than males which means less oxygen is transported in the blood to the working muscles. Body composition also affects VO_2 max with higher levels of lean tissues being associated with higher VO_2. The higher percent body fat of women compared to men negatively affects aerobic power since fat acts as dead weight which burdens the cardiorespiratory system because it contributes to the body weight that is moved during exercise but it is not metabolically active.

Endurance Rowing

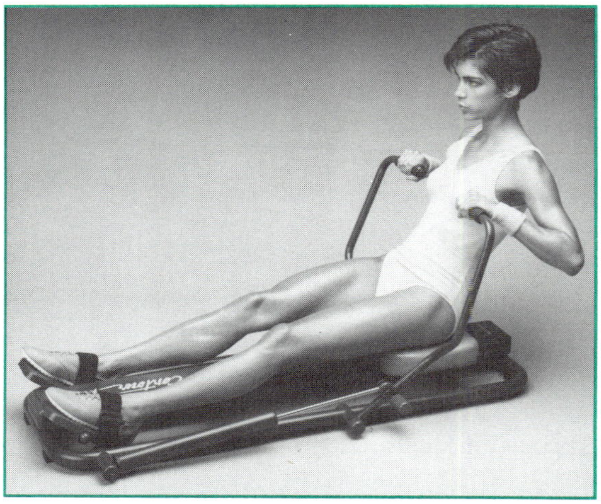

Figure 10.2. A women's cardiovascular system improves with aerobic exercise.

Sex differences also are evident in cardiovascular function, related to the smaller body size of women. Women tend to have smaller hearts than men; therefore, **stroke volume,** the volume of blood pumped with each heart beat, is less than in men. To compensate for the lower stroke volume, heart rate tends to be higher at a given workload in order to have the same amount of blood supplied to the working tissues.

Despite the differences in physiological function, men and women show similar adaptations to endurance training. In general, women are able to show improvements in VO_2 max, cardiovascular function, and in metabolism with aerobic training (Figure 10.2). Women, therefore, should follow an individualized training program which is based on the general training principles for aerobic fitness.

EXERCISE AND THE MENSTRUAL CYCLE

EFFECTS ON EXERCISE PERFORMANCE

Sex Steroids and Energy Metoblism

The female reproductive cycle is 23-35 days in length and it is divided into two phases; the **follicular phase**, from day 1 of menses to day 14, and the **luteal phase**, from ovulation (release of egg from ovary) to the onset of next menses. The menstrual cycle is regulated by the reproductive hormones, including **estrogen** and **progesterone**, which are produced by the ovaries. The blood concentrations of these female sex steroids fluctuate during the menstrual cycle; thus the follicular phase is associated with relatively low levels of estrogen and progesterone, and the luteal phase is associated with high levels of these hormones.

The female sex steroids have been shown to affect energy metabolism; therefore, exercise performance and metabolic responses during exercise may be influenced by the phase of the menstrual cycle. The majority of evidence indicates heart rate, ventilation, and oxygen uptake during maximal exercise are similar during the follicular and luteal phases of the strual cycle. The luteal phase, however, has been associated with greater endurance performance and lower blood lactate levels during submaximal steady state exercise. These responses suggest endurance performance is improved by the female sex steroids which are higher during the luteal phase.

EFFECTS ON REPRODUCTIVE FUNCTION

Endurance training has been associated with menstrual cycle problems, such as an irregular menstrual cycle or **oligomenorrhea** (menstrual periods once every 39-90 days), and the complete cessation of the menstrual period for 90 days or more, known as **amenorrhea**. The prevalence of amenorrhea varies from approximately 10% in swimmers and cyclists to as high as 40% in runners. The specific cause of amenorrhea is not known, however, there are multiple factors which predispose an athletic woman to this problem (Table 10.1). Low body weight and/or body fat seem to be an important predisposing factors since amenorrhea is more common in female athletes with low body weight such as runners compared to swimmers and cyclists who tend to have normal body weights. In addition, women with athletic amenorrhea often have a history of menstrual irregularities prior to their exercise training.

Causes of Amenorrhea

Factors Which Predispose a Female Athlete to Menstrual Cycle Problems

1. Weight loss	4. Dietary alterations	7. Emotional stress
2. Low weight	5. Nutritional inadequacy	8. Acute hormone alterations
3. Low body fat	6. Physical stress	9. Chronic hormone alterations

Table 10.1. From "Menstruation" by M.M. Shangold. In *Women and Exercise: Physiology and Sports Medicine* (p. 133) by M.M. Shangold and G. Mirkin (Eds.), 1988, Philadelphia: F.A. Davis Company. Copyright 1988 by F.A. Davis Company. Reprinted by permission.

The persistence of **menstrual cycle** problems can have serious health consequences. For example, if a woman experiencing oligomenorrhea is not ovulating, she may have an increased risk for developing breast cancer. Recent evidence suggests amenorrheic women experience reduced bone mineral density, perhaps related to low estrogen levels and a calcium deficient diet, both of which have been documented in amenorrheic athletes. The reduced bone density in these young women indicates they may be losing bone at rates similar to postmenopausal women, whereas they should still be building bone until age 35. This phenomenon has implications for bone health as musculoskeletal injuries, such as **stress fractures**, are more common in amenorrheic athletes compared to female athletes with regular menstrual cycles. Risk for osteoporosis, a bone disorder characterized by gradual bone loss and weakening of the skeleton, also may be increased in amenorrheic athletes. In fact, some young athletes have been diagnosed as osteoporotic with lumbar spine bone densities at levels similar to those of 50 year old women. One positive note is that athletic amenorrhea is reversible; that is, normal menses are resumed rapidly when the individual decreases exercise volume and/or gains weight. Hormone replacement, such as oral contraceptives, is another option for the amenorrheic athlete to restore menstrual function and to protect bone mass. Adequate dietary calcium intake also is critical for attaining peak bone mass and maintenance of skeletal health. Athletes taking hormone therapy should consume 1000 mg calcium per day, whereas those amenorrheic athletes with low estrogen levels require 1500 mg calcium per day to maintain calcium balance.

Amenorrhea is Reversible

ORAL CONTRACEPTIVE USE

Oral contraceptives (OC) are a combined form of synthetic estrogen and progesterone. The primary purpose of OC is to inhibit ovulation; although OC can have widespread systemic effects. The early forms of OC had detrimental effects on cardiovascular function and metabolism; however, recent OC formulations contain much lower doses of estrogen and progesterone and tend to have fewer side effects. An increase in body weight often is associated with OC use since estrogen increases fat deposition and progesterone enhances water retention. OC use may affect exercise performance as decreases in muscular strength and in maximal oxygen uptake have been reported with OC treatment. Recent evidence indicates energy metabolism during submaximal exercise is altered with OC use. Blood glucose levels and carbohydrate utilization were lower during walking for long durations in women taking OC compared to women with normal menstrual cycles. These findings suggest carbohydrate metabolism is impaired in OC users. Since carbohydrate is an important energy source for muscle metabolism and the nervous system, taking OC may be detrimental for exercise performance such as high intensity distance running. In summary, although OC use is a popular method of contraception, it may not be the best choice for normally menstruating women desiring optimal levels of exercise performance. As previously mentioned, amenorrheic athletes may find the benefits of OC therapy for protection of bone mass outweigh the potential detrimental effects on performance.

Negatives of OC

PREGNANCY

The increased participation in exercise by women has brought to light an additional concern about the safety of maternal exercise for the mother and the fetus. There are many physiological changes during **pregnancy** which increase the physical stress during exercise. Of utmost concern are the effects of exercise on the fetus who requires an uninterrupted supply of oxygen and nutrients for optimal growth and development.

MATERNAL RESPONSES

The average weight gain during pregnancy is 24 pounds, attributed to increased weight of the uterus, placenta, increased blood volume, and the fetus. Resting oxygen uptake also increases about 15% during pregnancy. The increase in body weight has a large effect on weight-bearing exercise which can require 20% or more energy during pregnancy. The efficiency of non-weight bearing exercise is not affected by pregnancy as oxygen uptake is not elevated during cycling exercise.

Please Be Seated

The hormone changes during pregnancy stimulate ventilation, apparently due to increases in tidal volume. This change does not affect greatly maternal exercise since ventilation is not a limiting factor for exercise performance in healthy individuals.

Circulatory adjustments to pregnancy include an increased blood volume (approximately 50%), an increase in cardiac output (liters of blood pumped per minute), and a decrease in peripheral resistance. In some individuals, pregnancy induces hypertension. The effects of posture on cardiovascular responses to exercise become particularly important during pregnancy. Decreases in venous return and cardiac output have been shown to be greater during supine exercise compared to lateral and seated positions. Additionally, a small percentage of pregnant women respond to the decrease in cardiac output during supine exercise with a decrease in blood pressure. These postural changes in cardiovascular function would be detrimental for the pregnant woman; thus, supine exercises should be avoided, especially in the later stages of pregnancy.

OUTCOMES

It has been speculated that physically fit women experience shorter labors than non-exercising counterparts. There is little scientific evidence to support this hypothesis since most studies did not report length of labor. A recent analysis of studies that examined the effects of exercise on pregnancy outcomes reported no significant differences in gestation length, body weight gain, or in birth weight between exercising and non-exercising groups. Additionally, values for these variables were within normal healthy ranges for both groups.

FETAL RESPONSES

Pregnancy and Exercise

There are several areas of concern for possible detrimental effects of maternal exercise on the developing fetus. Reductions in blood flow to the uterus and subsequent decreases in the supply of oxygen and nutrients to the fetus could result in suboptimal growth and hypoxic damage. Increases in maternal body temperature during exercise also could have a harmful effect on the fetus. Apparently, the fetus compensates for diminished blood flow during exhaustive exercise performed by the mother by increasing oxygen extraction. Animal studies show that despite decreases in fetal oxygen tension with increases in exercise intensity and duration, these values are maintained within an acceptable range.

Fetus in Distress

Fetal heart rate measured by Doppler monitoring has been used to detect fetal distress, although this technique can be difficult to interpret due to large variability in the data. Several studies have documented that fetal heart rate slows down during maternal exercise, but accelerates during recovery. This pattern of heart rate response during recovery may be a compensatory mechanism by the fetus for the bradycardia which occurs during exercise.

RECOMMENDATIONS

There is little evidence that exercise during pregnancy has a harmful effect on the mother or baby. In fact, obstetricians generally are in favor of women exercising and improving physical fitness during pregnancy.

Pregnant women wishing to exercise should follow the recommendations of their obstetrician. Depending on the initial fitness level, some women may be able to tolerate greater exercise stress than that outlined by the ACOG. The upper limits of safe exercise cannot be determined based on previous research, thus, it is better to follow the ACOG guidelines, which are well within the safe limits for normal pregnancies (Table 10.2).

ACOG Exercise Guidelines

1. Maternal heart rate should not exceed 140 beats per minute
2. Strenuous activities should not exceed 15 minutes in duration
3. Exercise should not be performed in the supine position after the fourth month of pregnancy
4. The valsalva maneuver and bouncy, jerky movements should be avoided
5. Maternal core temperature should not exceed 38° C.

Table 10.2. The guidelines for exercise established by the American College of Obstetricians and Gynecologists (ACOG) are written for the average woman and tend to be conservative in nature.

Finally, pregnant women should pay attention to their bodies and reduce exercise if discomfort, pain, and/or signs of vaginal bleeding occur. As their pregnancies progress, most women tend to slow down and modify their exercise programs to accommodate weight gains and postural changes.

Some Specific Suggestions for Pregnant Women

1. Do not begin an exercise program without consulting your obstetrician
2. Follow "safe" levels of exercise
3. Avoid overheating and dehydration
4. Avoid supine exercise

MENOPAUSE

Menopause refers to the duration of the last menstrual period, which, in actuality, is the biologic marker of the **climacteric**, the gradual change from reproductive to nonreproductive years in women.

Three Stages of Climacteric

1. Early climacteric from 35-45 years
2. Pre and post menopausal periods from 46-55 years
3. Late climacteric from 56-65 years.

The gradual change in reproductive function is brought about by a gradual decrease in the female sex steroids, estrogen and progesterone. Thus the late climacteric is characterized by symptoms associated with estrogen deprivation. In addition to its effects on reproductive function; estrogen has profound effects on cardiovascular and skeletal function; therefore, estrogen deficiency during the climacteric contributes to osteoporosis and coronary heart disease in postmenopausal women.

CARDIOVASCULAR FUNCTION

Age Takes Its Toll

In general, women experience an age-related decrease in cardiorespiratory fitness. This phenomenon is not related to menopause as maximal oxygen uptake (VO_2 max) in postmenopausal women was similar to that of premenopausal women of similar chronological age. Serum cholesterol levels, a primary risk factor for coronary heart disease, are related to menopause as indicated by higher total cholesterol and lower high density lipoprotein levels in postmenopausal women compared to their premenopausal counterparts.

OSTEOPOROSIS

Estrogen and You

Trabecular bone or spongy bone represents 20% of the skeleton, while the remaining 80% consists of **cortical bone** which is more compact and less metabolically active than trabecular bone. Peak bone mass occurs by age 35 in women, after which age-related bone loss occurs. By 80 years of age, women lose about 25% of cortical bone mass and 32% of trabecular bone mass. Estrogen deficiency in postmenopausal women may be the most important factor for bone loss which is accelerated after menopause. Osteoporosis is a skeletal disorder where excessive bone loss leads to increased fragility of the bones resulting in loss of height, and fractures of the wrist, hip and vertebrae as shown in Figures 10.3 and 10.4. Women receiving estrogen replacement therapy have fewer osteoporotic fractures as estrogen slows down the rate of bone loss. Thin, small-boned women, and Caucasian women tend to have a greater risk for osteoporosis. The risk for developing osteoporosis is increased by additional dietary and life-style factors listed on the following page (Table 10.3).

Three Principal Sites of Osteoporotic Fractures

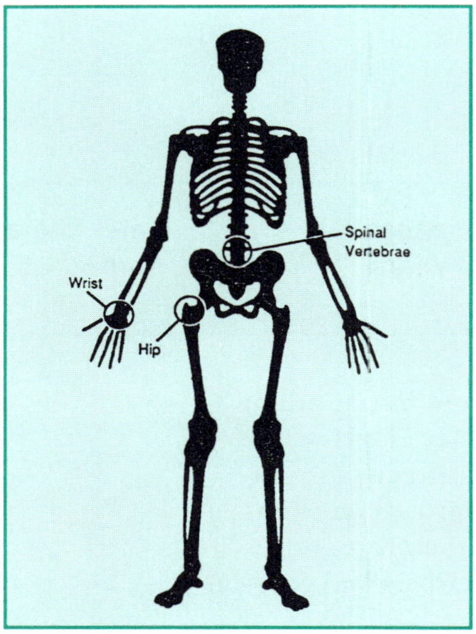

Figure 10.3. From *Women, Sport & Performance*, (p. 166) by C.L. Wells, 1991, Champaign: Human Kinetics Books. Adapted from the National Dairy Council (1984). Copyright 1991 by Christine L. Wells. Reprinted with permission.

Loss of Height with Development of the Dowager's Hump with Osteoporosis

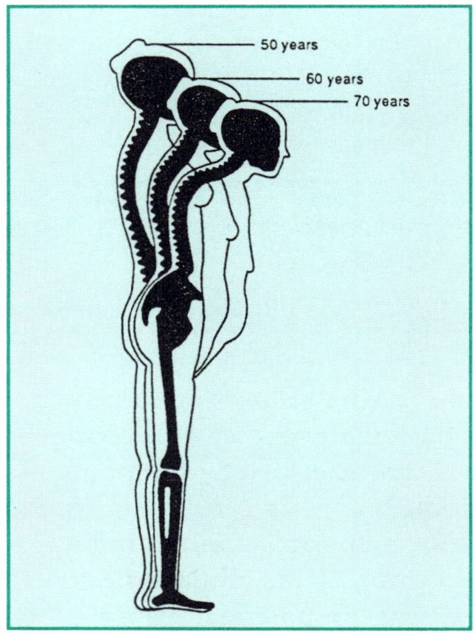

Figure 10.4. From Calcium: A Summary of Current Research for the Health Professional (p. 16), 1984, Rosemont, IL: National Dairy Council. Copyright 1984 by National Dairy Council. Reprinted with permission.

Risk Factors for Osteoporosis

1. Being a woman
2. Family history of osteoporosis
3. Being Caucasian or Asian, especially of Northern European descent
4. Low body weight
5. Small bone structure
6. Early menopause
7. Lack of calcium in diet
8. Lack of physical activity
9. Cigarette smoking
10. Alcohol and/or caffeine intake
11. High-protein diet (increases calcium excretion)

Table 10.3. Source: United States Department of Health and Human Services. (1986). *Osteoporosis: Cause, treatment, prevention* (NIH Publication No. 86-2226). Washington, DC: U.S. Government Printing Office.

Osteoporosis can be prevented by acquiring greater bone mass before the early climacteric period. Adequate calcium intake is necessary to achieve increases in bone mass. The Consensus conference on Osteoporosis conducted by the National Institutes of Health has recommended a calcium intake of 1000 mg per day for women with normal estrogen levels; however, estrogen-deficient women should increase their calcium intake to 1500 mg per day. Weight-bearing exercise is another important factor for building bone as the physical stress on the bones enhances bone mineralization and decreases the rate of bone loss. It is recommended that 40-50 minutes of aerobic weight-bearing exercise performed 3-4 times per week is adequate for skeletal maintenance. Some caution must be taken when prescribing exercise for women with osteoporosis. These individuals may have microfractures in trabecular bone which may be aggravated by strenuous exercise. These women, therefore, should participate in light to moderate exercise such as walking. Vigorous weight-bearing activities such as aerobic dance, jazz dance, and exercises that involve back flexion should be avoided.

NUTRITION AND THE EXERCISING FEMALE

IRON DEFICIENCY

Iron deficiency is a nutritional concern for young active women as iron intake in the diet tends not to be adequate for iron requirements. The average woman consumes about 11 mg of iron per day in the diet which does not meet the requirement of 15 mg of iron per day for menstruating women. Adult women have a higher iron RDA than males to compensate for losses of iron during menstruation and childbirth. Measurement of **ferritin** levels in the blood provides a good indication of iron stores in bone marrow. **Iron depletion**, the first stage of iron deficiency, is characterized by a decrease in serum ferritin levels. When iron deficiency continues, red blood cell formation is impaired, which is the second stage of iron deficiency. **Iron deficiency anemia** occurs when all the iron reserves in the body have been depleted resulting in the lowering of hemoglobin levels below 11 g/dl. A recent study found that 31% of female athletes were iron deficient, although this percentage was not different from non-athletic women. Since iron plays an important role in oxygen transport, iron deficiency anemia can adversely affect exercise performance, although most evidence indicates that the early stages of iron deficiency have a minimal effect on work performance. Increasing intake of iron, folate, and vitamin B12 will correct iron deficiency anemia. Heme iron, the form of dietary iron found in meat, fish, and poultry is better absorbed than nonheme iron found in eggs, milk, and plant foods. Recommendations for increasing iron intake in the diet are listed as follows (Table 10.4).

Put Iron In Your Life

Recommendations for Increasing Iron Intake

1. Eat more lean red meat or dark meat of chicken
2. Improve iron absorption from bread and cereal by avoiding coffee or tea with meals and drinking instead a source of vitamin C
3. Cook occasionally in cast iron skillets and pans
4. Eat poultry or seafood with dried beans or peas as the animal protein increases the absorption of iron in the vegetable

Table 10.4. From "Sports anemia": poor terminology for a real phenomenon, *Sports Science Exchange, 1* (6), (1988) by E.R. Eichner. Copyright 1988 by The Quaker Oats Company. Reprinted with permission.

CALCIUM INTAKE

The average calcium intake of women 19-50 years of age is 600 mg/day which is about 50% of the RDA for women 19-24 years of age and about 74% of the RDA for women 25 years and older. It is important for women to build as much bone as possible before age 35 as a preventive measure against osteoporosis. The National Institutes of Health recommends a calcium intake of 1000 mg/day for menstruating women and women taking estrogen; however, it should be increased to 1500 mg/day for women with low estrogen levels (i.e., postmenopausal women not receiving estrogen replacement therapy and amenorrheic women). Dairy products, fish, and shellfish are good sources of dietary calcium (Table 10.5). Individuals who avoid milk tend to have low calcium intakes.

Suggestions for Increasing Calcium Intake (without drinking milk)

1. Consume other dairy products such as yogurt and cheese
2. Use milk and cheeses in cooking (i.e., sauces, casseroles, desserts)
3. Eat vegetables that are good sources of calcium such as leafy vegetables, broccoli, and legumes

Women who have difficulty meeting the calcium RDA from dietary sources may consider calcium supplementations. As shown in Table 10.6, **calcium carbonate** contains the highest percentage of calcium. Therefore, supplements containing calcium carbonate have greater calcium content, and, generally are cheaper than supplements containing other calcium compounds.

Calcium Content in Various Foods

Food	Amount	Calcium (mg)
Yogurt, plain, lowfat	8 ounces	415
Skim Milk	8 ounces	302
2% Milk	8 ounces	300
Swiss Cheese	1 ounce	204
Cheddar Cheese	1 ounce	204
Turnip Greens cooked	1/2 cup	184
Processed American Cheese	1 ounce	174
Custard, baked	1/2 cup	150
Vanilla Ice Cream	1/2 cup	88
Broccoli	1/2 cup	68
Cottage Cheese creamed	1/2 cup	62

Table 10.5. Adapted from *Osteoporosis: A Guide to Prevention and Treatment, 1989* (pp. 81-85) by J.F. Aloia, 1989, Champaign, IL: Human Kinetics. Copyright 1989 by Leisure Press. Reprinted by permission. Sources: Consumer and Food Economics Institute (1976-1980). *Composition of Foods Handbook.* Nos. 8-1,4, 5, 6, 7. Washington DC: USDA Agriculture Research Service;Pennington, J.A.T., & Church, H. (1980). *Food Values of Portions Commonly Used* (13th ed.). New York: Harper & Row; Robinson, J., & Lawler, M.R. (1982). *Normal and Therapeutic Nutrition* (16th ed.). New York: McMillan;Schneider, H.A., Anderson, C.E., & Coursin, D.B. (1983). *Nutritional Support of Medical Practice.* (2nd ed). Philadelphia: Harper & Row.

Calcium Source and Content of Selected Calcium Supplements

Product Name (Manufacturer)	Calcium Source	Calcium Content %	Elemental Calcium/ Tablet (mg)
Tums Regular (Norcliff-Thayer)	Calcium Carbonate	40	200
Caltrate 600 (Lederle)	Calcium Carbonate	40	600
Biocal (Miles)	Calcium Carbonate	40	500
Os-cal (Marion)	Calcium Carbonate	40	500
Posture (Ayerst)	Tribasic Calcium Phosphate	39	235
Posture-D (Ayerst, with Vitamin D)	Tribasic Calcium Phosphate	39	600
Citracal (Mission Pharmaceutical)	Calcium Citrate	24	200
Calcium Lactate (Various Brands: Lilly, GNC, Nature's Bounty)	Calcium Lactate	13	85
Calcium Gluconate with Vitamin D (Lilly)	Calcium Gluconate	9	93

Table 10.6. Adapted from *Osteoporosis: A Guide to Prevention and Treatment, 1989* (pp. 59-64) by J.F. Aloia, 1989, Champaign, IL: Human Kinetics. Copyright 1989 by Leisure Press. Reprinted by Permission. Sources: E.K. Kastovp (Ed.) (1986). *Drug Facts and Comparision* (1986 ed.). St. Louis: Facts and Comparison (division of J.B. Lippincott).

EATING DISORDERS

Anorexia to Bulimia

Eating disorders are abnormal food intake patterns which stem from psychological disturbances. Two such conditions are **anorexia nervosa** and **bulimia**, both of which are primarily female diseases as 90-95% of all cases are women. Anorexia nervosa is estimated to affect from 1 to 5% of female adolescents, whereas bulimia affects approximately 10% of college-aged females. Anorexia nervosa is characterized by self-imposed starvation associated with substantial weight loss, at least 25% of original body weight. The anorectic is obsessed with food, has a distorted body image and participates in high levels of physical activity. Bulimics follow a binge-purge cycle, where large amounts of food eaten are eliminated by vomiting, and by the use of laxatives and enemas. Unlike the anorectic, the bulimic tends to have normal or near-normal body weight.

Some Signs That a Person May Have an Eating Disorder

1. Looks thin and keeps getting thinner
2. Wears layers of loose, baggy clothing
3. Fainting, blacking out
4. Frequent trips to the bathroom
5. Skips meals
6. Cuts food into small pieces
7. Eats large amounts of food

The following (Table 10.7) shows the physical consequences of anorexia nervosa and bulimia. The outcome of eating disorders can be extremely serious as 5-10% of patients die of complications such as cardiac arrest, extreme hypoglycemia, and suicide. Treatment for eating disorders involves nutritional and psychological rehabilitation.

It has been speculated that certain groups of female athletes suffer from eating disorders, specifically, women participating in those sports in which low body weight is associated with optimal performance, such as running, gymnastics, and ballet dancing.

Physical Consequences of Eating Disorders

Anorexia Nervosa
1. Emaciation
2. Dry skin
3. Lanugo
4. Loss of scalp hair and brittle nails
5. Cold extremities and impaired temperature regulation
6. Decreased heart size
7. Bradycardia
8. Hypotension
9. Edema
10. Osteoporosis

Bulimia
1. Tooth decay
2. Esophogus tears
3. Salivary gland enlargement
4. Aspiration pneumonia
5. Low potassium stores (hypokalemia)

Table 10.7. Adapted from "Eating Disorders" by J.L. Katz. In *Women and Exercise: Physiology and Sports Medicine* (p. 254) by M.M. Shangold and G. Mirkin (Eds.), 1988, Philadelphia: F.A. Davis Company. Copyright 1988 by F.A. Davis Company. Reprinted by permission.

Recent surveys have found female athletes engage in harmful weight control practices, including self-induced vomiting, laxative abuse, and use of diet pills. It was pointed out, however, that these weight loss behaviors are not synonymous with eating disorders, which stem from a serious psychological disturbance. Parents and coaches still need to be concerned since these weight control practices could jeopardize the athlete's health.

SUMMARY

Life-long Committment

Physical activity is an important contributor to health and fitness during all stages of a woman's life. While sex differences exist in muscular strength and cardiorespiratory endurance, females and males show similar training responses, thus women can benefit substantially from regular exercise. Moderate exercise during pregnancy is not contraindicated and tends to be supported by obstetricians. Weight-bearing exercise, adequate calcium intake, and estrogen replacement therapy are important ways for postmenopausal women to reduce their risk for osteoporosis. In certain individuals, intense endurance training is associated with menstrual cycle problems, although these conditions are reversible with decreased exercise volume. Amenorrheic women need to be aware of their increased risk for bone loss, particularly if dietary calcium intake is low. Oral contraceptives can be used to restore menstrual function and to protect bone mass in amenorrheic women.

Suggested Readings

Aloia, J.F. *Osteoporosis: A Guide to Prevention and Treatment*. Champaign, IL: Leisure Press, Chapters 1, 3, 6, and 8, 1989.

Consumer and Food Economics Institute. Composition of Foods Handbook. Nos. 8-1, 4, 5, 6, 7. Washington, DC: USDA Agriculture Research Service, 1976-1980

Kastovp, E.K. Drug Facts and Comparison (1986 ed.). St. Louis: Facts and Comparison

Leon, G.R. Eating disorders in female athletes. *Sports Medicine*. 12 (4): 219-227, 1991.

Lokey, E.A., Z.V. Tran, C.L. Wells, B.C. Myers, and A.C. Tran. Effects of physical exercise on pregnancy outcomes: a meta-analytic review. *Medicine and Science in Sports and Exercise.* *23* (11): 1234-1239, 1991.

Pennington, J.A.T., & H. Church. *Food Values of Portions Commnly Used* (13th ed.). New York: Harper & Row, 1980.

Robinson, H., & M. R. Lawler. *Normal and Therapeutic Nutrition* (16th ed.). New York: McMillan, 1982.

Schneider, H.A., C. E. Anderson & D. E. Coursin. *Nutritional Support of Medical Practice.* (2nd ed). Philadelphia: Harper & Row, 1983.

Shangold, S.M. and G. Mirkin. *Women and Exercise: Physiology and Sports Medicine*. Philadelphia: F.A. Davis Company, Chapters 6, 10, 11, 12, and 18, 1988.

Wells, C.L. *Women, Sport, & Performance: A Physiological Perspective.* (Second Edition). Champaign, IL: Human Kinetics Books, Chapters 5, 6, 7, 8, 9, 10, and 13, 1991.

CHAPTER

11

STRESS MANAGEMENT

Richard Fee

Learning Objectives

- Compare and contrast acute and chronic stress in terms of their effects on the human body.
- List the effects of stress on the immune, cardiovascular, gastrointestinal, muscular, and epidermal systems of the body.
- Compare and contrast major life change with daily hassles and uplifts.
- Describe the concept of Hardiness.
- Describe the stressful effects of noise on the body.
- Describe Type A behavior pattern and the health related changes which occur along with it.
- List the stressful effects of excessive caffeine and refined sugar in one's diet.
- List and describe various relaxation techniques.
- List and describe cognitive techniques for alleviating stress.
- Describe the unstressing effects of exercise.

Important Terms

acute stress
alarm phase
aldosterone
autogenic training
autonomic nervous system
B-cells
biofeedback training
caffeine
chronic stress
commitment
cortisol
decibels
endorphin
epinephrine
exhaustion phase
fight or flight
General Adaptation Syndrome (GAS)
gingivitis
hardiness
hostility
hypertension
journaling
norepinephrine
progressive relaxation
Raynaud's Syndrome
relaxation
resistance phase
resolution
social readjustmnet rating scale (SRRS)
social support
sympathetic nervous system (SNS)
T-cells
tension
tension signal
Type A behavior pattern
Type I stress
Type II stress
visualization

INTRODUCTION

What is stress? Stress is a normal part of our lives and as such can not be avoided. There are many definitions of stress. Stress is sometimes defined as an environmental event such as losing a family member, losing a job, or adding a new family member. Stress may be defined in terms of the body's reaction to life events such as a stress headache or upset stomach. When personal coping skills fail to meet environmental demands the resulting strain on the organism is also defined as stress. While there may not be complete agreement as to the precise definition of stress, most of us know the feelings of excessive stress or distress when we experience it.

Coping with Stress

A certain amount of stress adds zest and joy to life. Dr. Hans Selye termed this stress eustress or healthy stress. Stress which exceeds our coping skills may result in illness or even death. The key to healthy coping with excessive stress is learning to become aware of the signs of excessive stress and applying the concepts, techniques and skills contained in this chapter in our daily lives. Inventories #11, 14-18 in chapter 14 deal with stress.

BODY'S RESPONSE

Type I Stress

Type I stress or **acute stress** is a life event which requires a sustained physical response in order to survive. Some examples might be fleeing an assailant or getting out of the way of an oncoming truck. In each case there is the perception of a threat in an event, the mobilization of energy sources within the body, the expenditure of physical energy (fighting or fleeing) to successfully cope with the situation, and after the event the resolution of the stress response (Figure 11.1).

Notice that in our example there is a life event which is a trigger for the stress response and that the life event triggers a stress response because it is appraised as threatening to self. Indeed it is threat appraisal or perception which is the key to unlocking a stress response. When threat appraisal occurs a series of self protective reactions happens. Areas of the brain concerned with self preservation are activated and a "**fight or flight**" reaction is the result. The entire body is activated and readied for action (fighting or fleeing) by way of the **sympathetic nervous system (SNS)**. Sympathetic nerves travel from the brain to every organ system of the body providing a pathway for the body to be activated instantaneously. Harvard physiologist Walter Cannon coined the term "fight or flight" and studied it at the turn of this century.

Type I Stress (Acute Stress)

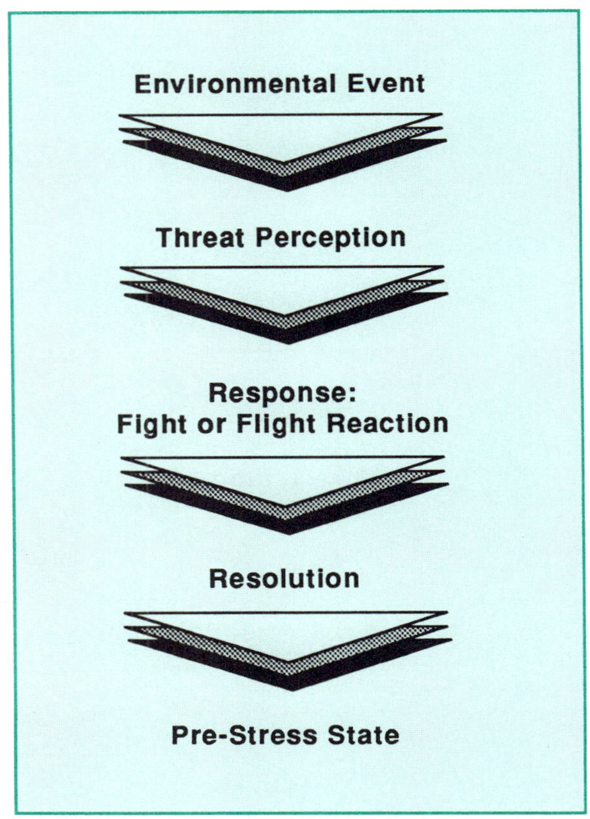

Figure 11.1 Sequence of events for Type I Stress.

Immediately the heart and breathing rate increase, blood pressure is elevated, pupils dilate, muscles tense, and the airways open. Adrenal glands, activated by the sympathetic nerve pathway activity, release large amounts of short term stress hormones, **epinephrine** and **norepinephrine**, into the blood stream. These hormones, also know as adrenalin and noradrenalin, act upon body organ systems to maintain the stress arousal initiated by the SNS. They also cause the body to release its stored fats and sugars into the bloodstream for the muscles to use as an energy source during fight or flight. At this time stress hormones also cause your body to elevate its manufacture of cholesterol many times over its normal rate. These changes in physiology will help one to survive a stressful life event by providing the readiness for fight or flight.

The Uptight Look

Following survival of the stressful event, there is a **resolution** of the stress reactions in the body. Responses return to normal through a built in homeostatic mechanism and the body returns to a prestress state. The actual act of fighting or fleeing (exercise) is crucial for resolution to occur.

Type II Stress (Chronic Stress)

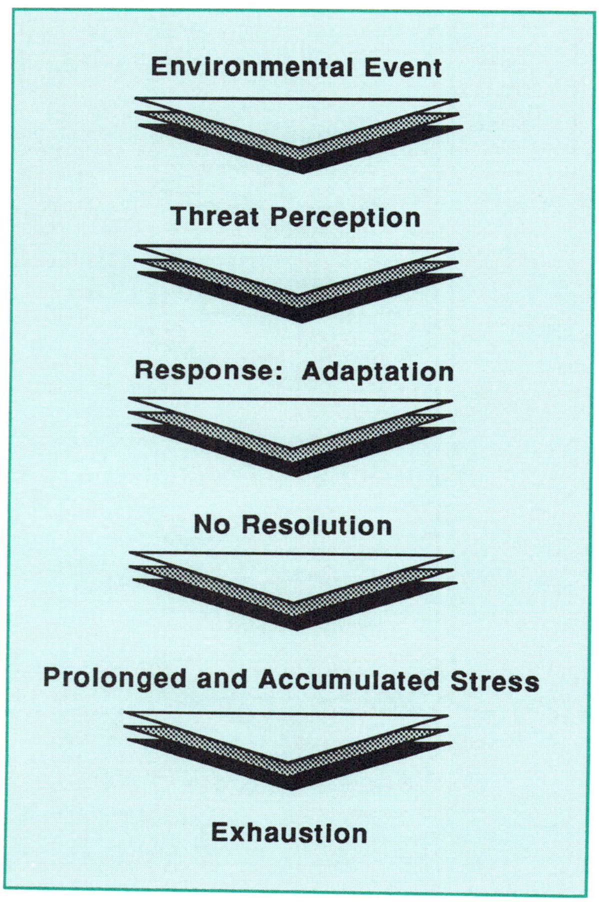

Figure 11.2. Sequence of events for Type II Stress.

Type II Stress

Type II or **chronic stress** begins similarly enough to an acute reaction but in this case the stress is of a different type. Chronic stressful life events or stressors are those that cannot be run away from or overcome by a physical fight. Therefore, because there is no physical response there is no immediate resolution to the event. The stress induced arousal within the body slowly subsides all the while the person experiences continued emotional and physical distress (Figure 11.2).

Chronic stressors threaten a person's beliefs, values, or social position and thus a person's psychological, philosophical, or sociological security not because of a physical threat. A person also may encounter chronic stress because of their personality, the way that they cope with life events or their nutritional practices. Environmental factors such as noise, crime, or economic conditions can be a source of chronic stress because when present these factors exert a continuing effect. However, the most profound chronic stressors involve human relationships and interactions. Dysfunctional relationships exert an exaggerated demand on personal resources.

Dr. Hans Selye was one of the first to study chronic stress. He found that during chronic stress there was a progression of events in a body through three distinct stages. Dr. Selye coined the term **General Adaptation Syndrome (G.A.S.)** to describe the physical changes associated with chronic stress. The first stage of the G.A.S. he termed the

alarm phase. In this stage there is a tremendous increase in bodily arousal, exaggerated sympathetic nervous system activity causing a fight or flight reaction, and increased secretion of **cortisol** from the adrenal glands. Cortisol's hormonal action releases the body's stores of energy for fight or flight. In this phase of the stress reaction the whole body is activated, thus no one organ system takes the brunt of the stress.

The Three Stages of G.A.S.

1. Alarm
2. Resistance
3. Exhaustion

As the stressful life event continues, the second stage, the **stage of resistance**, ensues. The body attempts to resist or adapt to the stressor thus the stress response is directed to a particular organ system rather than to the body as a whole and the generalized arousal in the body subsides. As the organ system responds to the ongoing stressor, it's function is altered, sometimes so drastically that the organ begins to malfunction. In late stages of the response, the organ may even begin to show signs of structural damage. After being stimulated by chronic stress for so long, the changes in the organ system pave the way for the last stage of the G.A.S., the stage of exhaustion.

In the third stage, the **stage of exhaustion**, the organ system has become totally fatigued through energy depletion caused by the stage of resistance. The organ system may then "shut down" or cease its function. The body makes a final attempt to survive as generalized arousal occurs and cortisol level elevates in the bloodstream again. Disability or death may occur depending on the organ system affected. Selye believed that the appearance of the exhaustion stage was caused by the depletion of a conceptual substance he referred to as adaptational energy. Selye believed that adaptational energy was consumed during the stage of resistance in order to physically cope with chronic stress. Because he believed that each person has only a limited store of adaptational energy, Selye taught that we should carefully guard our stores in order to avoid running out and facing the consequences of exhaustion.

In his writings Selye mentions a number of diseases he attributed to this mechanism. He referred to these disorders as diseases of adaptation. While the adaptation process certainly helps us cope with chronic stress it is maladaptive in that it is the cause of the ongoing disease processes associated with chronic stress. Selye also noted that a life event may be appraised in a positive or negative way, but that in either case the result is stressful. He was said to ask, "What do a kiss and a game of tennis have in common?" Can you figure out the answer? A description of the effects of chronic stress on important body systems follows. See if you can identify which system in your body responds to stress. What is your stress pathway?

The Stress Pathway

IMMUNE SYSTEM

This system is one of the most vital systems of the body. It has the power to defend us from invading microbes or from our own cells that have somehow become cancerous. When it is underreactive, cancers and infections may rage out of control in the body. When it is overreactive, allergies, arthritis, and autoimmune disorders can be the result.

Fortunately, the immune system functions very efficiently most of the time and we are well protected from many infectious diseases. Within the immune system are two classes of white blood cells (lymphocytes),

T-cells and **B-cells**. T-cells are able to attack bacteria and viruses directly and kill them by injection of toxic compounds. In fact, one type of T-cell is called a NK cell, a natural killer cell. B-cells protect us by producing antibodies against particular bacteria or viruses which we have been exposed to in the past. The antibodies cause the microbes to clump and thus become unable to reproduce or function. There are also suppressor T-cells which end the immune systems attack on bodily invaders when they have been destroyed and memory T-cells which remember previous invasions to provide an swift defense when reinvaded.

The effects of stress on the immune system happen through the release of stress hormones. Cortisol is known to cause the disappearance of certain types of lymphocytes and is thought to cause a reduction of antibody levels. Epinephrine also causes the loss of certain lymphocytes. **Endorphins** released from the pituitary during chronic stress can suppress the activity of NK cells. All of these situations will cause an inhibition of the immune system which may lead to increased susceptibility to infections.

ATTENTION: Brain and Immune System Communicating

It used to be thought that the immune system operated independently in the body. Exciting new research has shown that the immune system and the brain communicate and that the activities of one influence the activity of the other. The influence can enhance or inhibit immune function. Lymphocytes receive messages from the brain because they have receptors for many hormones produced by the brain that are released into the blood stream. Brain hormones bind to the receptor sites on the circulating lymphocytes and affect their activity. Likewise lymphocytes produce similar hormones which get into the brain's circulation and affect its activity.

The brain also may influence the activity of the immune system through the **autonomic nervous system**. Autonomic nerve pathways exist into the thymus gland and the bone marrow. The thymus gland is an endocrine gland which directs activity of the lymphocytes through hormonal activity and the bone marrow is an important site of blood cell production.

The name for the branch of science which studies the interconnections of the mind, brain and the immune system is psychoneuroimmunology. The mind's influence on the immune system through the nervous system is demonstrated by studies on the effect of mood on immunity.

Good and Poor Copers

A number of studies have indicated that depression or the feelings of helplessness and hopelessness are associated with markedly reduced immune function in humans. An interesting study examined the relationship of coping and natural killer cell activity. Samples of blood were taken from medical students and assayed for natural killer cell activity against bacteria. The students were divided into groups of "good copers" and "poor copers" on the evaluation of their professors. Students who were judged to be "good copers" had natural killer cells that aggressively attacked bacteria. The natural killer cells from the "poor copers" showed much less activity.

CARDIOVASCULAR SYSTEM

Vascular

Every artery has a wall of muscle surrounding it. This muscle is able to constrict and squeeze the blood in it raising the blood pressure, or it can relax with a resulting drop in blood pressure. The muscle is controlled by the autonomic nervous system and is also sensitive to levels of norepinephrine which cause it to constrict. While there are pressure sensors in the arterial system which help regulate blood pressure to keep it within normal limits their function can be overridden with repeated elevations of blood pressure during stressful life events. Thus blood pressure is allowed to creep up. Over a period of time, the pressure is maintained at the new higher level and high blood pressure or **hypertension** is the result. Another hormone released during chronic stress, **aldosterone**, causes the body to retain more and more water resulting in an increased blood volume and thus contributing to a higher blood pressure.

Up and Down of Blood Pressure

Blood vessels may also constrict excessively in the extremities of the body. Cold hands and feet are the result. In general, the colder the hands and fingers the more stress response that is being expressed through this system. In severe cases, the blood and nutrient flow is squeezed off by arterial spasms so completely that tissue in the fingers or toes may begin to die. This condition is known as **Raynaud's Syndrome.** With **relaxation** and/or biofeedback training, persons can learn to increase the blood flow and thus warm their hands voluntarily.

Stress and Cholesterol

Studies have also shown that stress elevates the levels of fats in the blood stream. It is known that stress specifically increases the internal manufacture and release of cholesterol several times its normal rate. If these fats are used for "fight or flight" such a response has survival value. However when there is no "fight or flight," fat in the blood stream may contribute to atherosclerosis or hardening of the arteries.

Cardiac

It is a universal experience that stressful situations make the heart beat faster. Anger is an emotion that speeds the heart rate; as does love. Stress hormones secreted by the adrenals affect heart rate, and the automonic nerves directly influence the heart's rhythm. It is normal for the heart to speed up during stress in order to meet the body's need for increased blood flow to working muscles and organs. However, a heart under stress may continue to work at an elevated pace long after the stress is over. Persons who respond to stress with a pronounced increase in heart rate describe the feeling as a pounding or racing heart. The heart may also begin to beat with an abnormal rhythm during stress. A higher heart rate at rest is also a sign of chronic stress expressed through the sympathetic portion of the autonomic nervous system.

My Heart Beats Faster

To make matters worse the coronary arteries feeding the heart muscle may begin to constrict during stress and reduce blood flow to the heart muscle at a time when it needs more blood flow. This event is apparently the result of the involvement of higher brain centers through the sympathetic nervous system. If this process occurs repeatedly over the years, it may lead to the diffuse loss of heart tissue setting the stage for eventual cardiac failure. Heart tissue weakened by years of stress is also easily damaged by the stress induced release of norepinephrine. This outpouring of norepinephrine combined with a weakened heart may cause a fatal arrhythmia. Coronary constriction may also cause angina, pain in the heart region caused by a lack of oxygen to the heart. If the coronary constriction is severe, it also may cause an irreversible tissue death or fatal arrhythmia. The end result is called a heart attack, otherwise known as a myocardial infarction.

GASTROINTESTINAL SYSTEM

Mouth

My Mouth is Dry

From one end to the other, the gastrointestinal system responds to stress. In the mouth antibody count is reduced in saliva of persons under stress. This opens the door for infections such as **gingivitis**, and allows some viruses held in check by immune activity to become active again. The result may be cold sores and oral ulcers.

Stomach

The lining of the stomach is somewhat like facial skin on the inside of the body. If we are angry, blood vessels dilate in the face and it turns red; if we are afraid, blood drains from the face and it turns pale. Similar events happen in the stomach and it has a marked ability to change color with emotional state. When a person is angry, the cells of the stomach lining are engorged with blood. In this state they are fragile and easily ruptured, resulting in erosion of the lining; a first step in ulcer formation. The emotion of anger is also associated with an increased output of digestive enzymes and acid which can then attack a damaged lining.

Avenue of Stress

If the dominant emotion is fear or disgust, the linings of the stomach pale as blood is shifted away. The output of gastric secretions decrease as well as activity of the stomach musculature. In general, digestive activity in the stomach is markedly slowed and may even come to a stop resulting in delayed emptying of the contents into the small intestine and a prolonged uncomfortable full feeling.

Intestines

In the small intestine, events under stress mirror what happens in the stomach in terms of blood flow and color, but to a lesser degree. The major change is one of changes in motility (peristaltic activity). Motility may be increased or decreased in the small intestine. Thus, the transport of nutritive material in the small intestine may be accelerated or delayed. Also the release of digestive enzymes may be altered. Since the small intestine is the major site for the absorption of nutrients and digested food into the bloodstream, stress can interfere with its absorption. Nutrients not absorbed here can be fermented by the normal bacteria living in the large intestine resulting in intestinal distress.

The large intestine serves to absorb water from its contents and act as a temporary storage depot. Again, stress may interfere with normal motility of the bowel resulting in bouts of constipation or diarrhea due to decreased or increased motility, respectively. With an increase in bowel activity cramps, flatulence and lower abdominal discomfort are common occurrences.

MUSCLES

Our muscles do the work of meeting our needs and expectations. When we think of doing something, it is our musculature which will get the job done. The muscular system can anticipate action through the process of thinking about doing something. Muscles to be used in the task begin to tighten in preparation for actual movement. **Tension** developed in this manner will tend to be maintained until the task is completed.

Stop Tensing Your Muscles

Our thoughts and feelings feed into this process of muscular tightening during stress. If one thinks "Run!", "I need to escape!" or "I've got to get out of here!"; the brain interprets these thoughts as literal commands for action, and the muscles needed will tense in anticipation of being used. If the actual movement is not performed the muscular tension will remain elevated for a long time contributing to the muscular stress. Thus, the body remains "braced" for action with the mind hyper-alert. Remember much of the stress we experience is Type II or chronic stress which we cannot physically fight or flee.

When a muscle group remains braced for a long period of time discomfort or pain may develop in the area. Muscular discomfort may develop for several reasons. Muscle bracing can interfere with blood flow into and out of an area reducing the amount of oxygen and nutrients reaching a muscle and allowing toxic waste products of muscle metabolism to build in the tissues. Inflammation may begin to develop in the tendons of muscles that are held tense. The by-products of inflammation can cause more pain and prolong the inflammation response.

EPIDERMAL SYSTEM

The skin is the largest organ of the body and it responds to stress in several ways. Within the layers of the skin is an electrical current with special characteristics. This current increases and decreases with changes in a person's emotional state and thus reflects in the skin the emotional state of the person. It can be measured from the surface of the skin using sensitive equipment for the purposes of lie detection or to come to an understanding of one's emotional responses to various environmental stimuli.

Your Touch is Electric

Another way that the skin responds to stress is through its blood vessels. Changes in local blood flow and circulation in the skin are the basis of stress induced skin disorders. In the case of certain forms of exema emotional stress is expressed by an increase in blood flow to an area resulting in the skin becoming swollen, red, and itchy. Often scratching the itchy patch of skin causes further increases in blood flow and thus more itching. A viscious cycle develops where the more one scratches, the more the skin itches and the subsequent scratching causes more skin responses.

The extremities are more frequently afflicted, especially the hands. Since emotional activity initiated the response, quieting the emotions through relaxation often helps to reduce the frequency of attacks and diminish the severity of symptoms. See suggested readings for more information about stress pathways.

SOURCES OF STRESS

PSYCHOLOGICAL

Type A Behavior Pattern

Faster
Faster
Faster

Do you often feel like there is too much to do and not enough time to do it in? Do you hate to wait in lines? Do you find it intolerable to drive behind someone you think is driving too slow? Do your feel compelled to accomplish tasks faster and faster? Do you often try to accomplish more in less time by doing two or more things at once? Do you feel guilty when you are not actively working on a project? Do you find yourself unable to feel comfortable when relaxing? Do you feel that competition is a motivator for much of your interactions with other human beings? Do you always eat and walk rapidly? Do you become irritated or even hostile when people or events interfere with your plans?

If you answered yes to most of these questions you may exhibit **Type A behavior pattern.** Attention was drawn to this behavior pattern by two cardiologists, Ray Rosenman and Meyer Friedman. They studied the behavioral traits of many men and found that some were associated with higher rates of death and disease from coronary artery disease. These behaviors are listed in the following chart.

Type A Behaviors

1. **Polyphasic behavior** - thinking or doing two or more things at once.
2. **Hurry sickness** - the inability to slow down, compulsion to do things faster and faster.
3. **Hard driving behavior** - the incessant need to accomplish more and more in less and less time.
4. **Hypercompetitive nature** - the compulsion to compete in any type of human interaction.
5. **Quantitative attitude** - the need to convert and evaluate all activities and possessions in terms of numbers.
6. **Hostile responses** - a feeling of frustration which often breaks down into diffuse hostility when thwarted.

A series of research studies confirmed that higher rates of coronary disease exists in those with Type A behavior pattern. Comparisons of Type A's with easier going Type B's revealed that difference existed between the two groups in the way that they responded to challenges or threats in terms of their cardiovascular systems.

When the Type A's were under stress, their cardiovascular responses were exaggerated in comparison to the responses measured in the Type B's. For example, changes involving increases in blood pressure, increases in stress hormone output, increases in platelet "stickiness" (propensity to form a blood clot), reduced blood clotting time, increases in heart rate and blood cholesterol occurred to a much greater extent in the Type A's.

Type A vs. Type B

When these types of changes occur regularly, they put a great strain on the cardiovascular system and predispose the person to higher rates of cardiovascular disease and death. Research comparing the rates of coronary artery disease and heart attacks between Typ A's and Type B's generally report higher rates of disease and death for the Type A's on the order of 3 to 5 times higher. Type A's generally experience more anginal pain and Type A women experience higher rates of hypertension.

Once scientists came up with a way to measure and study Type A behavior pattern, research attempted to find out if Type A behavior pattern was the cause of the cardiovascular reactions and illness or a pattern of behavior associated with the disease but not the cause of it. While early research focused on the cardiovascular differences between A's and B's after those differences had developed, later research among 3,500 healthy A's and B's indicated that the personality and behavioral differences between A's and B's precede the development of cardiovascular disease.

4 Better or 4 Worse

It is important to understand that Type A behavior pattern is a learned style of responding to environmental challenges. Therefore, intervention programs can be developed and administered which will reduce the rates of death and disability related to Type A behavior pattern. A four and one half year study of heart patients showed that the number of heart attacks could be cut in half and the death rate drastically reduced when patients received counseling aimed at changing Type A behavior in comparison to a similar group that only received advice on diet, exercise and treatment. Patients also reported improvement on a number of psychological scores.

Type A: Learned so Un-Learn

Another study looked at the role of behavioral intervention among healthy Type A's and found that these persons reported significant improvement in the areas of self esteem, self confidence, tolerance and interpersonal communications. While Type A's ascribe much of their success in life to their behavior patterns many researcher and therapists believe they are successful in spite of it.

Important skills for the Type A's to master include a relaxation technique of their choice, time management, task delegation, interpersonal communication, ego divestment from work roles, assertiveness training (so they learn the difference between assertiveness and aggressiveness), and cognitive stress management.

Hardiness

Some persons seem to go through life's stress and are often ill. Others seem to stay healthy in spite of high levels of stress and life change. In fact, some persons seem to thrive on stress that would be debilitating to others. In the late 1970's, Dr. Suzanne Kobasa began studying people who stayed healthy under stress in order to find out if there was some common thread which ran through the fabric of their lives. She found the common thread and named it "**hardiness**."

Stress is Down My Alley

After comparing those who become ill under stress and those who remained healthy, Dr. Kobasa found social and personality factors that separated the two groups. People who remained healthy were found to have developed a net of **social support**. Those who became ill reported that they had no support network of friends, family, co-workers, or persons with common interests to provide support during stressful times.

Dr. Kobasa found that the "hardy" individuals in her studies differed from those who became ill on three crucial psychological variables. Hardy individuals felt that they had some ability to modify or change events in their life; they felt a sense of control. They often reported feeling stimulated by stress and change; a trait Kobasa termed challenge. Further the hardy group reported a strong sense of involvement in the events of their lives: a trait Kobasa termed **commitment**. The pattern Dr. Kobasa found is sometimes referred to as the Three C's Hypothesis. Those who became ill often felt powerless to affect a life event; they felt a lack of control. The unhardy group reported feeling threatened by change instead of being challenged by it. Instead of being intensely involved in their own affairs, those who became ill felt a sense of alienation.

Dr. Kobasa's Three C's Hypothesis

1. Control	2. Challenge	3. Commitment

Dr. Kobasa believed that "hardiness" can be learned and so she has instituted a training program termed hardiness induction for those who are susceptible. She reported that after several months of training, significant reductions in blood pressure have been measured in the participants. The important point here is that persons in high risk groups can learn coping skills that will reduce the deleterious effects of stress on their bodies and minds.

Training Consists of Three Important Aspects

1. Focusing	2. Situational reconstruction	3. Compensatory self-improvement.

SOCIAL

Major Life Change

What do getting married, getting divorced, experiencing the death of a relative or friend, moving your place of residence, getting a jail term, getting a promotion, or the addition of a new member to a family have in common? All of the experiences are examples of major life change.

Life change requires that we to adapt or cope with the change. Our attempts to cope require appraisal of current life change, prediction of the success of efforts to cope by various methods, the selection of a course of action, and finally putting our plans into action. Thus, each event is a possible source of social stress.

Go with the Flow

Early attempts to study the effect of life change on human health looked for the "experiments of nature" such as floods, fires, earthquakes, storms, and even wartime disasters. While the events brought their own damage through physical trauma and damage to property, days later people experienced stomach complaints and high blood pressure as they attempted to cope with the stressful changes and worried about what exactly the future might bring.

Researchers, Holmes and Rahe, developed a checklist to help measure the amount of life change a person was expose to. A list of 42 common life events was compiled and used to represent the amount of life change and coping required buy each life event. Scores were simply the number of items checked. Later investigators attempted to quantify the amount of change and coping required by the same life events. It seemed apparent that some life events require greater amounts of change than others; thus a traffic ticket, while stressful, requires much less coping than the addition of children to a family. A scale ranging from 100 to 11 points was developed with two arbitrary reference points of 100 LCU's (Life Change Units) for death of a spouse and 50 LCU's for marriage. The rest of the life events were assigned specific point values by a panel of judges using the reference points of death of a spouse and marriage as a guide (see Inventory #11 on page 237).

The new checklist became known as the **social readjustment rating scale (SRRS)**. When it is used as a stress and illness research instrument, the repeated finding is that those persons who report high scores on the SRRS for the preceding 12 months have a higher than normal incidence of illness during the next year. See Inventory #11 on page 237 for a student version of the SRRS. Fill out the scale for yourself by adding the total value for all events which happened to you over the past 12 months. If you scored 150 points or less, you have low social adjustment stress. If you scored 300 points or higher, you have experienced high social adjustment stress in the past 12 months. You chances of becoming ill in the immediate future are higher than normal.

Score High and Fail

It is important to note that a high score on the SRRS is associated with an increased risk of disease, it is only an increased risk and the percentage of people who subsequently become ill is small. The SRRS does not predict who will become ill but only the probability of becoming ill. The situation is much like the prediction of deaths from auto accidents during a holiday weekend by safety experts. The number of people who will die from auto accidents can be predicted fairly accurately, but not the names of the victims.

Daily Hassles and Uplifts

This Always Happens to Me?

Some psychologists and health researchers believe that small daily life events or hassles have as great or greater impact on a person's physiological and psychological health as major life events. They wonder if little things like the light that won't turn green, the shoe string that breaks, the elevator that doesn't come, the check-out line that doesn't end, or the car in the lane ahead who won't move over are just as stressful as chronic events like divorce. These events can act like the "straw that breaks the camel's back" and become the final irritant that unleashes the expression of strong negative emotions in a person who is already under a lot of chronic stress.

On the other hand, a thank-you note, a smile from a friend, finding some lost money in a pocket, getting a good grade on a well written report, or a pat on the back can provide a much needed boost and leave our spirits lifted.

Richard Lazarus is a psychologist who has studied hassles and uplifts says that the most frequent hassles for college students are loneliness, trying to meet excessively high standards, and wasting time. In dealing with hassles, the key is to make sure that you don't waste too much energy dealing with them and to arrange your environment so you can avoid them if they bother you excessively.

It is also important to try to increase the frequency of uplifts. For example, if you provide an uplift for someone, they are likely to provide one for you in return. Sharing compliments, smiles, thank you's and hugs with friends, family and co-workers will mean more for you.

ENVIRONMENTAL

Noise

Noise is defined as unwanted sound. Thus what is music to one can be noise to another. Noise may induce stress directly through its effects on the central nervous system or indirectly acting as an irritant interfering with ongoing tasks.

Sweet Sound of Music

When sound waves enter the ear they are converted to electrical impulses and sent through nerves to the hearing centers of the brain. On the way, they pass through an area of the brain known as the reticular activating system causing an increase in muscle tension and sympathetic activity. In turn there are increases in heart rate, blood pressure and alertness. With chronic exposure to noise, blood pressure may become elevated enough to cause hypertension.

When noise is excessive, it can cause hearing loss ranging from temporary impairment to permanent loss. Sound waves are really alternating waves of pressure in the air. These waves of alternating pressure are measured in units known as **decibels**. As a sound gets louder or more intense its decibel reading increases. The louder the sound is, the greater the pressure against the eardrum and the delicate structures of the inner ear. Excessive pressure can damage these structures. Even very small speakers like those in headphones can generate enough pressure to damage the ear since they are very near to or in the ear canal. While hearing decrements occur with age it is known that elderly persons who have lived in very quiet environments have maintained acute hearing into old age.

It is important from a stress management and health viewpoint to reduce exposure to noise by reducing noise as possible at its source and if that is not possible to reduce the amount of noise reaching the ears by using ear covers or soft foam ear plugs.

Nutrition

While we may not realize it, substances in some food items can trigger stress responses inside the body. **Caffeine** is one of those substances. Caffeine is found in many dietary items including colas, coffee, soft drinks, teas (not most herbals), and chocolate. Caffeine is also found in many over-the-counter (OTC) medications. The effects of caffeine mimic a stress reaction in the body.

Caffeine acts to stimulate the release of stress hormones and is a stimulant to the central nervous system. It speeds the heart rate and elevates the blood pressure. Caffeine acts on the muscular system to increase tension in muscles especially in the facial regions. The jaw and temporal muscles are especially vulnerable to this effect. In other words, even if psychological or social stress levels are low, too much caffeine in the diet will make you feel as if you are having a lot of stress in terms of your internal reactions.

It is also important to note that caffeine is a drug which causes withdrawal symptoms when it is removed from a person's diet - a sign of dependency. The most common withdrawal symptoms reported are headache and fatigue. Amounts of caffeine in various products can be found in Table 11.1.

Amount of Caffeine in Various Products

Product	Caffeine in milligrams
Coffee, drip (5 oz.)	115
Coffee, perked (5 oz.)	80
Coffee, instant (5 oz.)	65
Coffee, decaffeinated (5 oz.)	3
Tea, brewed (5 oz.)	40
Tea, instant (5 oz.)	30
Tea, iced (12 oz.)	70
Colas (12 oz.)	45-30
Citrus sodas (12 oz.)	54-52
Dr. Pepper/Mr. Pibb (12 oz.)	59-40
No Doz	100
Vivarin	200
Anacin	32
Excedrin	65
Midol	32
Vanquish	32
Coryban-D	30
Triaminacin	30
Aqua-Ban	100
Maximum-Strength Aqua-Ban Plus	200

Table 11.1. Source: Ray, O. and Ksir, C., 1990, *Drugs, Society and Human Behavior*, Times Mirror/Mosby, St. Louis.

Another nutritional concern related to stress is the increasing intake of simple sugars and syrups in the American diet. While the percentage of simple sugars and syrups (which are increasingly used by food manufacturers) has increased, the percentage intake of complex carbohydrates has dropped dramatically.

Most whole sources of complex carbohydrates contain many of the vitamins and trace mineral needed by the body to turn the stored energy in food in to energy in your body; simple sugars and syrups do not. When your diet is high in simple sugars, the vitamins needed must be taken from other food sources as they are not able to be stored by the body. This may set the stage for a deficiency in the water soluble B vitamins.

The deficiencies in these vitamins appear similar to the symptoms of a stress reaction and situations of high stress raise the body's nutritional requirements. In addition the adrenal cortex, one site of stress hormone manufacture, is normally rich in vitamin C but chronic stress depletes the cortex of it vitamin C reserves.

1990 Dietary Goals for Americans

1. Eat a variety of foods.

Vegetables	3-5 servings
Fruits	2-4 servings
Breads, Cereals, Rice, Pasta ..	6-11 servings
Milk, Yogurt, Cheese	2-3 servings
Meats, Poultry, Fish, Dry Beans & Peas, Eggs, Nuts	2-3 servings

2. Maintain a healthy weight.
3. Choose a diet low in fat, saturated fat, and cholesterol.
4. Choose a diet with plenty of vegetables, fruits and grain products.
5. Use sugars only in moderation.
6. Use salt and sodium only in moderation.
7. If you drink alcoholic beverages do so only in moderation. (One drink a day for women and 2 drinks a day for men).

Table 11.2

Some persons reading this may be immediately tempted to go out and buy a "stress formula" vitamin supplement. Such a move is usually not necessary or recommended. Nutritionists instead recommend to eat a variety of whole foods including lots of fruits, vegetables, and whole grain products. Remember to reduce your consumption of fats to less than 30% of your daily caloric intake. Try to eat foods that are whole and close to their natural state, for example, a baked potato instead of fried potatoes or potato chips, or an apple rather than apple juice. This strategy will usually help you meet your dietary needs. If you are unsure if your diet meets all of your dietary needs, consult with a nutritionist. Check the dietary goals listed in Table 11.2 and complete Inventory #12 on page 239.

TECHNIQUES FOR REDUCING STRESS

RELAXATION

Practice Makes Perfect

Relaxation is one of the most powerful techniques available to provide protection from the harmful effects of uncontrolled stress. The term relaxation is defined as a reduction in tension, in this case muscle tension. Thus, when a person is truly relaxed the muscles will show a very low level of tension. Research into relaxation indicates that there is a naturally occurring phenomenon known as the "relaxation response." When the "relaxation response" occurs there are a series of changes which happen in the body, all of which are the exact opposite of the stress reaction. These changes alter the activity of the brain, endocrine, cardiovascular, gastrointestinal, and muscular systems in order to restore equilibrium after a profoundly stressful situation. Research demonstrates that persons who regularly elicit the relaxation response experience an internal stress reaction of much shorter duration when compared to normal. This means that the negative effects of repeated stressors will be much less likely to accumulate in the person who practices a relaxation technique regularly. The relaxation response can be triggered by a variety of relaxation and self regulation techniques, such as progressive relaxation, autogenic traning, biofeedback training and visualation.

Progressive Relaxation

Progressive relaxation, also known as neuromuscular relaxation, was developed nearly 60 years ago in the United States by a physician, Dr. Edmund Jacobson. Dr. Jacobson recognized the ability of muscle to tense in anticipation of movement, i.e. that if you think about moving a muscle or flexing a joint that muscle will tense up. Also Dr. Jacobson discovered the connection between muscle tension and emotions. He reported from studies on patients that it was impossible to be totally relaxed and anxious at the same time, i.e. the two conditions were incompatible states. He developed a relaxation technique based on a developed ability to perceive and release muscle tension.

One tenses and relaxes muscle groups progressing from one muscle group to the next while maintaining attention on the muscle group under training. When one tenses the muscle a **tension signal** is generated which is brought to awareness. As the person relaxes the muscle group, the tension signal leaves and awareness is focused on the feelings of tension reduction in the area. This is the feeling of relaxation. As skill is developed in the technique, one can recognize a tension signal with increasingly smaller levels of muscular contraction. Finally all attention is focused on the release of any tension in the body. One simply allows all of the tension to leave the body by passively focusing on specific muscle groups and letting go of any tension there.

Focusing on Relaxation

Persons who have developed skill in progressive muscle relaxation also find that they are more aware of tension in everyday activities of work and play. One is aware of tension at lower levels and can release it before it builds up to levels which might cause pain or dysfunction.

Six Specific Phrases (formula) Used in the Traditional Clinical Practice of Autogenics

1. My arms and legs are heavy.
2. My arms and legs are warm.
3. My heartbeat is calm and regular.
4. My breathing is calm and easy.
5. My solar plexus is warm.
6. My forehead is cool.

Autogenic Training

This anti-stress self regulation technique has its beginning in auto or self hypnosis. **Autogenic training** (self generated) grew out of the clinical hypnosis experience of Dr. Johannes Schultz of Germany in the 1930's. Dr. Schultz found that his patients developed profound sensory and physiological changes as they entered the hypnotic state. He thought that if he could teach his patients to enter a self induced hypnotic state and experience these changes it would have a beneficial effect on their health. The procedure he developed has the person repeat specific phrases with "passive concentration" on the body part that they are attempting to influence.

In the clinical training of patients, each phrase is worked on individually and in order until the patient can readily produce the desired feelings of heaviness, warmth, etc. then the next phrase is attempted and so on.

When the patient is able to relax and produce all of the desired feeling states, advanced meditative and visualization exercises may be prescribed which follow a regular sequence and provide an avenue for the patient to shed the residue of past traumatic events and get insight about one's personality valuable for continued psychological growth and health. The latter stages of training must be done under the guidance of a qualified therapist.

Calm and in Control

When autogenic training is used for stress management, usually only the first two phrases or formulae are used. A person who is "stressed out" but have not yet developed any stress related disorder, the regular practice of the first two phrases of autogenic training balances the effects of stress and allows one to feel calm and "in control." The feelings of heaviness and warmth are correlated with decreases in muscle tension and increases in skin temperature, a good indication that the person is relaxing. Usually feelings of warmth and heaviness will generalize or spread to all parts of the body.

Biofeedback Training

Long ago yoga adepts found that as they practiced their discipline, marked physiological and psychological changes occurred in their bodies. They experienced that for every psychological state there is a corresponding change in the physical activity of the body. Much later during some brain wave research, Dr. Joe Kamiya had student research subjects guess if their brains were showing alpha or beta brain waves. He found that if he gave them feedback about the correctness of their guesses their accuracy rapidly improved as they developed an awareness of their brain wave state. Further research by Kamiya showed that some of his students could alter their brain waves at will and produce either pattern upon demand after developing brain wave awareness.

Alpha or Beta Waves

Whether the beginnings of **biofeedback training** stem from ancient yoga or recent electronics, self awareness is one of the keys to successful biofeedback training. Biofeedback training uses electronic equipment to sense, amplify, and display or feedback faint biological signals from a person's body. A person can use this information to develop an awareness of their body activity being monitored, the first step toward self control.

As bodily activity awareness develops, one can begin to sense internally how the body's activity is changing and in what direction. Information from the biofeedback machine provides instantaneous moment by moment feedback about the accuracy of one's internal sensations. Soon one is able to connect changes in body activity with changes in thoughts and emotional feelings. This is an important step because the connection between thoughts and feelings and bodily activity is a two way street. The biofeedback trainee learns that by changing thoughts and feelings there is a resulting change in bodily activity. Through continuing practice this mind/body pathway becomes strengthened and the learned control becomes stronger. The desired bodily response becomes more automatic.

Time to Warm-Up

Biofeedback training is terminated when the person is able to produce the desired response with access to feedback from the biofeedback machine while they are being monitored by the machine. Usually a goal is set at the beginning of training and when the person has achieved this goal then training is discontinued. Goals are set in terms of criterion behaviors such as being able to raise the temperature of the finger of a hand to 95 degrees fahrenheit or to be able to show a 1 degree increase in skin temperature per minute. A common goal for facial muscle tension is to be able to relax the muscles of the face to 1 microvolt (millionth of a volt) of muscle activity. Once a person learns the skills needed to warm their hands or relax their muscles they no longer need the biofeedback equipment as the skill is theirs to practice.

Biofeedback Units Come in Three Grades or Levels of Complexity and Sophistication

1. **Home training units.** These are small compact relatively inexpensive units which are fairly rugged. While they are not as accurate or sensitive as the more advanced units they can provide enough information about what's going on inside the body to be useful for home practice away from the clinic or lab. These units range in price from $30.00 to $300.

2. **Clinical trainers.** These units are more sensitive and can provide a wider variety of tones, lights and meter readings. These units range in price from $300.00 to $1,000.00.

3. **Research quality.** These units are very sensitive and pricey! They feature computerized feedback displays provide an astounding variety of feedback forms. If you think you might benefit from biofeedback training, consult your local university or college health education, psychology, or education programs to find available biofeedback training on your campus.

The types of biofeedback machine that are in most common use are the thermal units which measure skin temperature, EMG (electromyograph) units which measure muscle tension, EDR (electrodermal) units which measure activity in the sweat glands on the palms of the hands, and EEG (electroencephalograph) units which measure surface brain electrical activity.

Visualization

Visualization is a self regulation technique based upon the concept that sensing what you want to happen will allow those responses in your body to occur by association or previous experience. Think back to a recent happy experience in your life. For a little while sit back and allow yourself to re-experience that time. Involve all you your senses, things you saw, sounds you heard, smells in the air, feelings you experienced. Make the experience as vivid as possible; try to really get into it. Do this little experiment now, then resume reading.

What happened during your experiment? As you remembered the experience were you able to vividly sense it as you did when it happened? Do you feel somehow different now in your feelings or thoughts? Did some of that happy feeling from the past linger on affecting your current mood and experience? An important thing to remember is that pleasant memories can influence our moods as well as unpleasant ones.

Sweet Smell of Success

What you have experienced is the basis of visualization. Besides using material based on memories, scripted material in the form of text, audio tapes, video tapes, spoken words might also be used.

COGNITIVE METHODS

Cognitive methods of stress management reduce a person's stress by examining and altering the ways in which a person appraises or evaluates stressful life events. Its a way of checking out if the ways in which one evaluates and responds to life events is appropriate, useful and healthy. Its been described as "getting a check up from the neck up."

While there are many cognitive techniques there are some methods which are easy and effective to put into practice in everyday life.

Scale

10	Worst Possible Experience
9	
8	
7	
6	
5	
4	
3	
2	
1	Very Contented

1 to 10 Scale

One of the simplest is to apply a 1 to 10 scale to the stressful life event which has happened. One represents a high level of contentment and satisfaction with life. Ten represents the worst possible event which has happened in your lifetime.

Now rate your current problem on this scale. Is it as bad as you first appraisal? Can you cope with it? What options do you have available now to deal with the situation?

Wants versus Needs

Another method involves becoming aware of wants and needs in our lives and making sure we don't confuse the two. When wants are confused for needs and they are not attained a person feels as if they are in a mortal conflict. Imagine you haven't had any water for several days. You would be very thirsty, dehydrated, and seriously close to death! That is a need. You need water in order to survive. People die when their basic survival needs aren't met.

Now imagine that your sweetheart tells you they need some space and want to cool off the relationship. Does it feel like your going to die? Do you need that person and that relationship? Or did you want the relationship to work out and it didn't? Did you want the person to want you as much as you wanted them? That is a want. Another way to look at the situation is to substitute the word prefer, as in "I would prefer that we were still together, and that is not possible now." Ken Keyes suggests that when a person expresses a preference for something the emotional tie to it is lost and that person is free to preference something else.

Time Projection

The time projection method asks us to examine our stressful life event from a vantage point in the future - maybe a month, 6 months, or several years from now. Ask yourself how important will this event be in a month or 6 months or 2 years from now. The answer is usually that the life events that seems so worrisome right now will seem a lot less stressful when seen from the vantage point of a later date.

Two Rules for Stress Management

1. Don't sweat the small stuff.
2. It's all small stuff.

"When you can't fight and you can't flee - FLOW."

From Cardiologist, Robert Eliot, Author of *Is It Worth Dying For?*

Self Talk

Author Mark Twain once said "I'm an old man and have known a great many troubles, but most of them never happened." He was referring to the fact that most of us can create a lot of stress in our minds worrying about events that have yet to occur. Examine thoughts you have (self talk) about anticipated life events and see if they help you plan or only serve to increase anxiety, worry, and stress arousal. If your self talk is productive, good. If not, use the subverbal command STOP (thought stopping). It may be necessary for you also to stop what you are doing and remove yourself from the environment associated with the negative self talk. Do not allow the negative self talk to continue. Why continue with negative self talk when you might hold other thoughts in your mind?

Just Say Stop

Affirmations

Affirmations are positive statements that people use to create a new point of view or to change an attitude. Affirmations are repeated several times daily and are a powerful form of self talk. Examples might be "I choose to relax daily", "I love and accept myself just as I am", "I love and accept _____ (person's name) just as they are", or "I care for myself with regular exercise." Affirmations are written as if the behavior has already occurred and in the present tense. The book *Creative Visualization* by S. Gawain is a good starting point for those not familiar with affirmations. (See suggested readings.)

Think Positive

JOURNALING

Keeping a **journal** is an excellent way to diffuse some of the unwanted stress. A journal is a series of regular notes that you write to yourself. Putting your thoughts and feelings about the events in your life in a journal or diary can help you cope in a number of ways.

Benefits of Journaling

1. It provides a healthy release for feelings which might come out in a harmful way otherwise.
2. It allows you to become aware of specific stressors in your life. You may decide to eliminate certain events or modify aspects of your life so as to avoid unnecessary stressors.
3. It provides a record of your thoughts and feelings that is very important for self understanding and self growth. Students who keep journals often remark that while they get immediate relief from stressful feelings by journaling, important self growth comes from reading the entries that they wrote months ago in order so see who they were and find out who they are becoming.
4. It provides insight into how you interact with your immediate life environment.
5. It allows you to become aware of the truly important things in your life so you can prioritize commitments and eliminate truly unimportant ones.
6. It provides an important boost to your immune system. Studies with university students showed that those whose entries related to their feelings about stressful life events showed a long lasting (up to 6 weeks) improvement in immune function and visited their doctor's office less often. Students who did not write about their feelings did not receive these benefits.

Healer Bernie Seigel, M.D. author of the book *Love, Medicine, & Miracles*, mentioned that once when he re-read his journal he became aware that something was missing. He had only written about his negative feelings and had left out all of the positive joyous events and feelings that he had experienced. He related that this realization was an important lesson for him and that the validation of positive feelings was every bit as important for self growth as the validation of negative feelings.

HUMOR

Everyone has experienced the pleasant uplifted mood that lingers on after a good laugh. Who hasn't said "What I need now is a good laugh!"? After some humor our problems seem less overwhelming and our step is a little lighter. There are numerous clinical reports about the healing power of laughter and its health enhancing benefits. Probably the most widely known story relating to laughter and healing concerns author Norman Cousins.

Cousins was diagnosed with a terminal arthritic spine disease, ankylosing spondylitis. He was "given" a 1 in 500 chance of recovery from his ailment. He chose to take that one chance and cured himself through a process which involved regular doses of humor. Because of pain he was unable to sleep but he found that 10 minutes of belly laughter produced 2 hours of uninterrupted sleep. He used reruns of Candid Camera and old Marx Brothers movies in order to accomplish his funny business.

Laugh and the World Laughs with You

We know that some of the internal effects of laughter include the release of endorphins, whose effects include potent pain relief and mood elevation. Other reports indicate that positive emotions such as laughter stimulate portions of the immune system. Cousin later remarked that a good bout of belly laughing is similar to the effects of mild exercise; a process he termed "internal jogging".

Some therapists include the use of humor as a first rate coping mechanism used by mature healthy happy people. Some hospital and nursing homes now regularly prescribe a dose of humor for their patients. They set out special humorous materials, books, magazines, cartoons and movies. Some even provide stand up comedians for their group!

Humor Helps

1. Taking some time for yourself to read a book of humor.
2. Go see a funny movie or rent a funny video.
3. Ask your friend to tell you new jokes they have heard and share your new ones with them.
4. Find some humor in everyday life.

EXERCISE

If your mind is stressed out and your body is filled with stress hormones and tension, you need the "fight or flight" fix - exercise. Since stress gets your body ready to fight or flee, some exercise is just what the body needs in order to get back to normal.

Any kind of movement is helpful when you are experiencing unwanted stress. Exercise reduces tension in the muscles and helps to reduce stress hormones and fats released into the blood stream from the stress response during rest. After exercise is over a relaxation response occurs which slows the heart rate, reduces blood pressure and in general gets the body back to normal, but when feeling stressed follow this chart.

When Feeling Stressed

1. Go for a walk.
2. Play a game of frisbee or racquetball.
3. Climb some stairs.
4. Go to the gym for a workout.
5. Ride a bike.
6. Go out dancing.
7. Go for a jog.

If you exercise on a regular basis rather than just when you feel stress you will strengthen every system of your body. You will find that there is less of you (fat tissue) to be carried around and more of you (lean tissue) to do the carrying. You will find that you have more energy to get through the day in part because more energy is being stored and muscles are stronger and more efficient.

Change Your Mood: Exercise

Regular exercise is also associated with mood elevation and has been used in part or whole as a treatment for depression. In fact, in a prospective study of thousands of women initially mentally healthy who were followed up for several years, the best predictor of which women became depressed at the end of the study was a lack of exercise. Because of the internal chemical changes induced by regular exercise you will feel better in terms of mood.

The Exact Mechanisms are Not Known, but at Least Three Have Been Implicated

1. An increase in endorphin levels.
2. An increase in brain catecholamines.
3. Diversion of thoughts from problems and concerns.

The sense of health, vitality, and well being reported by those who exercise regularly has been an inspiration for many to begin exercise programs.

Making your exercise fun is important. Do something that you like to do. If you make you exercise competitive in nature (against someone else or yourself) or use your exercise program to build your ego, your program will begin to generate stress and it will lose its effectiveness. Keep your exercise program noncompetitive and ego void.

Remember to follow the guidelines for a healthy exercise program given in Chapter 5 of this book. If you are over 40 and have been sedentary for some time, seek the evaluation of a physician before beginning an exercise program (see Inventory #13 on page 241).

MUSIC

An Easy Pill to Swallow

It is said that "Music hath charms to soothe the savage beast." Many of us have discovered that listening to quiet flowing music when we are frazzled or stressed-out, quiets and calms our bodies and minds. A favorite piece of music can provide a sense of continuity and connection in our lives when life events seem to be changing too fast or disjointed. Baroque music is said to be particularly calming and is reported to facilitate concentration and retention of material.

One hospital did a study on persons undergoing cardiac catheterization procedure and found that music reduced stress, pain, and anxiety during the traumatic procedure. The study also found that different types of music worked better for different ages of persons. As you might have guessed teens responded well to rock music.

Listen to music with a faster beat can energize a person and get us "up" for the tasks we have to accomplish. It provides a rhythm to help one accomplish physical work and a distraction to discomforts associated with exertion and daily problems. Through the experience of music we can elevate our mood or calm ourselves down. We need only to listen.

SUMMARY

We experience stress responses as a natural consequence of a built-in "fight or flight" survival mechanism. In modern society however the ability to alleviate our stress by physical means has been removed by changes in culture. The resulting chronic stress arousal has alter body function and is implicated in numerous disease states. Certain social and personality factors combine to increase stress arousal and resulting disease.

When it is desirable, stressful life events may be altered or avoided. When it is not possible to control stressful life events, one can modify excessive stress arousal through the use of exercise, relaxation and cognitive techniques.

It is Important To Remember Two Truths About Stress Management

1. If one cannot control the events of one's life, one can control one's reactions both internal and external.
2. "Knowing and not doing is the same as not knowing" (Chinese fortune cookie proverb).

Suggested Readings

Asterita, M.F. *The Physiology of Stress*. New York: Human Sciences Press, Inc., 1985.

Eliot, R. and D. Breo. *Is It Worth Dying For?*. New York: Bantam Books, 1984

Freidman, M. and H. R. Rosenman. *Type A Behavior and Your Heart*. New York; Knopf, 1974.

Ganong, W. F. *Review of Medical Physiology*. Norwalk: Appleton & Lange, 1989.

Gawain, S. *Creative Visualization*. New York: Bantam Books, 1985.

Gawain, S. *Living in the Light*. SanRafael, CA.: Whatever Publishing, Inc., 1986.

Girdano, D. A., G. S. Everly, and D. E. Dusek. *Controlling Stress and Tension: A Holistic Approach*. Englewood Cliffs, NJ: Prentice Hall, 1990.

Keyes, K. *a conscious person's guide to relationships*. St. Mary, KY.: Living Love Publications, 1979.

LeShan, L. *How to Meditate*. New York: Bantam Books, 1980.

Locke, S. and D. Colligan. *The Healer Within*. New York: Mentor, 1987.

Mason, J. L. *Guide to Stress Reduction*. Berkley, CA.: Celestial Arts, 1985.

Millman, D. *Way of the Peaceful Warrior*. Tiburon, CA.: H J Kramer, Inc., 1984.

Pelletier, K. *Mind as Healer, Mind as Slayer*. New York: Delta, 1977.

Rice, P. L. *Stress and Health*. Monterey, CA.: Brooks/Cole, 1987.

Seigel, B. S. *Love, Medicine & Miracles*. New York: Harper & Row Pub, 1986.

Selye, H. *Stress Without Distress*. Philadelphia: Lippincott, 1974.

Williams, R. *The Trusting Heart*. New York: Random House, 1989.

CHAPTER 12

EXERCISE, MOTIVATION AND ADHERENCE

Steve Houseworth

Learning Objectives

- Understand the role of exercise in people's lives.
- Understand reasons people engage in and withdraw from exercise.
- Comprehend the effect of expectancy and outcomes/results upon motivation to maintain exercise.
- Understand perceptual and environmental barriers to initiating and maintaining exercise.
- Define and understand motivation.
- Understand the effect of self-efficacy and self-esteem upon motivation.
- Understand the role of locus of control upon motivation and exercise behavior.
- Understand the influence and value of social support upon exercise motivation and maintenance.
- Understand the nature of and factors which contribute to exercise addiction.
- Understanding possible methods for working with exercise addiction.

Important Terms

belief systems
cognitive dissonance
environmental barriers
exercise addiction
exercise motivation
expectancies
locus of control
motivation
perceived need
perceptual barriers
pleasure principle
relative outcome
self-efficacy
self-esteem
social facilitation

IMPORTANCE OF MOTIVATION TO EXERCISE

NATURE OF MOTIVATION

The purpose of this chapter is to present an understanding of how motivation operates, specifically within a framework of exercise/health behavior.

Motivation is a term that can be used in many contexts to refer to many seemingly disparate items. The motive for someone to embezzle money is quite different from the motive for someone to purchase a particular car. Also, building up the necessary motivation to confront someone on an issue is quite different from the motivation to try learning a new skill.

Actually, this tremendous versatility of application comes from the fact that motivation is a basic psychological construct which is an essential ingredient of human behavior. In simple terms **motivation** is "anything that impels a person to action." Defined in this way, motivation can develop from desiring rewards, avoiding punishments, needs for social affiliation, and sating physiological drives.

For our purposes motivation will be considered as a cognitive construct. That is, something people evaluate, consider and determine. This is opposed to a more mechanistic or biological approach. **Exercise motivation** is the specific name ascribed to the need, desire, importance and actual participation in exercise and/or health related behaviors. Exercise motivation assumes that people perceive a reason for exercise and evaluate the importance of exercise, probably from many different perspectives.

Some Exercise Motivation Perspectives

1. Physical attractiveness
2. Physical effort of working and sweating
3. Developing physical attributes such as strength, endurance and flexibility
4. Overall health and wellness
5. Disease prevention.

RELATIONSHIP OF EXERCISE MOTIVATION TO EXERCISE/HEALTH BEHAVIOR

We know that exercise attrition rates are quite high, which means that this cognitive process of evaluating the importance of exercise is both increased and decreased by the influence of other factors. Real life constraints are quite different from the theoretical propositions found in textbooks. The reality is that motivation to exercise becomes entangled with factors such as getting the kids off to school, constraints of a demanding job, feelings of achieving desired results, and enjoyment of an exercise activity.

So, the relationship of exercise motivation to exercise/health activities is: people will exercise and exhibit health behaviors to the degree they are motivated, and this involves both internal and external factors.

Get Motivated

Another important point is that motivation is dynamic, not static. Someone can be quite motivated to exercise after the kids are off to school, but not as motivated if tempted with a conflict of going out to breakfast with a friend. This holds true for remaining on a diet or for exercising five days a week (maybe only two this week, I'm a little sore). Ultimately, exercise motivation is something which must become part of a life-style; something which is an inherent part of one's value system. As part of one's value system exercise motivation can then be as flexible and diverse in directing and accounting for behavior as is general motivation (Figure 12.1).

Circular Effect of Self-Esteem, Self-Efficacy and Locus of Control

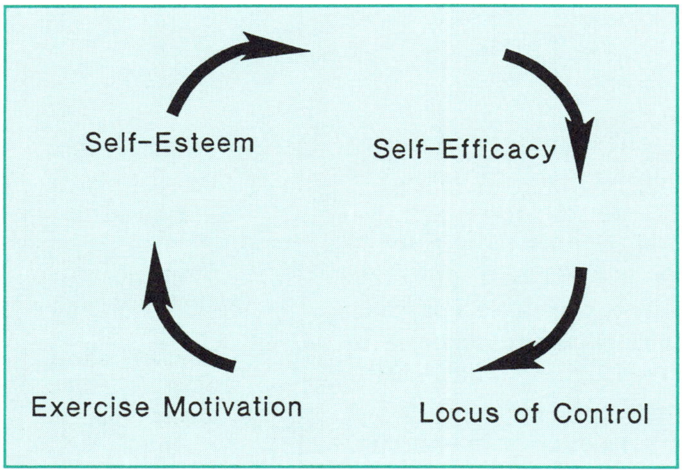

Figure 12.1.

WHY PEOPLE INITIATE EXERCISE

FUNCTIONAL REASONS

People exercise for a combination of functional reasons. That is we all have the ability and the drive to exercise and these functional reasons are an important determinant of exercise motivation.

Some Functional Factors

1. Human nature
2. Perceived needs
3. Belief systems or knowledge base
4. Conscious determination or will

Although this section is devoted to initiating exercise behavior, these same factors can also contribute to a lack of or attrition from exercise.

Investigating the Influence of Functional Factors for Initiating Exercise Will Provide

1. Insight for motivational strategies
2. Techniques for helping people maintain exercise

Your Beliefs: Fact or Fiction

Exercise is a part of human nature. Just watch children at play, adults in recreation programs or out for a walk. Exercise is enjoyable, soothing, stimulating. It satifies physical, emotional, and psychological needs. However, people also learn to modify many behaviors, including exercise behavior. Both under exercise and over exercise are extreme forms of modified behavior which are not completely natural or healthy. For example, while some people are unhealthy because they underexercise, others are unhealthy because they overexercise.

The ability for people to modify behavior leads to exercise motivation due to a **perceived need**. While Sumo wrestlers perceive the need to gain weight for their performance, housewives may perceive the need to lose weight and have the endurance to complete a hectic day. The key is one's perception, which can either match reality or conform to fantasy. An anorexic perceives the need to lose more weight which is not reality but is a fantasy belief which is acted upon (conformed) due to the perceived need.

Belief systems aid people in initiating behavior because of one's knowledge base or how much they know and the accuracy of their information. However, just as perceived needs may not match reality, beliefs can be based more upon myths than on accurate knowledge. Consider the myth of spot reducing exercises. Performing leg-lifts to lose weight from the thighs certainly is not effective nor based upon accurate knowledge, but is believed by many people. So, learning specific information can be a motivational factor. Evidence linking consistent exercise with longevity is an example of knowledge which can instill an exercise ethic or belief system such as: "Exercise can help me live healthier, longer."

Each of these functional explanations are sufficient but not necessary to explain why people initiate exercise.

Understanding and recognizing these sufficient and necessary components can provide a common thread, an integrity for understanding exercise initiation, maintenance and attrition.

The Necessary Component is a Conscious Decision, a Focus and Determination, a Will to Act Upon...

1. an innate exercise drive
2. a perceived need to exercise
3. a belief system leading to exercise.

ROLE OF EXPECTANCY

For whatever combination of functional reasons people initiate exercise we, as humans, expect results. Hopefully, results from exercise will match our beliefs or knowledge base. For example, an overweight executive begins an aerobic exercise program expecting to lose fat, gain muscle, look and feel better. In short, people often expect exercise to help build their bodies in more ways than oat bran, vitamin enriched, whole wheat bread. Thus, a slight variation from our belief/knowledge base is our **expectancies.**

Examine Your Reason For Exercising

Expectations will depend upon the reasons people have for exercise. Specifically, if you expect to lose body fat percent, you expect to see less fat in the future. If you expect not to be so tired after a day of work, you expect to have more energy at the end of the day and not have sore muscles. This point may seem evident but is extremely important for understanding why people initiate and maintain exercise.

MAINTAINING EXERCISE PROGRAMS

EXPECTANCIES VERSUS OUTCOMES

Ideally, outcomes will match expectancies which strengthens desire or will, what we recognize as motivation. However, when outcomes do not match expectancies, a psychological dilemma exists and something has to give. Either belief systems change and/or knowledge bases are modified. That is, people learn from and adapt their perspective based upon their experiences. Positive experiences in which outcomes match or exceed expectancies can result in: "I'm feeling better than I thought I would. I can maintain this program!" However, negative experiences in which outcomes do not match expectancies can result in: "This is more work than I ever expected and I have an extra set of exercise clothes to wash as well!"

Such psychological dilemmas are termed **cognitive dissonance** because what people hold as true is not coming true. For example, someone begins cycling to lose weight. Appetite increases due to exercise and this person doesn't lose weight for a month. The cognitive dissonance between expectations (exercise loses weight) and reality (caloric balance) can reduce this person's motivation to maintain exercise. However, if they have gained the knowledge from someone like you, that weight loss is gradual and their appetite might increase for a few weeks, they could maintain their motivation. Consequently, the more outcomes match expectancies, the stronger the link between desire/motivation and actual behavior. That is people will persist or maintain their exercising.

BARRIERS TO MAINTAINING EXERCISE PROGRAMS

Outcomes Need to Match Expectations

Barriers are factors which interfere, impede, deter and prevent action or behavior. Generally we can group barriers into two classes: Environmental and Perceptual.

Environment

Physical factors which are outside of oneself are **environmental barriers**. Examples include: cold or hot weather, job constraints, family constraints, location, convenience and time.

These environmental barriers can overlap or have a cumulative effect. For example, a parent has a demanding job. Weekends are the time to relax and for kids to have their sport games. The health club or available gym is across town and parents do not have the time to travel that distance. These are reasons why home exercise equipment has sold quite well in recent years. People can exercise at home and at their convenience.

Perceptual

While environmental barriers are real constraints, **perceptual barriers** are inconsistencies between the acutal situation and one's interpretation/perception of the situation.

Perceptual Barrier Examples Would Include Differences Between

1. Expectancy and outcome
2. Relative outcome - how much of a benefit is enough to be worth the effort
3. Perceived value of self

Similar to environmental barriers, perceptual barriers can overlap or have cumulative effects. Consider a family with both husband and wife working and with kids to take to school. The husband may perceive that getting up at 6:00 a.m. to exercise for 30 minutes will be too tough and probably not worth the effort. The wife may feel too tired after work to exercise.

Expectancy and outcome have been discussed already; however, a question each person must decide is if the benefits are worth the costs. In other words, is what I get (outcomes) really worth the cost? This is **relative outcome.**

Relative Outcome Can Be Evaluated on Several Levels

1. What is it worth for the type of exercise?
2. What is it worth for the effort, pain, exertion?
3. What is it worth for the social stimulation?
4. What is it worth for the time investment?

Evaluated positively, exercise can be maintained and evaluated negatively, exercise can be reduced or ceased. Consequently, a key component of exercise motivation is establishing specific, meaningful and attainable goals. Goals which exceed time constraints, effort/exertion or desire simply reduce motivation and exercise adherence (Table 12.1).

Effect of Goal Types Upon Motivation Level

Goal Type	Motivation
Specific Reasonable Desirable Challenging	Increase motivation
Unrealistic Time constraints Too difficult Too easy	Decrease motivation

Table 12.1

Perceived Value of Self

If people begin exercise programs to improve themselves in some ways, an underlying feature is that people - everyone - have certain beliefs or perceptions about their worth or status. This is **self-esteem.** How each person regards him/herself can also greatly influence exercise adherence. So, if self-esteem is enhanced the prospects of maintaining exercise are improved, while prospects of attrition could increase if self-esteem is not maintained or enhanced (Table 12.2).

Effect of Self-Esteem Upon Motivation

Self-Esteem	Motivation
High Self-Esteem	Higher Motivation
Low Self-Esteem	Lower Motivation

Table 12.2

From the perspective of most physical/health practitioners, the link between exercise and positive self-esteem seems quite logical, while the link between exercise and decreases in self-esteem may not seem so logical. After all, why would a person not feel better about his/herself if exercise helps build strong bodies more ways than oat bran, vitamin enriched bread? The answer lies in factors which influence self-esteem. **Self-efficacy** and **locus of control** are two such factors as shown in Figure 12.1 on page 186.

Self-efficacy refers to one's feelings of accomplishment or degree to which one can perform. While improvements in fitness usually develop improvements in self-efficacy, feelings of accomplishment can be dampened if goals/expectations are not satisfied. If a novice exerciser cannot complete an entire 15 minute aerobic session, feels like a klutz, or has no short term goals which indicate progress toward long-terms goals, then self-efficacy and subsequent motivation to continue exercise will diminish.

Locus of control refers to feelings of being in charge and control, direction of an activity. Examples would be (a) relying too much on direction and support from an exercise director and (b) depending upon friends for transportation to the aerobic studio. Inclement weather, going away for vacation, or other temporary interferences could easily be sufficient excuses

Example of a Strong Locus of Control

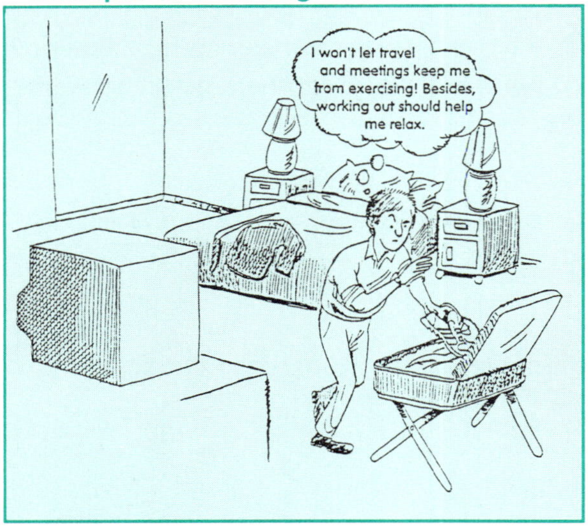
I won't let travel and meetings keep me from exercising! Besides, working out should help me relax.

Figure 12.2.

to cause attrition. However, someone who takes charge of their exercise & does not let situations impede their exercise routine has a strong locus of control (Figure 12.2).

Similarly, the ability to exercise well or to endure discomfort may not be developed well and locus of control (the ability of oneself to work through discomfort) would be low. Consequently, a low locus of control could lead to feelings of helplessness and despair, resulting in sporadic exercising or attrition. However, someone who takes charge of their exercise and does not let situations impede their exercise routine, has a stong locus of control. Emil Zatopek, the great Checkoslovakian distance runner is an example of someone with a strong locus of control. While in the army, he would run in place in full fatigues while on guard duty, rather than let the situation dictate that he could not run overdistance in running gear.

Social Support

Humans are social creatures who can be influenced greatly by the presence of others. Certainly, the family unit is a prime example of social support influence for learning and maintaining behaviors. **Social facilitation** describes the effect of the presence of others upon behavior. This effect can be positive or negative. Exercisers tend to maintain exercise with social support from others and dropout of exercise if social support is lacking.

Find a Workout Partner

For example, a spouse being willing to accommodate exercise times by adjusting the dinner schedule or simply not complaining about resulting inconveniences could be tremendous support. However, being unyielding and complaining sends the opposite signal, leading to attrition. Thus, people should be encouraged to involve significant others in their exercise life-style, to discuss adjustments in daily family schedules, and to be supportive by recognizing the effort and discipline needed to exercise.

Exercising with Others can be a Tremendous Motivational Boost

1. Know they are not alone
2. See others are taking the time
3. Say to themselves "If they can be committed, so can I"
4. Form commitments or informal contracts which they want to honor or uphold

Consider a group of about 20 middle aged to senior male runners who exercise regularly and meet every Sunday morning. Some run longer, some shorter, and smaller groups of 3-5 form. But barring acute sickness or being out of town, they meet at 7:00 a.m. sharp every Sunday all year long.

If someone is late, that person must catch up. They are serious, committed, bonded and expect if someone wants to be in the group, that person will informally commit themselves to the group. The same process occurs to a lesser or greater extent with mall-walkers and groups in which the person who misses a workout buys a steak dinner for everyone else in the group.

This sort of social support can be extended to another level. Making deals, bets, verbal commitments such as "You drive to aerobics this week and I'll drive next," is a form of informal contracting. Certainly, a commitment in the form of, "Exercising with someone else really helps the time fly by. Let's get together on a regular basis," can provide direct commitment and social support.

Part of your role as a professional is to initiate social support groups, partnerships, car pools, informal contracting, and family support. You can do this in several ways. Consider having orientation sessions in which you present these ideas to exercisers. Locate on a map where people live, perhaps with a number code so exercisers can form car pools and off-day/weekend exercise groups (Figure 12.3).

Support Systems to Maintain Exercise

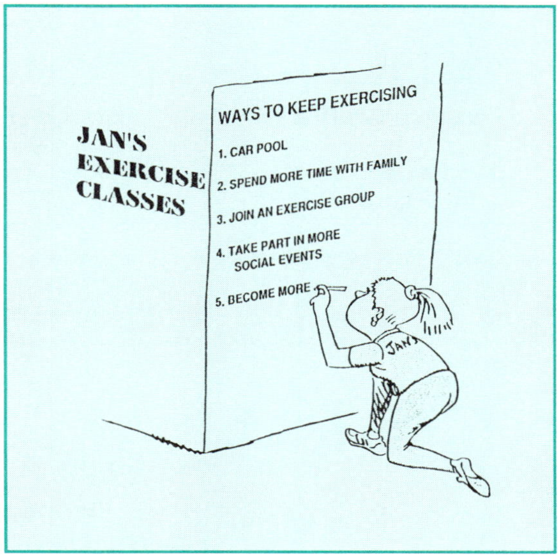
JAN'S
EXERCISE
CLASSES
WAYS TO KEEP EXERCISING
1. CAR POOL
2. SPEND MORE TIME WITH FAMILY
3. JOIN AN EXERCISE GROUP
4. TAKE PART IN MORE SOCIAL EVENTS
5. BECOME MORE
JAN

Figure 12.3.

EXERCISE ADDICTION

Positive or Negative Addiction

Exercise addiction is the reverse of exercise attrition and is probably the more pernicious problem. Rather than a lack of commitment or not enough motivation, exercise addiction is a problem of overcommitment or too much motivation. Just as phobias are irrational fears, addiction to exercise can be irrational; believing that more is always better or that even the slightest deviations from a training program will upset one's entire life.

CAUSES

Our culture contains many value systems and ethics which form a motivational seed bed for exercise addiction. People who become addicted to running, tennis, swimming or aerobics probably have incorporated one or more of these social components into their personal value system, then take it to an irrational or illogical extreme.

Consider the Following Ethics/Value Systems

1. Work ethic
2. Personal gratification
3. Comparison with others
4. Glory through abuse

Positives and Negatives for Each Ethic/Value System

Ethic/Value	Positive	Negative
Work Ethic	"Work Smart"	"Work Hard"
Personal Gratification	"Exercise Feels Good"	"More is Necessary"
Comparison with Others	"Others are great examples."	"I need to be like or exceed others."
Glory Through Abuse	"A little soreness won't stop me."	"I'll never stop or give in."
	Mental Toughness	Irrational Toughness

Table 12.3.

Work Ethic

On the positive end of the spectrum, the work ethic can promote beneficial exercise through such daily and household activities as mowing the lawn, raking leaves, or walking the dog. Accomplishing work while exercising can be a powerful motivator.

No Pain More Gain

On the negative end of the spectrum this ethic embodies the ideal that the harder you work the better you will become and the more benefits you will receive. "No pain, no gain" and "More pain, more gain" could be slogans for this work ethic. People with an overdeveloped work ethic could believe, "If exercising 20 minutes three times a week is the basic formula, then doubling this will be twice as good." While exercising more does produce more benefits, double benefits are not guaranteed. Also, considered in isolation from specific goals, and proper rest and without long-term objectives, the work ethic exercise addict is motivated for the sake of doing work rather than the purposefulness of that work. One suggestion for these overworkers is to instill a working smart ethic to complement their working hard ethic. This means to consider training specificity, short-term and long-term goals and, cost-benefit ratios.

Personal Gratification

It Feels Good

Personal gratification can contribute to exercise addiction through a basic psychological principle called the **pleasure principle**. Once a person finds an exercise or sport they enjoy the satisfaction of pursuing it at all costs becomes a reality. Similarly, losing fat and looking better is quite gratifying and can lead to the "More exercise will help me look better" or, "More exercise is necessary for remaining this way" syndrome. Runners, cyclists, swimmers, and people involved in other aerobic activities over many years know the tremendous pleasure of being able to continue, to keep going, to be active. It just feels good.

The key is to keep the pleasure in perspective. Understand that running, aerobics, tennis, cycling are only one source of enjoyment in life. Also, if exercise addiction leads to injury due to overuse, the pleasure can be reduced drastically or could cease.

Comparison with Others

Testimony how great athletes train can be very motivational. Stories of unique if not bizzare training methods, exercises and diets of Olympians, professional and other elite athletes can be quite inspirational. Children can view these athletes as role models and want to work just as hard to be a great athlete. Examples of Seniors who started swimming as a hobby and eventually completed an endurance swim or competed in the Ironman Triathlon can provide hope and direction for other Seniors. Similarly, and more practically, aerobic exercisers and mall walkers can compare themselves to friends/acquaintances. "Peggy hasn't missed a day in over two years" and "Phil goes hard from the start" are standards with which others can be compared.

Set Goals But Be Realistic

High achievement oriented individuals can easily become addicted by striving to meet or exceed these standards. However, not everyone has the same physical abilities and not everyone's body responds to the same exercise in exactly the same way. Be sure to explain that each person should exercise appropriately for themselves. While one person may be able to train with high intensity and low duration, another person may train best with high duration and low intensity. Trying to match or exceed the performances of others is great for competition. However, training for competition is quite different than exercising for health and fitness.

Determining the level and variation of exercise best for each person comes with time and experience. A general rule and great motivational strategy is: Gradually progress from lower to higher levels of exercise intensity. This ensures each person is ready to advance, and they have already succeeded at lower levels, increasing self-esteem, efficacy and intrinsic motivation. Consider two women: Jennifer, who has been exercising only a few months, and Maria, who has been exercising for three years (Figure 12.4). Jennifer perceives Maria as a great role model, but might not realize the progress necessary for Maria to achieve her exercise level. Explaining to Jennifer the slow, gradual progress of Maria's three years of exercise would help place her goals in perspective.

Exercise Progression

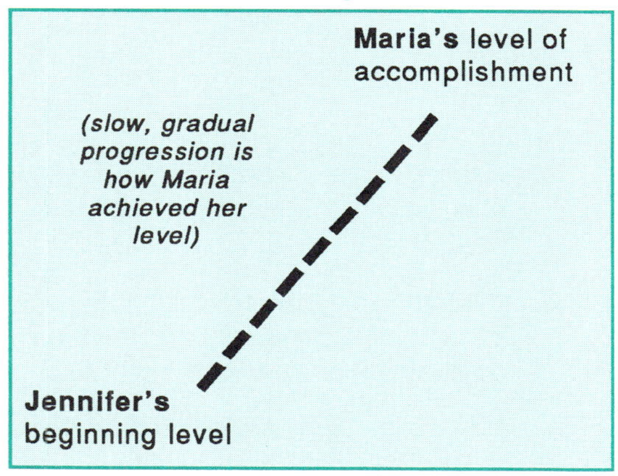

Figure 12.4. Gradual exercise progression as part of long term goals and comparison with others.

Glory through Abuse

The belief that disciplining the body and mind through punishment - physical work - is the basis for this ethic. "Harry never complains, even though I know he is hurting" and "Jackie is so tough, she doesn't know the meaning of quit" are examples. Harry and Jackie revel in viewing themselves or having others view them as sacrificers. The more pain and punishment, the more they can endure and overcome, the more glorious their personal development or stature in the eyes of others.

We all do this from time to time and call it "mental toughness." However, the line is drawn from "mental toughness" to irrational toughness when being tough is seen as necessary for self improvement and necessary to repeat the experience regularly.

Be Realistic and Careful

Explain to exercisers that the fine line between being mentally tough enough to exercise rather than not work through pain/discomfort is crossed when the exercise is more important than long-term health or goals. For example, someone who has finally increased to jogging 3 miles without stopping may still need to walk during some workouts. Just because our bodies have performed at one level does not mean we are capable of performing at that level every time. Even world record holders do not match world records each time out, no matter how mentally tough they are. Helping people understand this can improve their motivation greatly.

WORKING WITH EXERCISE ADDICTION

While exercise addiction is real, the numbers of people affected and the extent of addiction are not known. Also, while some basic suggestions are available, exercise/fitness leaders must be aware that addiction to exercise could be the result of deeper psychological or emotional factors which should be handled by other professionals. This begins to enter the clinical arena within which specific technical training and experience is required. So, specific psychological and emotional treatment should be left to trained professionals.

Here are some general recommendations for helping people keep their exercise in perspective.

Recommendations to Keep Exercise in Perspective

1. ***Encourage exercising with others of lower ability*** from time to time. This can help exercise addicts to realize how advanced they are, possibly attenuating any obsessive or irrational drives.
2. ***Encourage periodic 1 to 2 week breaks***. Many top endurance athletes simply take time off after a season or at regular intervals. This forces people to do other things and allows their bodies to recover from stresses of long-term training.
3. ***Vary exercise activities periodically***. Change from aerobics to swimming or from running to cycling. Not only will this provide a break from routine, it is great for the body because varying activities trains different muscles. Often, people find they become healthier and feel better by varying exercise rather than exercising in only one way.
4. ***Develop other hobbies and interests***. Just as we enjoy the company of many people, yet are most committed to a few, so also can we be most committed to exercise, yet have many other interests. This provides not only a mental diversion but a goal orientation diversion to which people can be motivated, lessening any motivational obsession with exercising.
5. ***Set and follow specific goals for exercising***. One part of these goals should be regular periods of rest. Writing out goals also allows others to review them to determine their appropriateness. I recall a story about Steve Prefontaine who as a college freshman set the challenging but unrealistic goal of running better than the world record for the mile. His coach worked with him to realize how fast he would need to run each interval of the mile in order to accomplish this. The result was that Prefontaine revised his goals to a more appropriate level. Fitness and exercise leaders can serve this same function, evaluating exercise intensity, duration, etc. and providing feedback for the most appropriate exercise level.

Suggested Readings

Benyo, R. *The Exercise Fix.* Champaign, IL: Human Kinetics Publishers, 1990.

Dishman, R. (Ed.). *Exercise Adherence: It's Impact on Public Health.* Champaign, IL: Human Kinetics Publishers, 1988.

Duda, J.L. and M. K. Tappe, Personal investment in exercise among adults: The examination of age and gender-related differences in motivational orientation. In A. Ostrow (Ed.), *Aging and Motor Behavior*, 239-256. Indianapolis: Benchmark Press, 1989

Kimiecik, Jay (Ed.). A practicioner's guide to exercise motivation. *Journal of Physical Education, Recreation and Dance*, September, 33-48, 1991.

Maer, M.L. and L. Braskamp, The motivation factor: A theory of personal investment. Lexington, MA: D.C. Health, 1986.

Rejeski, W.J. and E. A. Kenney. *Fitness Motivation: Preventing Participation Dropout.* Champaign, IL: Human Kinetics Publishers, 1988.

Sallis, J.F. & M. F. Hovell, Determinants of exercise behavior. *Exercise and Sport Science Reviews*, 18, 307-330, 1990.

U.S. Public Health Service. Healthy People 2000: National Health Promotion and Disease Prevention Objectives. Washington, D.C., U.S. Government Printing Office, 1990

CHAPTER

13 PREVENTING FITNESS-RELATED INJURIES

Carole Zebas

Learning Objectives

- Distinguish the difference between acute and overuse injuries in fitness related activities.
- Identify some of the common acute injuries and their causes in fitness related activities.
- Identify some of the common overuse injuries and their causes in fitness related activities.
- Describe other fitness related problems such as blisters, muscle cramps, muscle soreness, and nerve impingement.
- Describe and distinguish between heat exhaustion and heat stroke.
- Describe and distinguish between hypothermia and frostbite.
- Identify and describe the training errors that are responsible for overuse injuries.
- Identify and describe the anatomical factors which predispose fitness participants to potential injury or impairment problems.
- Describe those precautions which can be used to prevent fitness related injuries.

Important Terms

Achilles tendinitis
acute injury
anterior knee pain
blister
bursitis
calcific bursitis
chondromalacia patella
chronic injury
compartment syndrome
dislocation
fatigue fracture
fracture
frictional bursitis
frostbite
genital irritation
heat exhaustion
heat stroke
hypothermia
iliotibial band friction syndrome
load-deformation curve
low back pain
muscle cramp
muscle soreness
osteoarthritis
overuse injury
patellar tendinitis
patellofemoral pain
periostitis
plantar fasciitis
runner's knee
sciatica
shin splints
sprain
stitch-in-the-side
strain
stress fracture
subluxation
tendinitis
tibial stress syndrome
tibial stress fracture
ulnar neuropathy

INTRODUCTION

Anyone who has ever engaged in a sport or fitness related activity probably has experienced a few aches and pains along the way. Many of these aches and pains may have been nagging or annoying, but they were not severe enough to prevent participation in the activity for any length of time. Others, on the other hand, may have been more severe and required special treatment and care. While some injuries occur "accidentally," others are preventable. It is the purpose of this chapter to explore the reasons why injuries occur, what injuries are common to fitness related activities, and how injuries can be prevented.

Accidents are Preventable

ACUTE VERSUS OVERUSE INJURIES

Injuries usually are divided into two major categories, acute and overuse. A single event injury is classified as an **acute injury**. For example, running on an uneven surface and suddenly turning the ankle may result in an ankle sprain. An injury which takes a long time to develop is referred to as an **overuse** or **chronic injury**. For example, an aerobics dance participant may develop a stress fracture in the foot from poor body mechanics or exercising on a concrete floor over an extended period of time. Most of the fitness related injuries fall into this category.

ACUTE INJURIES

Acute injuries of the musculoskeleton system involve the bones, joints, ligaments, muscles and tendons. Bones can be fractured, subluxed, or dislocated. Joints and ligaments are sprained, and muscles are strained. Generally, acute injuries are unavoidable. The only prevention is common sense and safety first (e.g., wearing protective equipment when needed, warming-up before an exercise bout).

Sprained vs. Strained

Fractures

Fractures are breaks in a bone. They are more common in contact sports than in fitness related activities because of the direct and high forces generated. However, a fitness exercise participant could incur a fracture by twisting or falling awkwardly. In any case, this potentially is a serious injury and should be diagnosed and treated by a qualified medical person. The greatest danger in fracture injuries lies in the damage that could result to the surrounding soft tissues (e.g., ligaments, nerves, skin, muscles, tendons). The most common anatomical sites for fractures in fitness exercise participants are the ankle, lower leg, wrist, lower arm, and finger.

You Fracture Me

Subluxations/Dislocations

A **subluxation** is a partial separation of two bones at the joint. Usually there is an immediate "popping" back into place after the separation. A **dislocation**, on the other hand, is a complete disjoining of the bones at the joint site. Falling on an outstretched arm might cause a subluxation or dislocation. The most common sites for this injury are the shoulder, fingers, and patella (kneecap). Just as in the fracture, a dislocation may cause damage to the surrounding structures. In fact, the signs and symptoms of a fracture and dislocation are similar. There usually is an observable deformity, swelling, tenderness to touch, bruising, and loss of function. The first aid treatment for both fractures and dislocations is to immobilize the injured limb by splinting, elevate the limb to reduce the swelling, and transport the person to a medical facility. Healing may take up to six weeks depending upon the severity of the fracture.

Sprains

A **sprain** involves a stretching or tearing of the ligamentous fibers that connect bones to bones. The severity of the injury depends upon the number of fibers affected and the amount of functional stability lost in the joint. Sprains usually are caused by a sudden twisting movement or awkward turn. For instance, running on uneven terrain may result in an inversion ankle sprain. The anatomical sites most affected are the ankle, wrist, elbow, shoulder, and knee.

Mild to Severe

The severity of a sprain may be described as mild, moderate, or severe. A mild sprain involves the stretching or tearing of less than 25% of the fibers or a partial tearing of the ligament away from its attachment site. A moderate sprain involves up to 50% of the fibers. In both cases, the joint remains relatively stable with little loss of functional mobility. A severe sprain consists of more than 50% of the fibers being torn, or a fragment of the bone being torn away, and loss of joint stability.

The most obvious symptoms of a sprain are pain upon movement, swelling, and tenderness. In more severe cases, hemorrhaging may be visible and the joint will be unstable. In the less severe sprains, immediate treatment is rest, ice, compression, and elevation (RICE). The following table provides a more detailed explanation of the RICE treatment.

The R. I. C. E. Treatment

Rest	Stop using the injured part for at least 24-48 hours. Do not participate in any fitness activities which could aggravate the condition.
Ice	Use ice for the first 24 hours to decrease the bleeding from the injured blood vessels. Apply for 20-30 minutes, then warm for 15 minutes for the first 2-3 hours. Then apply for 30 minutes every hour for the next 2-3 hours.
Compression	Use a support wrap or compression bandage to control the swelling and reduce the bleeding.
Elevate	Raise injured part to help drain excessive fluid and reduce pain. Keep elevated for 24-48 hours.

Table 13.1.

Gentle range of motion exercises are important for the healing process, and should be begun after the initial swelling has subsided. More severe ankle sprains should be treated by medical personnel. Mild sprains may take anywhere from 1-2 weeks to heal, moderate sprains from 2-4 weeks, and severe sprains from 4-8 weeks or more.

Strains

A **strain**, sometimes called a pull, refers to the stretching or tearing of a muscle or its tendon attachment. This probably is the most common fitness related injury. An acute strain may be caused by a sudden twisting motion or moving in an awkward manner. For example, lifting too heavy a weight may cause you to use an unorthodox move in performing the lift. More often, strains are caused by inadequate or faulty warm-up techniques, fatigue, tenseness, prolonged exposure to cold, insufficient recovery from a previous injury, or working a previously injured muscle. Aerobic dancers who use heavy hands or other weights in their hands may become tired, thus making them susceptible to shoulder strains. On the other hand, they may move the arms through a range of motion too quickly and develop an acute shoulder strain. Likewise, swimmers who train improperly may suffer an overuse strain to the rotator cuff muscles. The muscles of the body most frequently affected are found in the lower back (paraspinals), back of the leg (hamstrings and gastrocnemius), front of the leg (quadriceps), hip (flexors and adductors), and shoulder (rotator cuff).

Warming-Up is the Key

Strains are classified in the same manner as sprains. That is, the severity depends upon the percentage of fiber involvement and the amount of mobility present. The most severe type of strain also can be a rupture. The symptoms and signs are pain on movement, loss of function, discoloration, weakness, stiffness, and spasms. In the instance of a rupture, a sudden pain may be felt and an indentation or defect in the muscle may be noticeable. This is a more common condition in older fitness participants whose muscles and tendons may not be as flexible as younger participants. Treatment, too, is similar to a sprain so follow RICE (See Table 13.1), plus, mild stretching exercises, and anti-inflammatory medication such as ibuprofen are the main forms. Any mild or moderate strain which does not heal in a reasonable length of time should be attended to by medical personnel. Severe strains should always be checked by a medical person. A major consequence of improperly treated strains, and especially those where bleeding has occurred, is the formation of scar tissue. When fibers are torn, blood fills the spaces between the muscle fibers. As the blood clots, it is turned into connective tissue, and then gradually into scar tissue. The muscle elasticity is compromised causing an increased risk of re-injury. Healing time varies anywhere from 1-6 weeks, or several months in severe cases.

Strain to Rupture to R.I.C.E.

OVERUSE INJURIES

Overuse injuries are chronic type injuries, usually caused by repetitive events that have occurred over time. This major class of injuries most often is associated with fitness related activities. The constant pounding of the leg and foot on the ground in running or aerobic dancing, the repetitive

Be Careful When Stretching

overload stresses of weight lifting, or the pressure on the hands when holding onto bicycle handlebars are examples of potential problem areas for fitness exercise participants. Also, stretching and strengthening exercises potentially can create dangerous situations. This is due to the stresses placed on the neck and lower back areas.

The body reacts to excessive repetitive activity, pressure, friction, or external trauma by causing an inflammatory response. The structures most affected are the tendons, bursa sacs, periosteum, or bone and cartilage. The other reaction to repetitive stresses is the stress fracture. The lower legs and feet most often are affected here. A description of the common inflammatory conditions, with a look at specific fitness related examples, is covered later in the chapter.

Tendinitis

Rest Ice Support and Heat

Tendinitis is an inflammation of the tendon or tendon sheath. It is caused by a constant and repetitive strain on the tendon structure which causes microtears and bleeding. This, in turn, produces the inflammation. It is characterized by pain and tenderness at the attachment site or along the tendon and by pain around the attachment when the muscle contracts. The most common sites for this overuse injury are the Achilles tendon, elbow extensor tendon, patellar tendon, and hip adductor tendon. (See Achilles tendinitis discussion on page 204. The general treatment for tendinitis is rest, ice, support, heat after the acute phase when the swelling has subsided which usually takes 48-72 hours after, and anti-inflammatory medication such as ibuprofen to reduce the swelling and pain. Be sure to take the medication only as directed on the bottle or by a physician.

Connective Tissue Inflammation

There are three kinds of connective tissue that often are implicated in fitness related injuries. They are the fascia, iliotibial band, and retinaculum. All are fibrous type membranes that either cover, support, or separate other tissues. Sometimes they act as extensions of the tendon or ligament structures, so they respond in a similar manner. Specific examples of plantar fasciitis, iliotibial band syndrome, and knee pain are described more fully later in this chapter.

Bursitis

Bursitis is the inflammation of a bursa sac. Bursae are small sac-like structures filled with fluid. They are found between a bone and a tendon, between two tendons, between a tendon and the skin, or between a bone and the skin. Their function is to reduce friction and reduce stress. When a structure such as the Achilles tendon repeatedly moves over the bursa site, the bursa may become irritated and inflamed. Other sites which may be irritated in fitness related injuries are the knee, hip, shoulder, and heel. This particular type of bursitis is called **frictional bursitis**.

Another form of bursitis occurs in older participants who have performed repetitive motions over a long period of time. Sometimes calcium deposits from an overused tendon may penetrate the bursa causing a **calcific bursitis**. Pain, tenderness and swelling are symptoms of most bursitis cases. The primary treatment for this condition is rest until the pain has subsided. Ice may be used initially, with heat being used after the first 24 hours. A compression bandage may be used to relieve pressure. Sometimes the bursa needs to be aspirated, but that should be done only by qualified medical personnel.

Periostitis

The periosteum is a bone covering. When it becomes irritated and inflamed the condition is known as **periostitis**. A common site for this disorder is the lower leg around the medial portion of the tibia. Pain, tenderness, and swelling at the site of the injury characterize this condition. The treatment for this is similar to all the inflammatory conditions, that is, rest and heat over the site. If this is not taken care of properly, stress fractures may develop. (See shin splints page 206).

Next: Stress Fracture

Arthritis

Located on the joint surface of a bone is cartilage. Articular cartilage functions to absorb impact shocks and to reduce wear and tear on the bones. However, because it has no blood supply, it cannot repair itself once it has been damaged. When the cartilage becomes damaged, as it could with activities requiring repeated impacts, it repairs itself with scar tissue. This is a degenerative condition called **osteoarthritis.** It usually is noticeable in older adults or those individuals who have had repeated cartilage damage. Individuals who have this condition usually complain of pain and morning stiffness. A clinical examination might reveal joint changes such as abnormal movement, tenderness, crepitus (grinding sound), and possibly muscle atrophy. (See knee pain, page 204).

Not all fitness participants are susceptible to this condition. However, if the condition exists, load on the affected joints must be reduced. This can be done by doing alternate aerobic activities such as cycling or swimming. It also is important to maintain good range of motion in the joints, muscle flexibility and muscle strength.

Stress Fractures

A **stress fracture**, also known as a **fatigue fracture,** is a slight crack in the bone caused by repeated stresses. (Figure 13.1). The body is a remarkable machine which has the ability to become stronger when stresses are placed on it. It builds new bone and removes old bone at the point of the stress. If the stresses occur more rapidly than the building process, a breakdown occurs. As the breakdown occurs, pain begins and continues to intensify as long as the stresses continue. There is tenderness to the touch on both sides of the fractured site. Sometimes the condition previously described as periostitis will be a precursor to stress fractures. This condition requires rest and the care of qualified medical personnel.

Stress Fracture

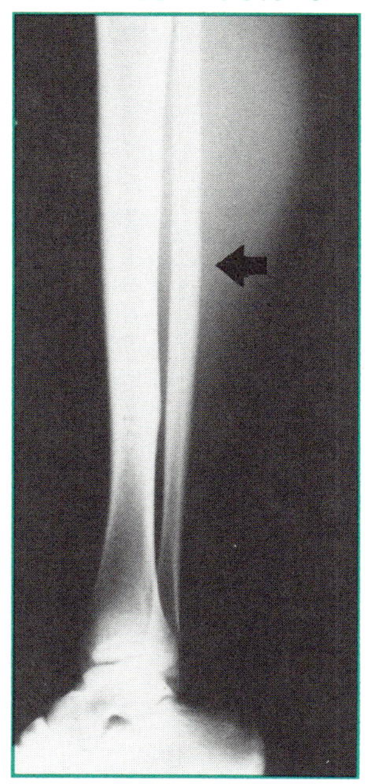

Figure 13.1. Notice the raised shaded area indicating a fatigue or stress fracture.

MECHANISMS OF INJURY

Warning: Tissues Under Stress

To better understand the mechanism of injury, or how an injury occurs, we must first define the two main sources, internal and external. External sources are things that come from outside the body such as stepping in a hole, colliding with another person or object, falling down the stairs, slipping on the ice, or letting a weight fall on your foot. Internal sources are things that come from within the body. They involve body structures such as the muscles, ligaments, tendons, and various connective tissues. For example, an awkward movement or sudden turn may cause a muscle strain. Other internal sources mainly include the repetitious nature of the activity (e.g., running), posture imbalances (e.g., unequal strength in a muscle group), or anatomical factors (e.g., excessive pronation of the foot). Some additional anatomical factors are described in Table 13.2.

It is no secret that along with the fitness boom came the inevitable injury problems. Researchers in the field of biomechanics, exercise physiology, and health have tried very hard to explain how injuries occur, especially the overuse injuries. Internally, this has been explained by describing how the various tissues react under loads or stresses.

In the field of biomechanics or engineering, the strength of a material is determined by how much "give" that material can withstand before failure as a load is placed upon it. This best can be illustrated with the **load-deformation curve** shown in Figure 13.2. As a load is placed on a tissue, it begins to deform. Depending on the type of tissue, the type of load, and how fast it is applied, the deformation ("give") will continue until the load is released. Provided the load has been released within the region designated as the elastic region, the tissue will return to its original shape. Take, for example, a muscle being stretched. The muscle will continue to "give" as long as you continue to stretch it. When you stop stretching, the muscle tends to return to its original shape. If the load continues to be applied beyond the region into the inelastic region, the tissue loses some of its ability to return to its original shape. Up to a point, this may cause no problem and may even be desirable. When attempting to improve range of motion (flexibility) in the joints of the body, applying loads which reach into the elastic zone are desirable. However, there comes a point of failure where there is no returning back to the original shape. When this point is reached, the tissue fails (e.g., rupture, fracture).

Load-Deformation Curve

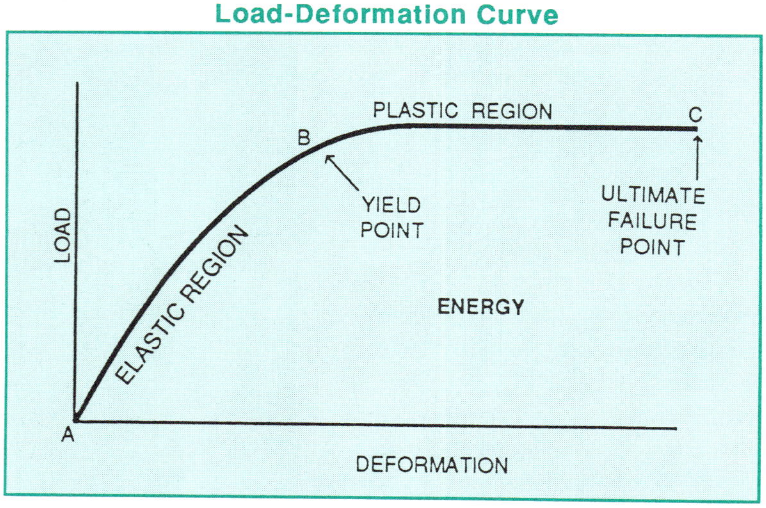

Figure 13.2. Modified from M. Nordin and V. H. Frankel: *Basic Biomechanics of the Musculoskeletal System, 2nd edition*. Philadelphia, Lea and Febiger, 1989. Reprinted with permission.

In overuse injuries, the repeated nature of the activity causes an overloading on the system. Fortunately for humans, there are warning signals when the system is being overloaded. Those signals are pain, soreness, and inflammation. If the warning is heeded and rest is given to

Anatomical Factors Predisposing One to Injury

Condition	Description	Potential Problems
Leg Length Discrepancy	one leg shorter than the other	low back pain, hip pain, one foot pronates, other supinates
Excessive Pronation	extreme rolling to medial side of the arch (flat-footed appearance)	more weight on the first toe and posterior tibial tendinitis on stretched tissue at the ankle, knee pain (medial), tibial stress syndrome (medial), posterior tibial tendinitis, hip bursitis, Achilles' tendinitis, plantar faciitis
Excessive Supination	extreme rolling to lateral side of the arch	lateral ankle sprains, shin splints, iliotibial band syndrome, trochanteric bursitis, peroneal tendinitis, plantar faciitis, stress fracture, Achilles' tendinitis, calf muscle strain
Flat Arches	see excessive pronation	
High Arches	see excessive supination	
Genu Valgus	knock-kneed appearance	medial knee pain tightness on lateral side of leg
Genu Varus	bow-legged appearance	lateral knee pain tightness on medial side of leg
Excessive Q-Angle	angle formed by intersecting the line extended from the patellar tendon and the line of the femur	knee pain, patellar tendinitis
Functional Equinnus	limited function of ankle dorsiflexion due to muscle imbalance of gastrocnemius and soleus	medial arch pain, posterior leg fatigue, plantar fasciitis, shin splints
Tibial Torsion	an outward turning of the tibia in relation to the femur	knee pain
Femoral Torsion	an inward turning of the femur in relation to the tibia	knee pain, chondromalacia

Table 13.2.

re-strengthen the tissues, further and more critical injuries may be prevented. The factors which make the tissues susceptible to injury are the intrinsic and extrinsic factors. Individuals vary in the amount of overloading their tissues can withstand. It all depends on how the intrinsic and extrinsic factors which cause the injuries are eliminated. A discussion of general injury prevention techniques can be found later in this chapter.

COMMON FITNESS RELATED INJURIES

The discussion up to this point has centered around acute and overuse injuries in general. This section will describe specific fitness related injuries and why they occur. This will be followed by a section on the prevention of overuse injuries.

KNEE PAIN

Weak Knee

The knee is the most often injured part of the body in fitness related activities. This is not so surprising when one considers that the legs are under constant stress in any of the many aerobic and conditioning activities. It is not difficult to understand why running and aerobic dance activities make the knee so vulnerable to injury. However, it may be surprising to some to know that other fitness related activities involving the stair climbing machine, stationary cycling, and weight lifting also cause knee problems. For instance, while using the stair climbing machine, technique is important. Hyperextending the knee at the bottom of the down phase stroke places undue stress on the knee joint. Likewise, cyclists are susceptible if the saddle height is set too low or the gears are set too high. The angle of pull of the quadriceps is compromised and causes stress on the knee joint.

In general, there are three conditions labeled as knee pain. They are **"runner's knee"**, **chondromalacia patella**, and **patellar tendinitis** (Table 13.3).

ACHILLES TENDINITIS

10 Times Body Weight

The Achilles tendon is the common tendon for the gastrocnemius and soleus muscles. It attaches to the heel bone and is active as the foot moves in plantarflexion and dorsiflexion. It has been estimated that the forces on this tendon can be up to 10 times body weight during running. This is to be expected with aerobic dancers, too, and the forces may even be more than that. Training errors such as increasing mileage/workouts suddenly, overtraining, excessive hill running, and running on hard surfaces have been implicated as the major causes of **Achilles tendinitis.** Stresses on the tendon can cause small microtears which in turn cause the inflammation characteristic of this condition. The second most common cause of Achilles tendinitis, according to some researchers, is excessive pronation of the foot. When the foot rolls to the inner border of the foot, the Achilles tendon is stretched. Other causes of this condition are improper footwear, and lack of flexibility in the calf muscles.

Runner's Knee	Chondromalacia Patella	Patellar Tendinitis
The most common knee injury among runners is sometimes referred to as **patellofemoral pain.** It is characterized by soreness and discomfort around the kneecap (patella) and the retinaculum (fibrous band lying on either side of the knee and forming part of the joint capsule). The quadriceps and patella act as a pulley system to increase the effectiveness of knee extension. When some condition forces the tracking of this system to go awry, a great deal of pres-sure is built up between the kneecap and the end of the femur bone of the upper leg. Those individuals who excessively pronate (weight shifts to the inner borders of the feet) tend to be more susceptible to this condition. Also, those who have a muscle imbalance in the quadriceps muscle group, especially the vastus medialis, tend to experience this overuse injury.	When the vastus medialis is weaker than the other vasti muscles of the quadriceps group, it prevents the group from contracting as one unit. When the pressure on the back side of the patella becomes extreme, a wearing away of the underlying bone can occur. This causes a crepitus (grinding sound) when bending at the knee. Others consider it to be a more severe form of "runner's knee". (Note: The term chondromalacia is being replaced by the term **anterior knee pain** in recent literature on injuries.)	This is a common condition of runners and aerobic dance participants because of the bouncing action required in the activity. As the foot lands on the ground, the quadriceps muscle must contract eccentrically to soften the impact. The eccentric contraction causes the quadriceps muscle to lengthen, thereby pulling on the patellar attachment. Repeated pulling causes a tenderness at the tendinous attachment.

Table 13.3.

ILIOTIBIAL BAND SYNDROME

The iliotibial band is connective tissue which runs down the outside of the leg from the hip to the knee. It is an extension of the tensor fascia latae and gluteus maximus muscles. When certain underlying conditions are present, friction between the band and the knee bone cause irritation. This is called the **iliotibial band friction syndrome.** Some of those underlying conditions of an anatomical nature are limb length discrepancies, bowlegs, and high arches. Other causes are excessive downhill running, running on a cambered (uneven or slanting to one side) road, and wearing shoes worn out on the lateral side (outside) of the foot.

Run-Down on Injuries

LOW BACK PAIN

Low back pain takes many forms. If a fitness participant makes a sudden turn or unexpected movement, the low back may be affected. Usually this is in the form of a muscle strain. If the injury is an overuse injury, it could be related to pre-existing poor postural problems. More often than not, however, low back pain is the result of weak abdominal muscles and hip flexor muscles, or inflexibile hamstring muscles and hip extensor muscles. A good example of where muscle weaknesses may cause low back pain is in weight lifting. Take for instance the bench press. If a heavy weight is lifted and the abdominals are weak, there is a tendency to "arch" the back. Repeated arching of the back makes it susceptible to a strain. Similar back "arching" can occur in someone performing leg lifts or straight-leg situps. Even daily activities such as driving a car, sitting, or lifting can cause low back pain if they are performed incorrectly or for sustained periods of time.

Strengthen those Muscles

Arching is for Monuments

Another form of low back pain is **sciatica.** The large nerve which runs from the lower back, over the buttocks, and down the leg is sometimes compressed from tight muscles or muscle spasms. At other times, a slipped disc may be responsible for the compression. This causes a pain down the leg, some tingling, and maybe a numbing affect. Things which could aggravate this condition are the impact of running or aerobic dance, knee problems, a limb length discrepancy and overpronation. Among weight lifters and fitness participants who use rowing machines, this is a potential problem. Much of this can be related directly to poor technique.

PLANTAR FASCIITIS

A band of tissue called the plantar fascia runs from the heel to the toes and supports the bottom of the foot. When weight is placed on the arch, it flattens causing a pull at the calcaneal (heel bone) attachment. If the pull is repeated over time, the attachment area becomes irritated and inflamed from the small microtears which have been building up. This is a condition called **plantar fasciitis.** Sometimes a heel spur is formed making the foot feel bruised. Usually the pain is at the site of the heel where it feels like a "stone bruise." Runners who overpronate or train improperly are susceptible to this injury. Too, runners and aerobic dancers who train on hard surfaces are prone to this injury.

SHIN SPLINTS

Shin splints is a term that no longer is popular among medical personnel and athletic trainers because it cannot be defined precisely. At one time it was used to describe pain along the tibia (shin bone). However, now this condition has been given a variety of names.

Names for Shin Splints

1. Tibial stress syndrome
2. Tibial stress fracture
3. Periostitis *(inflammation of the bone covering)*
4. Compartment syndrome *(swollen muscles cutting off the blood supply)*

They either involve the muscle and tendon sheath (e.g., anterior tibialis muscle or posterior tibialis muscle), the bone, or the bone covering (periosteum). Of the previously mentioned varieties, the compartment syndrome is least likely to be present in fitness participants. In all of the cases, tenderness, pain, and inflammation occur somewhere along the tibia bone. The anatomical structures are unable to keep up with the constant stresses and they break down.

Shin splints is the most common aerobic dance injury, but also has been found to affect runners. Training errors, hard surfaces, and excessive pronation have been known to cause this condition. It is especially prevalent in fitness participants who have just begun a program and overdo the first few conditioning bouts.

MISCELLANEOUS FITNESS RELATED INJURIES

There are several injuries or disorders that are related to fitness participation, but do not fall under the classification of musculoskeletal injuries. A brief description of the most commonly encountered of these injuries will be discussed in this section with an emphasis being placed on prevention techniques.

Practice Prevention

BLISTERS

Blisters are a collection of fluid under the outer layer of the skin produced by repeated friction or pressure against the skin. Hot and humid weather seems to provide a more favorable setting for blisters. Most blisters are found on the feet or hands.

Precautions to Preventing Blisters

1. Wear socks that are clean, free from holes, and are of the correct size
2. Break in new shoes gradually
3. Protect sensitive skin with adhesive plaster
4. Wear shoes that fit snuggly
5. Use powder in shoes if socks are not worn, or use powder or gloves on hands before gripping equipment such as weights.

MUSCLE CRAMPS

Muscle cramps are painful involuntary contractions of a muscle. They seem to occur more frequently when the weather is hot, the exercise bout is long, and large amounts of fluid are lost from the body. The leg is the most common site for this condition, but the stomach area also is affected frequently. Prevention consists of proper training progression, warming-up prior to exercise, drinking plenty of fluids prior to exercise (especially electrolyte drinks when exercising in the heat), and eating foods high in potassium (e.g., bananas, citrus fruits,fresh vegetables).

Price of Fitness

MUSCLE SORENESS

Muscle soreness is a painful condition usually brought on by eccentric muscle contractions or negative work. Running downhill or lifting weights (especially during the return to position phase) are examples where the muscles must go through a lengthening to control the movement. In untrained individuals who suddenly take up an exercise program, muscle changes in the form of "ruptures" occur. It is thought that these ruptures occur in the Z-discs of the muscle and in the muscle capillaries. The onset of pain occurs anywhere from 24-72 hours after the onset of exercise. Aside from the discomfort, it causes no real damage. Prevention lies in gradual progression of an exercise program and avoidance of excessive eccentric work until the muscles have become conditioned to the training.

STITCH-IN-THE-SIDE

Warming-Up Helps

A **stitch-in-the-side** is a pain under the ribs usually occurring on the right side of the body. The causes of this pain really are not known, but it has been suggested that improper warm-up and a lack of oxygen supply to the diaphragm are precursors to this condition. Prevention lies in warming-up properly and stretching, taking deep breaths before an exercise bout, and avoiding flatulent (gas-producing) foods before exercising.

NERVE RELATED INJURIES

Nerve impingement syndromes can occur with fitness activities. Sciatica probably is the most common. It was discussed earlier with overuse musculoskeletal injuries. Two other injuries are associated with cycling. One is **ulnar neuropathy** and the other is a **genital irritation.** Ulnar neuropathy affects the nerve that runs down the outside of the arm and hand. When a cyclist leans forward on the handlebars, pressure is placed on the hands. After prolonged riding, the pressure may cause a numbness in the hand where the nerve is being compressed. Prevention of this condition is to pad the handlebars or change positions occasionally during the exercise bout.

Change Positions

Genital irritation can occur in cyclists whose saddles do not fit properly. The irritation may take the form of chafing, nerve impingement (males especially), or ischial bursitis (females especially). Adjusting the seat to the proper height can be used as prevention techniques for these conditions.

A summary of some common prevention suggestions for specific overuse injuries are listed in Table 13.4.

HEAT RELATED INJURIES

The hypothalamus gland, located in the brainstem, is the "thermostat" for the body. It senses extreme changes in temperature within the body. The normal body temperature is 98.6 degrees Fahrenheit, but it can range from 91.6 degrees to 105.6 degrees for short periods of time with very little damage to the system. However, in the case of heat, when temperatures within the body rise excessively high, the hypothalamus reacts by causing the blood vessels to vasodilate. The sweat glands are activated to produce a cooling affect on the body.

Prevention of Common Fitness Related Injuries

Injury	Prevention
Achilles Tendinitis	Use a heel lift in shoe • Get shoe orthotics • Avoid sudden increases in mileage or routines • Avoid exercising on hard surfaces • Avoid excessive uphill running • Buy shoes with good rearfoot control • Stretch lower leg muscles (gastroc/soleus) • Strengthen lower leg muscles
Hamstring Strain	Stretch the hamstring muscles before and after exercising • Strengthen hamstring muscles equally
Iliotibial Band Syndrome	Use orthotics for unequal leg lengths • Buy shoes with good cushioning • Avoid excessive downhill running • Avoid running on cambered hills/roads
Knee Pain	Strengthen quadricep muscles equally • Stretch the hamstring muscles before and after exercising • Stretch the iliotibial band before and after exercising • Buy shoes with good shock absorption and rearfoot control • Avoid exercising on extremely "soft" surfaces • Avoid excessive downhill running • Avoid knee hyperextension movements
Low Back Pain	Use orthotics for excessive pronation • Use heel lifts for unequal leg lengths • Strengthen abdominal and lower back muscles • Stretch the hip flexors (iliopsoas) • Stretch the lower back muscles • Avoid banked surfaces • Reverse directions in running activities • Do low impact aerobic routines
Misc. Foot Problems (blisters, corns, ingrown toe nails)	Buy good fitting shoes • Avoid wrinkled socks in shoes • Avoid undue pressures on toes
Muscle Cramps	Drink plenty of fluids before and during activity • Avoid overexertion • Eat foods high in potassium
Muscle soreness	Stretch before and after activity • Avoid excessive "negative" work • Gradually increase intensity of exercise
Nerve Impingement	Use padding when necessary • Change body positioning periodically • Adjust seat on bicycle
Plantar Faciitis	Use shoe orthotics to compensate for any foot abnormality • Strengthen anterior and posterior muscles of lower leg equally • Buy shoes with good arch support, shock absorption, and rearfoot control • Avoid exercising on hard surfaces • Avoid sudden increases in intensity of exercise • Do low impact aerobic dance routines
Shin Splints	Strengthen lower leg muscles • Stretch lower leg muscles before and after exercising • Buy shoes with good shock absorption and rearfoot control • Avoid exercising on hard surfaces • Avoid excessive hill running • Avoid prolonged exercise on banked surfaces • Avoid excessive mileage or prolonged routines in the early stages of an exercise program • Do low impact aerobic dance routines
Stress Fractures	Use a heel lift for unequal leg lengths • Strengthen lower leg muscles equally • Buy a shoe with good shock absorption • Avoid exercising on hard surfaces • Avoid intensive and excessive mileage or prolonged routines in earlier stages of a program • Do low impact aerobic dance routines

Table 13.4.

Heat Stress Index

TOTAL of Temperature (°F) + Humidity (%)	Zone
Equals 160 or less	Safe
Equals 161-175	Caution
Equals 176-190	Dangerous
Equals 191 or more	Extremely Dangerous

Figure 13.3. Any combination of humidity and temperature adding up to 160 or less is considered safe to exercise. (Institute for Aerobic Research, 1979.)

A more problematic situation arises when changes in heat are accompanied by changes in humidity. The combination of high temperatures and high humidity can make exercising extremely risky because many of the body's cooling mechanisms are inhibited. To avoid the risk, an exerciser should consider the heat stress index shown in Figure 13.3. Any combination of air temperature and relative humidity adding up to 160 or less would be a safe environment in which to exercise. Combinations above 190 would be extremely dangerous.

HEAT EXHAUSTION

Heat exhaustion is most likely to occur on hot, humid days, during the times of the day when the sun is directly overhead, or when the air is still. Exercise participants become dehydrated causing the blood volume to drop. Because the muscles and cardiovascular system need the blood flow, the skin is denied its share. That is why the characteristic signs of heat exhaustion are profuse sweating, cool and moist skin, rapid and weak pulse, weakness, dizziness, headache, and nausea.

HEAT STROKE

Danger: Body Shutting Down

Heat stroke results from extremely high body temperatures, and should be considered a death-threatening situation. The body's ability to cool itself has failed because the evaporation mechanism for dissipating body heat shuts down. The signs and symptoms of heat stroke are hot and dry skin, flushed skin, rapid and pounding pulse, elevated blood pressure, and deliriousness.

To prevent heat related injuries from occurring, a fitness participant should be acclimatized slowly to the heat conditions, lightweight and "airy" clothing should be worn, plenty of fluids should be taken, and the heat stress index should be checked before beginning the exercise bout.

COLD RELATED INJURIES

Body temperatures drop when heat losses become greater than heat production. When body temperature falls below 90 degrees Fahrenheit, the body responds by closing down the circulation to the skin and by shivering. If the situation continues, the regulatory system fails, respiration becomes difficult, the heart begins to fibrillate, and death may be imminent.

HYPOTHERMIA

When fitness participants exercise in cooler air temperatures, cooler winds, and wet conditions, they may be vulnerable to **hypothermia.** This occurs when the exerciser begins removing outer clothing in response to the perspiration generated during the activity. The signs and symptoms are shivering, vague and slurred speech, incoherence, stumbling, muscle rigidity, discolored skin, and drowsiness.

FROSTBITE

Study the Chill Factor

As outdoor temperatures become colder, the body is susceptible to **frostbite** injuries. When the body becomes chilled, the fluids around the skin turn to ice crystals. In the early stages of frostbite, there is a redness to the skin, some swelling, and numbness. As the severity of the condition increases, more damage is done to the underlying tissues of the body. The severity will depend on the temperature, wind factor, humidity, and length of exposure. Because of their prominence on the body, the ears, nose, fingers, and toes are most vulnerable to frostbite.

To prevent cold related injuries from occurring, several things can be done. Layers of clothing should be worn with the outer layers being wind and water proof. Mittens for the hands, muffs for the ears, and cotton socks next to the skin are best. Acclimatization to cooler temperatures should take place if possible. Eat properly to account for the increased metabolic activity. Avoid alcohol and nicotine. Check the wind chill chart (Table 13.5) before exercising.

Wind-Chill Chart

Wind MPH	**Temperature** (Fahrenheit)																				
Calm	**40°**	**35°**	**30°**	**25°**	**20°**	**15°**	**10°**	**5°**	**0°**	**–5°**	**–10°**	**–15°**	**–20°**	**–25°**	**–30°**	**–35°**	**–40°**	**–45°**	**–50°**	**–55°**	**–60°**
5	35°	30°	25°	20°	15°	10°	5°	0°	–5°	–10°	–15°	–20°	–25°	–30°	–35°	–40°	–45°	–50°	–55°	–65°	–70°
10	30°	20°	15°	10°	5°	0°	–10°	–15°	–20°	–25°	–35°	–40°	–45°	–50°	–60°	–65°	–70°	–75°	–80°	–90°	–95°
15	25°	15°	10°	0°	–5°	–10°	–20°	–25°	–30°	–40°	–45°	–50°	–60°	–65°	–70°	–80°	–85°	–90°	–100°	–105°	–110°
20	20°	10°	5°	0°	–10°	–15°	–25°	–30°	–35°	–45°	–50°	–60°	–65°	–75°	–80°	–85°	–95°	–100°	–110°	–115°	–120°
25	15°	10°	0°	–5°	–15°	–20°	–30°	–35°	–45°	–50°	–60°	–65°	–75°	–80°	–90°	–95°	–105°	–110°	–120°	–125°	–135°
30	10°	5°	0°	–10°	–20°	–25°	–30°	–40°	–50°	–55°	–65°	–70°	–80°	–85°	–95°	–100°	–105°	–115°	–120°	–130°	–140°
35	10°	5°	–5°	–10°	–20°	–25°	–35°	–40°	–50°	–60°	–65°	–75°	–80°	–90°	–100°	–105°	–115°	–120°	–130°	–135°	–145°
40*	10°	0°	–5°	–15°	–20°	–30°	–35°	–45°	–55°	–60°	–70°	–75°	–85°	–95°	–100°	–110°	–115°	–125°	–130°	–140°	–150°

Little Danger (40°–20° at 20–40 mph) | **Increasing Danger** (Flesh may freeze within one minute) | **Great Danger** (Flesh may freeze within 30 seconds)

* *Winds above 40 mph have little additional effect.*

Table 13.5. Exercising in extremely windy and cold conditions is dangerous. Source: National Oceanic and Atmospheric Administration

PREVENTION OF MUSCULOSKELETAL INJURIES

Overuse injuries can be traced to four major causes: training errors, anatomical misalignments, improper shoes, and unsuitable exercise surfaces. To prevent these injuries from occurring, we must avoid the things that cause them.

Suggestions for Preventing Overuse Injuries

1. **Avoid training errors.** Start a new program slowly and progress slowly. Avoid any sudden changes in the training schedule like training longer or at a higher intensity. High intensity training over a long period of time also is not desirable. The body needs time to recover from the exercise bouts. It should be mentioned that returning to exercise after an injury or illness should be done slowly.

2. **Warm-up before a bout.** A proper warm-up before participation is essential. Using cold muscles is not only inefficient, but makes one more susceptible to sprain and strain type injuries. (See Chapter 7)

3. **Flexibility.** Maintain good range of motion in all joints and good stretchability in all muscles. This, too, will avoid sprain and strain injuries. (See Chapter 7)

4. **Muscle strength and balance.** Strength is the foundation for all performance, and ultimately for the prevention of most injury problems. Of particular importance is an equal balance of strength in antagonistic muscle groups (e.g., hamstrings, quadriceps) and in contralateral (e.g., right leg gastrocnemius and left leg gastrocnemius). (See Chapter 8)

5. **Techniques.** Many injuries can be prevented by simply performing the activity correctly. Seek expert help in performing unfamiliar activities. With fitness related activities, attention to postural alignment is of utmost importance.

6. **Surfaces.** Avoid exercising on extremely hard or soft surfaces. Impact forces are increased greatly. Also, in running, avoid cambered or uneven surfaces. Excessive hill running should be avoided.

7. **Wear the proper shoes.** Most shoe stores now have sales people who are knowledgeable in shoe design and what is best for your needs. Those people who are excessive pronators (feet roll inward) generally have flat arches. They need shoes with good arch supports and good rearfoot stability. People who are supinators (feet roll outward) need shoes with good cushioning. Also buy shoes designed for your activity. Cross-trainers are especially desirable.

8. **Wear orthotics.** If you have an anatomical misalignment these devices in shoes help to correct misalignment problems. They should be prescribed by a qualified person such as a podiatrist (foot doctor) or orthopedist (bone doctor).

9. **Consider cross training.** Get involved in other activities to avoid stressing the same anatomical structures.

10. **Common sense and safety first should prevail.**

Suggested Readings

Griffith, H. W. *Complete Guide to Sports Injuries.* Tucson: HP Books, Inc., 1985.

Hafen, B. Q. *First Aid for Health Emergencies.* St. Paul: West Publishing Company, 1981.

Morris, A. F. *Sports Medicine: Prevention of Athletic Injuries.* Dubuque: Wm. C. Brown Publishers, 1984.

Peterson L. and P. Renstrom. *Sports Injuries: Their Prevention and Treatment.* Chicago: Year Book Medical Publishers, Inc.,1986.

Roy, S. and R. Irvin. *Sports Medicine: Prevention, Evaluation, Management, and Rehabilitation.* Englewood Cliffs: Prentice-Hall, Inc., 1983.

Schneider, R. C., J. C. Kennedy, and M. L. Plant. *Sports Injuries: Mechanisms, Prevention, and Treatment.* Baltimore: Williams and Wilkins, 1985.

Southmayd, W., and M. Hoffman. *Sports Health: The Complete Book of Athletic Injuries.* New York: Quick Fox, 1981.

Zebas, C. and M. Chapman. *Prevention of Sports Injuries: A Biomechanical Approach.* Dubuque: eddie bowers publishing, inc., 1990.

CHAPTER

14 INVENTORIES FOR FITNESS AND HEALTH PROMOTION

Contents

1) Hamstring Flexibility 215
2) Iliopsoas Flexibility 217
3) Adductor Flexibility 219
4) Shoulder Flexibility 221
5) Shoulder and Upper Arm Flexibility 223
6) Upper Back Flexibility........................ 225
7) Abdominal Flexibility 227
8) Sit and Reach 229
9) Posture Assessment 231
10) Health Risk Appraisal 233
11) Stress Inventory 237
12) Nutrition Survey 239
13) Exercise Survey 241
14) Relaxation Survey 243
15) Stress Symptom Checklist 245
16) Guidelines for Effective Stress Management..... 247
17) Type A/B Behavior Evaluation 249
18) Hostility Evaluation 251
19) Body Fat Assessment 253
20) Waist/Hip Ratio (WHR) 257
21) Ideal Body Weight 259
22) Caloric Balance 261
23) Diet Analysis Software 265
24) One Mile Walk Test 267
25) Adult Fit-N-Dex 269
26) Personal Wellness Life-Style Plan 271
27) Strength Assessment 273
28) Exercise Log 277
29) Resistance Training Workout Records 279
30) Fat, Fiber and Sodium Log 281

HAMSTRING FLEXIBILITY

Inventory 1

Name ______________________ Date ______________

Before beginning a stretching program, it is wise to assess where you are in terms of flexibility. Remember there is no such thing as overall flexibility. Flexibility is specific to a joint. You may be flexible in one area of the body but not another. It is, therefore, important to consider doing a battery of screening tests to assess your flexibility.

A screening session for flexibility should be conducted before an exercise program is begun. Determine where your strengths and weaknesses are. If you are not flexible enough in certain areas of the body, plan a program of stretching exercises to improve those areas. See Chapter 7 for exercise examples. Test yourself periodically to assess your current status.

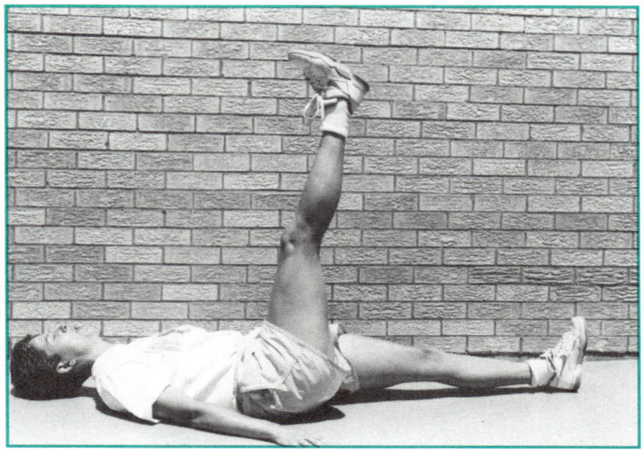

DIRECTIONS: The person lies on the ground with both legs extended. Keeping one leg on the ground with the knee straight, the opposite leg is raised as high as possible so that the leg and body form a 90 degree angle. If a 90 degree angle cannot be achieved the test has been failed. Repeat the test on the opposite leg. The entire test should be repeated three times and the best score recorded.

Hamstring Scoresheet

Week	Pass	Fail	Date:
1			Strengths:
2			
3			
4			
5			Weaknesses:
6			
7			
8			
9			Goals:
10			
11			
12			

ILIOPSOAS FLEXIBILITY

Inventory 2

Name ______________________ Date ______________

DIRECTIONS: The iliopsoas is an important hip flexor muscle. It's function is to bring the thigh forward in such activities as running. On the other hand, this muscle must be flexible to allow the thigh to swing backward. If it is tight, it inhibits a full range of motion about the hip. A simple pass-fail test for assessing the flexibility of this muscle is demonstrated. The subject being tested lies on a table so that the legs extend over the edge. One of the legs is grasped below the knee with both hands and drawn up toward the chest. The opposite leg should remain in its original hanging position. If it moves upward, the iliopsoas is considered to be tight on that side and the test has been failed. Repeat the test on the other leg.

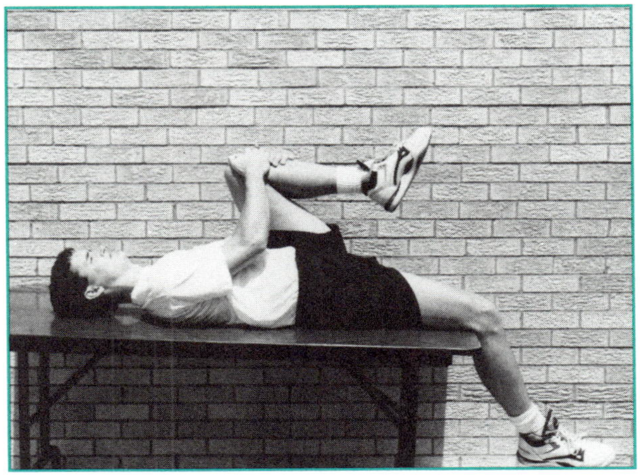

Iliopsoas Scoresheet

Week	Pass	Fail
1		
2		
3		
4		
5		
6		
7		
8		
9		
10		
11		
12		

Date:
Strengths:
Weaknesses:
Goals:

ADDUCTOR FLEXIBILITY

Inventory 3

Name ______________________ Date ______________________

DIRECTIONS: The flexibility of the adductor muscles (groin) may be tested in a seated position. The subject being tested sits on the ground with the soles of the feet touching each other and placed about 6 inches from the groin as shown. The knees are pushed toward the ground. If the knees cannot be pushed to within 2 inches of the ground, the test has been failed.

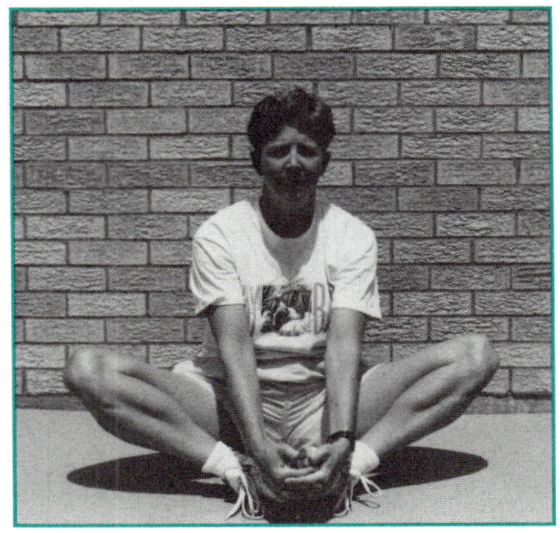

Hamstrings Scoresheet

Week	Pass	Fail
1		
2		
3		
4		
5		
6		
7		
8		
9		
10		
11		
12		

Date:

Strengths:

Weaknesses:

Goals:

SHOULDER FLEXIBILITY

Inventory 4

Name ______________________ Date ______________

DIRECTIONS: One test for shoulder flexibility calls for the subject to lie on the ground. The chin and toes should remain on the ground for the entire test. The arms are grasped behind the back and lifted upward as demonstrated. The ideal position is for the arms to form a 45 degree angle with the body. If this cannot be done, the test is considered to have been failed.

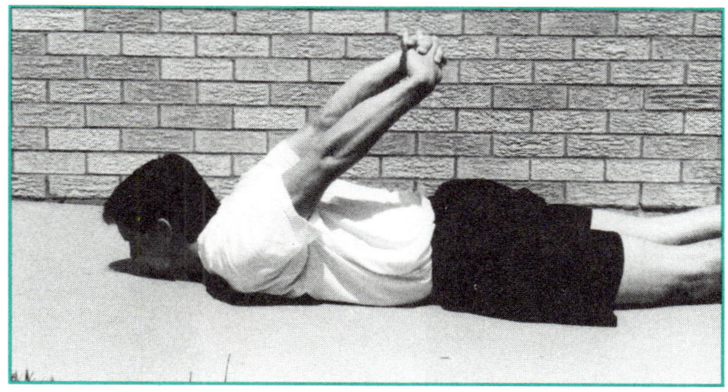

Shoulder Scoresheet

Week	Pass	Fail
1		
2		
3		
4		
5		
6		
7		
8		
9		
10		
11		
12		

Date:
Strengths:
Weaknesses:
Goals:

SHOULDER AND UPPER ARM FLEXIBILITY

Inventory 5

Name ______________________ Date ______________

DIRECTIONS: Grasp the hands on each side of the body behind the back. One hand reaches up under the shoulder blade while the other hand reaches over the top of the shoulder blade. If the fingers do not touch, the test has been failed.

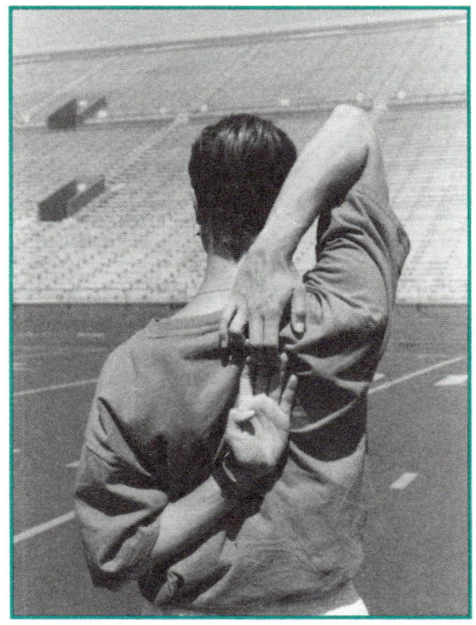

Shoulder and Upper Arm Scoresheet

<table>
<tr><th>Week</th><th>Pass</th><th>Fail</th><th>Date:</th></tr>
<tr><td>1</td><td></td><td></td><td rowspan="4">Strengths:</td></tr>
<tr><td>2</td><td></td><td></td></tr>
<tr><td>3</td><td></td><td></td></tr>
<tr><td>4</td><td></td><td></td></tr>
<tr><td>5</td><td></td><td></td><td rowspan="4">Weaknesses:</td></tr>
<tr><td>6</td><td></td><td></td></tr>
<tr><td>7</td><td></td><td></td></tr>
<tr><td>8</td><td></td><td></td></tr>
<tr><td>9</td><td></td><td></td><td rowspan="4">Goals:</td></tr>
<tr><td>10</td><td></td><td></td></tr>
<tr><td>11</td><td></td><td></td></tr>
<tr><td>12</td><td></td><td></td></tr>
</table>

UPPER BACK FLEXIBILITY

Inventory 6

Name ______________________ Date ______________________

DIRECTIONS: The flexibility of the upper back may be assessed by using a test called the plough. The subject being tested lies on the ground and attempts to draw the legs over the head as demonstrated. The object is to touch the toes to the ground while keeping the legs straight. If the toes do not touch the ground, the test has been failed. NOTE: If there are any existing back or neck problems, this test should not be performed.

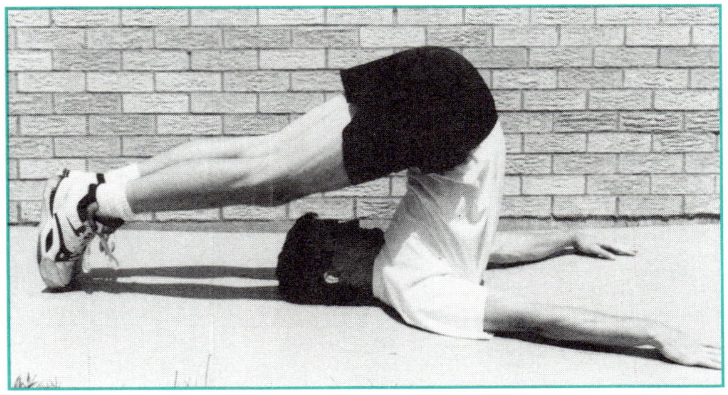

Upper Back Scoresheet

Week	Pass	Fail	Date:
1			Strengths:
2			
3			
4			
5			Weaknesses:
6			
7			
8			
9			Goals:
10			
11			
12			

ABDOMINAL FLEXIBILITY

Inventory 7

Name ______________________ Date ______________________

DIRECTIONS: The subject being tested lies on the ground and attempts to raise both outstretched arms off the ground. Both feet should remain in contact with the ground throughout the test. A second person holds a ruler or yardstick in an upright position near the center of the shoulder. The height the upper body is lifted off the ground is measured in inches. Three trials should be given with the best score recorded.

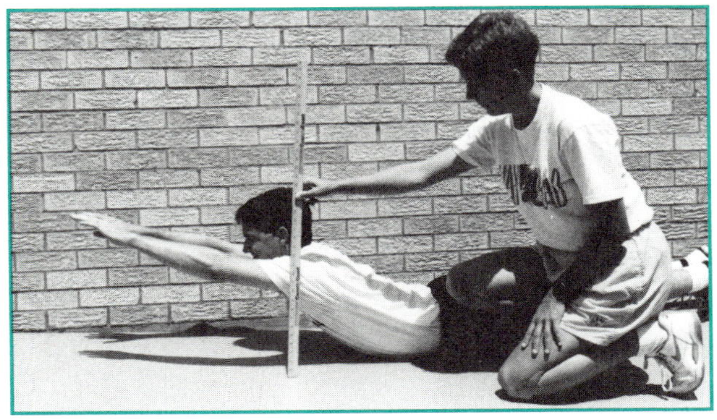

How to Score

High	Average	Low
>10"	6-10"	<6"

Abdominal Scoresheet

Week	Pass	Fail	Date:
1			Strengths:
2			
3			
4			
5			Weaknesses:
6			
7			
8			
9			Goals:
10			
11			
12			

SIT AND REACH

Inventory 8

Name ______________________ Date ______________________

DIRECTIONS: The sit and reach test is used to assess the flexibility of the hamstrings muscle group and the muscles of the lower back . The person being tested is seated with the legs extended and the feet at a 90 degree angle to the ground. The person administering the test holds a ruler or yardstick against the upper sole of the shoe and horizontal to the floor. The person performing the test bends at the waist, keeps the knees straight, and reaches forward with both hands. The score is the number of inches reached beyond the toes. If the person cannot reach to or beyond the toes, measure the number of inches from the hands to the soles of the shoes. This score will be a negative score. The entire test should be repeated three times with the best score being recorded.

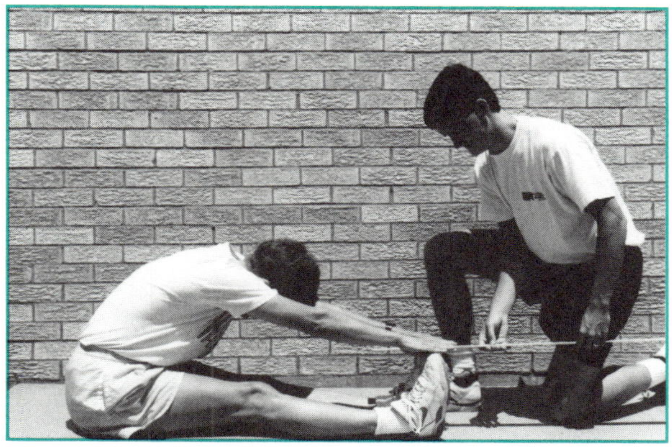

How to Score

High	Average	Low
>8"	2-8"	<2"

Sit and Reach Scoresheet

Week	Pass	Fail	Date:
1			Strengths:
2			
3			
4			
5			Weaknesses:
6			
7			
8			
9			Goals:
10			
11			
12			

POSTURE ASSESSMENT

Inventory 9

Name ______________________ Date ______________

DIRECTIONS: Good posture implies proper alignment of body parts for the purpose of producing maximum functional efficiency in movement activities. Improper relationships of body parts often lead to stress in some part of the body. Minor deviations in postural alignment are common in the general population. These should not be cause for undue concern, and performances are unlikely to be affected in most activities. The major concern lies in the possibility of pain or fatigue occurring due to stress. Pain most likely would occur in running which is a repetitive activity. Postural malalignments such as unequal leg lengths or pronated feet can precipitate painful conditions. Major deviations should be referred to an orthopedist or a podiatrist. These conditions may require special care for the proper functioning of the body parts.

Posture may be assessed quickly and efficiently in several ways. One way is to use some form of a grid as the background. A brick wall can provide such a grid. The position of the head, shoulders, hips, knees, and feet can be viewed in relation to the lines on the grid (Figure A). Use Posture Evaluation on page 232 as a guide for assessing front or back postural alignment.

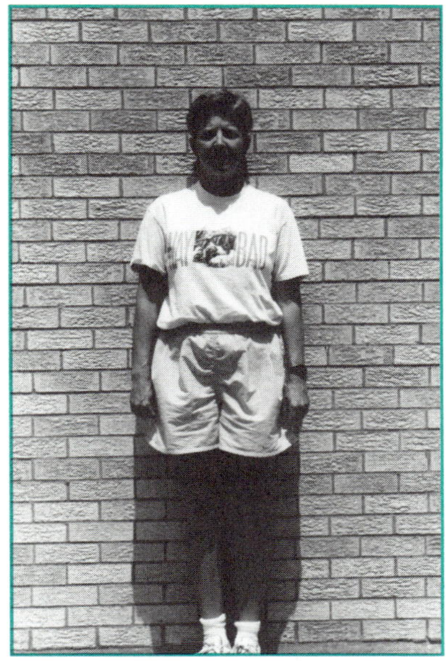

Figure A. Posture analysis using brick wall as a grid.

Body Alignment for Aerobic Dance Exercise

Viewing the subject from the side also is valuable. A plumb line (a weight suspended at the end of a string) can be used to determine side view alignment. The string should be held above the head and allowed to drop to the ground. Good alignment would cause the plumb line to intersect the ear, shoulder, hip, back of the knee, and front of the ankle. See Posture Evaluation on page 232 as a guide for assessing side view postural alignment. NOTE: The less clothing worn, the better the view of the body.

In the erect standing position, the pelvis is aligned with the knees and the rib cage. The knees are relaxed and aligned over the arches of the foot. The abdominals and gluteals are tightened so they align over the feet. The head rests comfortably over the shoulders with the eyes looking straight ahead (Figure B). Figure C is an example of someone whose shoulders are hunched forward and the hips are thrown forward. (In kinesiology terminology this is known as a backward or posterior pelvic tilt.) Figure D shows another "extreme" position. Here the pelvis has been thrust backward (forward or anterior pelvic tilt) giving the appearance of a "sway back." The misaligned positioning of the body structures creates stresses on the joints and muscles of the body and cause the body to fatigue more quickly than normal.

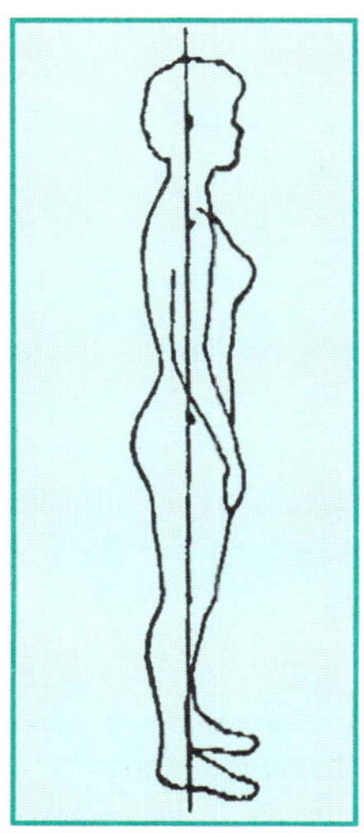

Figure B. Good body alignment.

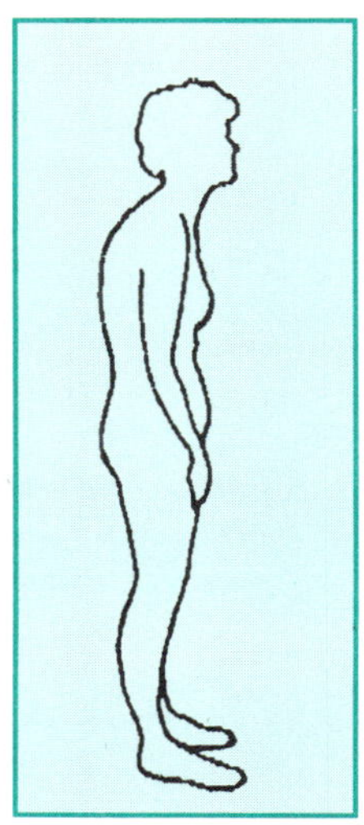

Figure C. Hunched shoulders, backward pelvic tilt.

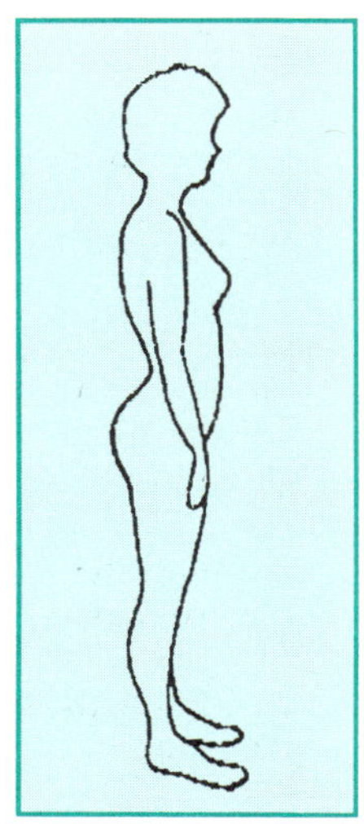

Figure D. Foward pelvic tilt, sway back.

Arch of Foot Assessment

To determine the shape of the arch of the foot, a simple barefoot "water" test can be performed. Simply wet the bottom of the foot (e.g., stepping out of the shower) and step onto a surface where the imprint will be left. The higher the arch, the less the amount of imprint left on the surface over the arch area (Figure E). Use the following Posture Evaluation for assessing your arch.

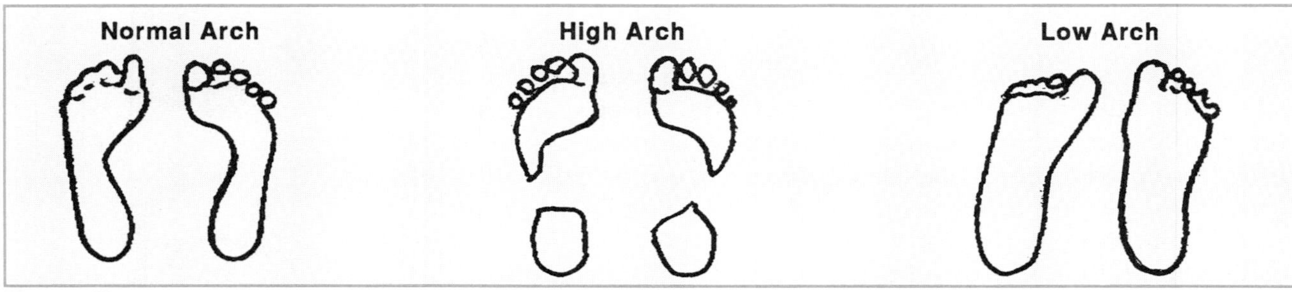

Figure E

Check the items which best describe your posture.

Posture Evaluation

Body Part	Condition	
Head and Neck (front/back)	◯ Aligned over spinal column	◯ Tilted to right or left
Head and Neck (side)	◯ Ear in line with shoulder	◯ Tilted forward or backward
Shoulders (front/back)	◯ Level with each other	◯ One shoulder higher than another
Spine (front/back)	◯ Straight	◯ Curved to right or left
Hips (front/back)	◯ Level with each other	◯ One hip higher than another
Trunk and Lower Back (side)	◯ Shoulders aligned over hips ◯ Arched back	◯ Hunched shoulders
Abdomen (side)	◯ Flat	◯ Protruding
Knees and Lower Legs (front/back)	◯ Straight ◯ Bowed out	◯ Knock knees
Knees and Lower Legs (side)	◯ Straight	◯ Hyperextended
Ankles and Feet (front/back)	◯ Toes pointed straight ahead ◯ Toes pointed outward	◯ Heel perpendicular to floor
Arches	◯ Normal ◯ High	◯ Low

HEALTH RISK APPRAISAL (HRA)

Inventory 10

Name ______________________ Date ______________

DIRECTIONS: This sample questionnaire is from a microcomputer based software program titled *Healthier People Version 4.0* (IBM PC, XT, or AT compatible). The software package is designed as an educational tool. It shows you choices you can make to keep good health and avoid the most common causes of death for a person your age and sex. This health risk appraisal is not a substitute for a check-up or physical exam that you get from a doctor or nurse. It only gives you some ideas for lowering your risk of getting sick or injured in the future. Users with little or no computer experience can begin processing HRAs within a few hours and can add customized questions to the basic questionnaire, as well as a personalized message to the reports. The program provides participant reports highlighting the health risks affecting life expectancy and pinpointing particular risks the individual can control. A group report is also available to assess the health status of an organization's employees and to help set priorities for health promotion efforts. In addition to the *Healthier People* software program, users receive a camera ready copy of the questionnaire and a 532 page manual. The manual has extensive documentation of the program's structure and risk calculations, and step by step operating instructions, including how to customize the questionnaire and reports.

The software for this HRA is available for $150 plus $5 for insurance/shipping. For additional information call *eddie bowers publishing, inc.* 1-800-747-2411.

Please put your answers in the empty boxes. (Examples: [X] or [125])

1. SEX	1 ☐ Male 2 ☐ Female
2. AGE	☐ Years
3. HEIGHT (Without shoes) (No fractions)	☐ Feet ☐ Inches
4. WEIGHT (Without shoes) (No fractions)	☐ Pounds
5. Body frame size	1 ☐ Small 2 ☐ Medium 3 ☐ Large
6. Have you ever been told that you have diabetes (or sugar diabetes)?	1 ☐ Yes 2 ☐ No
7. Are you now taking medicine for high blood pressure?	1 ☐ Yes 2 ☐ No
8. What is your blood pressure now?	☐ / ☐ Systolic (High number)/Diastolic (Low number)
9. If you *do not* know the numbers, check the box that describes your blood pressure.	1 ☐ High 2 ☐ Normal or Low 3 ☐ Don't Know
10. What is your TOTAL cholesterol level (based on a blood test)?	☐ mg/dl
11. What is your HDL cholesterol (based on a blood test)?	☐ mg/dl
12. How many cigars do you usually smoke per day?	☐ cigars per day
13. How many pipes of tobacco do you usually smoke per day?	☐ pipes per day
14. How many times per day do you usually use smokeless tobacco? (Chewing tobacco, snuff, pouches, etc.)	☐ times per day

15. CIGARETTE SMOKING
How would you describe your cigarette smoking habits?

1 ☐ Never smoked ☛ Go to 18
2 ☐ Used to Smoke ☛ Go to 17
3 ☐ Still Smoke ☛ Go to 16

16. STILL SMOKE
How many cigarettes a day do you smoke?

☐ cigarettes per day ☛ Go to 18

☛ GO TO QUESTION 18

17. USED TO SMOKE
a. How many years has it been since you smoked cigarettes fairly regularly?

☐ years

b. What was the average number of cigarettes per day that you smoked in the 2 years before you quit?

☐ cigarettes per day

18. In the next 12 months how many thousands of miles will you probably travel by each of the following?
(NOTE: U.S. average = 10,000 miles)
a. Car, truck, or van: ☐ ,000 miles
b. Motorcycle: ☐ ,000 miles

19. On a typical day how do you USUALLY travel?
(Check one only)

1 ☐ Walk
2 ☐ Bicycle
3 ☐ Motorcycle
4 ☐ Sub-compact or compact car
5 ☐ Mid-size or full-size car
6 ☐ Truck or van
7 ☐ Bus, subway, or train
8 ☐ Mostly stay home

20. What percent of the time do you usually buckle your safety belt when driving or riding?

☐ %

21. On the average, how close to the speed limit do you usually drive?

1 ☐ Within 5 mph of limit
2 ☐ 6-10 mph over limit
3 ☐ 11-15 mph over limit
4 ☐ More than 15 mph over limit

22. How many times in the last month did your drive or ride when the driver had perhaps too much alcohol to drink?

☐ times last month

23. How many drinks of alcoholic beverage do your have in a typical week?

(Write number of each type of drink)
☐ Bottles or cans of beer
☐ Glasses of wine
☐ Wine coolers
☐ Mixed drinks or shots of liquor

☛ *(MEN GO TO QUESTION 33)*

WOMEN

24. At what age did you have your first menstrual period?

☐ years old

25. How old were you when your first child was born?

☐ years old
(If no children write 0)

26. How long has it been since your last breast x-ray (mammogram)?	1 ☐ Less than 1 year ago 2 ☐ 1 year ago 3 ☐ 2 years ago 4 ☐ 3 or more years ago 5 ☐ Never
27. How many women in your natural family (mother and sisters only) have had breast cancer?	☐ women
28. Have you had a hysterectomy operation?	1 ☐ Yes 2 ☐ No 3 ☐ Not sure
29. How long has it been since you had a pap smear?	1 ☐ Less than 1 year ago 2 ☐ 1 year ago 3 ☐ 2 years ago 4 ☐ 3 or more years ago 5 ☐ Never
★ 30. How often do you examine your breasts for lumps?	1 ☐ Monthly 2 ☐ Once every few months 3 ☐ Rarely or never
★ 31. About how long has it been since you had your breasts examined by a physican or nurse?	1 ☐ Less than 1 year ago 2 ☐ 1 year ago 3 ☐ 2 years ago 4 ☐ 3 or more years ago 5 ☐ Never
★ 32. About how long has it been since you had a rectal exam? ☛ *(WOMEN GO TO QUESTION 34)*	1 ☐ Less than 1 year ago 2 ☐ 1 year ago 3 ☐ 2 years ago 4 ☐ 3 or more years ago 5 ☐ Never
MEN ★ 33. About how long has it been since you had a rectal or prostate exam?	1 ☐ Less than 1 year ago 2 ☐ 1 year ago 3 ☐ 2 years ago 4 ☐ 3 or more years ago 5 ☐ Never
★ 34. How many times in the last year did you witness or become involved in a violent fight or attack where there was a good chance of a serious injury to someone?	1 ☐ 4 or more times 2 ☐ 2 or 3 times 3 ☐ 1 time or never 4 ☐ Not sure
★ 35. Considering your age, how would you describe your overall physical health?	1 ☐ Excellent 2 ☐ Good 3 ☐ Fair 4 ☐ Poor
★ 36. In an average week, how many times do you engage in physical activity (exercise or work which lasts at least 20 minutes without stopping and which is hard enough to make you breathe heavier and your heart beat faster)?	1 ☐ Less than 1 time per week 2 ☐ 1 or 2 times per week 3 ☐ At least 3 times per week
★ 37. If you ride a motorcycle or all-terrain vehicle (ATV) what percent of the time do you wear a helmet?	1 ☐ 75% to 100% 2 ☐ 25% to 74% 3 ☐ Less than 25% 4 ☐ Does not apply to me

★38. Do you eat some food every day that is high in fiber, such as whole grain bread, cereal, fresh fruits or vegetables?	1 ☐ Yes 2 ☐ No
★39. Do you eat foods every day that are high in cholesterol or fat such as fatty meat, cheese, fried foods, or eggs?	1 ☐ Yes 2 ☐ No
★40. In general, how satisfied are you with your life?	1 ☐ Mostly satisfied 2 ☐ Partly satisfied 3 ☐ Not satisfied
★41. Have you suffered a personal loss or misfortune in the past year that had a serious impact on your life? (For example, a job loss, disability, separation, jail term, or the death of someone close to you.)	1 ☐ Yes, 1 serious loss or misfortune 2 ☐ Yes, 2 or more 3 ☐ No
★42a. Race	1 ☐ Aleutian, Alaska native, Eskimo or American Indian 2 ☐ Asian 3 ☐ Black 4 ☐ Pacific Islander 5 ☐ White 6 ☐ Other 7 ☐ Don't know
★42b. Are you of Hispanic origin such as Mexican-American, Puerto Rican, or Cuban?	1 ☐ Yes 2 ☐ No
★43. What is the highest grade you completed in school?	1 ☐ Grade school or less 2 ☐ Some high school 3 ☐ High school graduate 4 ☐ Some college 5 ☐ College graduate 6 ☐ Post graduate or professional degree
★I.	A ☐ B ☐ C ☐ D ☐ E ☐ F ☐ G ☐ H ☐ I ☐ J ☐ K ☐ L ☐
★II.	A ☐ B ☐ C ☐ D ☐ E ☐ F ☐ G ☐ H ☐ I ☐ J ☐ K ☐ L ☐

Last Name	First Name	M.I.
Address	City State	Zip

STRESS INVENTORY

Inventory 11

Name______________________________ Date______________________

DIRECTIONS: Following is a list of events.* Circle the number next to the life event that has happened to you in the past year. When you've gone through the entire list, add up your score. The higher the total score the more stress you have experienced (see scoring interpretation on next page).

Life Event	Point Values	Life Event	Point Values
Death of a spouse	100	Change in work responsibilities	29
Divorce	73	Son or daughter leaving home	29
Marital separation	65	Trouble with in-laws	29
Jail term	63	Outstanding personal achievement	28
Death of close family member	63	Spouse begins or stops work	26
Personal injury or illness	53	Starting or finishing school	26
Marriage	50	Change in living conditions	25
Fired from work	47	Revision of personal habits	24
Marital reconciliation	45	Trouble with boss	23
Retirement	45	Change in work hours, conditions	20
Change in family member's health	44	Change in residence	20
Pregnancy	40	Change in schools	20
Sex difficulties	39	Change in recreational habits	19
Addition to family	39	Change in church activities	19
Business readjustment	39	Change in social activities	18
Change in financial status	38	Mortgage or loan under $10,000	17
Death of a close friend	37	Change in sleeping habits	16
Change to different line of work	36	Change in number of family gatherings	15
Change in number of marital arguments	35	Change in eating habits	15
Mortgage or loan over $10,000**	31	Vacation	13
Foreclosure of mortgage or loan	30	Christmas season	12
		Minor violations of the law	11
		Score	

* If you are a full-time student or under 25, use the Student Questionnaire that follows. If you are borderline between these two life phases, take both and use the higher score.

** An updated version might be "Mortgage or loan payment more than 25 percent of salary."

Inventory is from Holmes, T.H. and R.H. Rahe. The Social readjustment rating scale. *Journal of Psychosomatic Research.* 11:213-218, 1967. Used with permission of Pergamon Press Ltd. Oxford, England.

STRESS INVENTORY FOR STUDENTS

Name____________________ Date____________________

DIRECTIONS: Following are events that occur in the life of a college student. Circle the number next to the life event that has happened to you in the past year. When you've gone through the entire list, add up your score. The higher the total score the more stress you have experienced.

Life Event	Point Values	Life Event	Point Values
Death of a close family member	100	Problems with your boss or professor	25
Jail term	80	Outstanding personal achievement	25
Final year or first year in college	63	Failure in some course	25
Pregnancy (to you or caused by you)	60	Final exams	20
Severe personal illness or injury	53	Increased or decreased dating	20
Marriage	50	Change in working conditions	20
Any interpersonal problems	45	Change in your major	20
Financial difficulties	40	Change in your sleeping habits	18
Death of a close friend	40	Several-day vacation	15
Arguments with your roommate (more than every other day)	40	Change in eating habits	15
Major disagreements with your family	40	Family reunion	15
Major change in personal habits	30	Change in recreational activities	15
Change in living environment	30	Minor illness or injury	15
Beginning or ending a job	30	Minor violations of the law	11

Inventory is from Holmes, T.H. and R.H. Rahe. The Social readjustment rating scale. *Journal of Psychosomatic Research.* 11:213-218, 1967. Used with permission of Pergamon Press Ltd. Oxford, England.

Score ______

Scoring Interpretation

Low Stress	Moderate Stress	High Stress
149 & below	150-300	301 & above

If you scored less than 150 pts you are experiencing low stress from adjustment to life events and change. Continue with you regular lifestyle.

If you scored 150 to 300 pts you are experiencing moderate stress from adjustment to life events and change. Recognize that extra demands will be made on your coping skills. Practice a relaxation technique to reduce the effects of stress reactions on your body and mind.

If you scored over 300 pts you are experiencing severe stress from adjustment to life events and change. Recognize that extraordinary demands will be made on your coping skills. Regularly practice a relaxation technique to reduce the effects of stress reactions on your body and mind. Utilize the cognitive methods as outlined in Chapter 11 such as affirmations or managing self talk in order to cope with the stressful demands of life change.

NUTRITION SURVEY

Inventory 12

Name ______________________ Date ______________

DIRECTIONS: Choose an answer for each item which most accurately reflects your behavior.

1. I drink - cola or caffeinated soft drink beverages (12 oz. portion) per day.
   a. 2 or less
   b. 3-4
   c. 5-7
   d. 7 or more

2. I drink at least ___ cups of coffee or tea per day (excluding herbal tea).
   a. 2 or less
   b. 3-4
   c. 5-7
   d. 7 or more

3. When I eat chocolate, I eat __ (per day):
   a. one average sized bar (1 oz.) or less
   b. 1-2 bars
   c. 2-3 bars
   d. 3 or more bars

4. I eat a donut or pastry as my only breakfast food besides a beverage.
   a. 2 or less times/week
   b. 3-4 times/week
   c. 5-6 times/week
   d. every day

5. I usually eat pastries or other foods high in quick energy as my only lunch.
   a. 2 or less times/week
   b. 3-4 times/week
   c. 5-6 times/week
   d. every day

6. I use ___ teaspoons of refined sugar per day.
   a. 4 tsp. or less
   b. 5-8 tsp.
   c. 9-15 tsp.
   d. 16 or tsp.

7. I add salt to my food at meals (total shakes of a table salt shaker).
   a. 10 or less
   b. 11-20
   c. 20-30
   d. 31 or more

8. I smoke tobacco cigarettes:
   a. I don't
   b. less than a pack/day
   c. 1-2 packs
   d. more than 2 packs

9. I am exposed to the sidestream smoke of others around me.
   a. not at all
   b. less than 1 hr./day
   c. 2-4 hrs./day
   d. more

10. When I am around even minimal cigarette or cigar smoking my eyes or nose become irritated.
    a. never true
    b. seldom true
    c. usually true
    d. always true

Interpretation

Items 1, 2 & 3 deal with the amount of caffeine that you consume in a day. Remember that an intake over 250 mg is enough to cause physical stress symptoms on an otherwise stressless day. Caffeine is a substance which can cause a dependency so it is wise to be aware of and reduce your intake of caffeine.

Items 4, 5 & 6 have to do with the amount of highly refined carbohydrates and simple sugars in your diet. The more of these substances that you consume the greater the likelihood that you will experience a rapid rise in blood sugar followed by a rapid fall leaving you feeling weak and shaky. These foods also are not good sources for the vitamins needed to change sugars into energy. A good dietary practice is to eat whole fruits and vegetables whenever possible. Also pastas (spaghetti, noodles, and macaroni), rice and whole grain breads provide the energy and nutrients needed to pursue an active lifestyle.

Item 5 provides insight into your sodium (salt) intake. Remember that each shake of a salt shaker provides about 100 mg of sodium, one tenth of your daily requirement for sodium. Remember that many processed food products are high in sodium. Be aware of your sodium consumption and limit it if it is excessive.

Items 8, 9 and 10 deal with cigarette smoke, a stressor and source of nicotine, a potent stimulant. Effects of nicotine are dose related so exposure to cigarette smoke should be strictly limited at all times. Be assertive and speak out when you are being unnecessarily exposed to tobacco smoke.

EXERCISE SURVEY

Inventory 13

Name ______________________ Date ______________

DIRECTIONS: Choose an answer for each item which most accurately reflects your behavior.

1. I usually jog or run:
   a. every day
   b. 3 or more times per week
   c. 3 or less times per week
   d. less than once a week

2. I play tennis, racquetball, handball, or other racquet sports:
   a. every day
   b. 3 or more times per week
   c. 3 or less times per week
   d. less than once a week

3. I swim, bicycle, walk briskly, skip rope, attend step aerobics or other aerobic classes or dance intensely:
   a. every day
   b. 3 or more times per week
   c. 3 or less times per week
   d. less than once a week

4. I incorporate some muscular strength and endurance building exercises such as isometric, resistance of body weight, or resistance against a force (weight lifting machines or resistance bands, etc.) into my workout:
   a. every day
   b. 3 or more times per week
   c. 3 or less times per week
   d. less than once a week

5. I do calisthenics, stretching exercises, or yoga:
   a. every day
   b. 3 or more times per week
   c. 3 or less times per week
   d. less than once a week

6. The length of my average workout is:
   a. 45 min. or more
   b. 30 min. to 44 min.
   c. 15 min. to 30 min.
   d. 14 min. or less

7. The intensity of my workout compared to "all out" effect is:
   a. 100% - 75%
   b. 75% - 50%
   c. 50% - 25%
   d. 24% or less

8. I take the stairs instead of an elevator or an escalator:
   a. usually true
   b. often true
   c. sometimes true
   d. never true

9. I try to park some distance from my job so I can exercise walking in to work and back to my car:
   a. usually true
   b. often true
   c. sometimes true
   d. never true

Interpretation

Items 1 through 3 have to do with the development of cardiovascular fitness and endurance. Remember to exercise 3 to 5 times a week in order to maintain fitness.

Item number 4 stresses the importance of having a muscular strength and endurance component in your exercise program. Strength training is important to help you get through daily activities with less fatigue, define your body contours and develop a sense of body awareness.

Item number 5 highlights the importance of maintaining flexibility. A flexible body is less easily injured during exercise and the activities of everyday living. Remember that many fitness activities reduce flexibility so experts suggest that you stretch after warming up and after your workout ends.

Items 6 and 7 deal with the intensity and duration of exercise. Guidelines suggest a duration of exercise session from 15 to 30 minutes for healthy cardiovascular functioning and an intensity within the 50% to 75% range for maximum benefits. Levels of exercise intensity which regularly exceed 75% can cause exercise related problems while levels less than 50% will provide much slower gains. Learn to calculate your target heart rate and use it as a guide during aerobic exercise.

Items 8 and 9 are examples of opportunities for incorporating extra exercise into your daily life. Whenever you can take the stairs instead of the elevator, walk up and down the escalator, take the long way when walking instead of short cuts, etc. Be active and try to do a little extra whenever you can.

RELAXATION SURVEY

Inventory 14

Name ______________________________ Date ________________

DIRECTIONS: Choose an answer for each item which most accurately reflects your behavior.

1. I usually spend some time with a hobby:
   a. at least once a day
   b. 3 to 5 times a week
   c. 3 to 5 times a month
   d. never

2. I usually spend some time just listening to quiet music:
   a. at least once a day
   b. 3 to 5 times a week
   c. 3 to 5 times a month
   d. never

3. I usually spend some time in exercise such as tennis, swimming, golf, etc.:
   a. at least once a day
   b. 3 to 5 times week
   c. 3 to 5 times a month
   d. never

4. I usually spend some time with muscle relaxation techniques such as progressive muscle relaxation, etc:
   a. at least once a day
   b. 3 to 5 times a week
   c. 3 to 5 times a month
   d. never

5. I usually spend some time watching T.V. or videos:
   a. at least once a day
   b. 3 to 5 times a week
   c. 3 to 5 times a month
   d. never

6. I usually spend some time with mental relaxation techniques such as meditation, autogenic training or visualization:
   a. at least once a day
   b. 3 to 5 times a week
   c. 3 to 5 times a month
   d. never

7. At night I usually sleep:
   a. 4 hours
   b. 6 hours
   c. 8 hours
   d. 10 hours

8. I usually take some time to remember a tranquil pleasing thought:
   a. at least once a day
   b. 3 to 5 times a week
   c. 3 to 5 times a month
   d. never

Interpretation

The answers to items 4 and 6 provide the strongest evidence that you are in fact relaxing. Remember that relaxation is defined as a reduction in muscle tension and studies have shown that the techniques mentioned in items 4 and 6 reliably provide relaxation. The more often that you practice these techniques the easier relaxation will come and the deeper it will be.

The answers to items 2 and 8 provide more evidence that you are relaxing. While the accumulated evidence is not as strong for these practices as for relaxation techniques, they are commonly suggested by stress management experts as effective techniques and employed successfully by many persons as part of an effective stress management program.

Remember that exercise, item 3, is a high arousal state that is not relaxation. The relaxation response comes after the end of the exercise session.

Sleep, item 7, is a necessary function in order to be healthy but cannot take the place of relaxation for stress management.

The remaining items refer to diversion rather than to relaxation. They are just as likely to produce stressful arousal as relaxation and cannot be counted on for reliable relaxation.

If you are highly stressed you may need to practice relaxation once or twice a day to achieve stress and symptom reduction. When you have developed skill in relaxation then you are on you way to experiencing some sense of peace and tranquility from these techniques.

STRESS SYMPTOM CHECKLIST

Inventory 15

Name ______________________ Date ______________

DIRECTIONS: The following list contains signs and symptoms commonly associated with stress. Check the ones which you experience under stressful life conditions. Can you identify your stress pathway?

Cardiovascular
- [ ] Cold hands, fingers or toes
- [ ] Heart palpitations
- [ ] Increased blood pressure
- [ ] Rapid erratic pulse
- [ ] Faintness
- [ ] Migraines

Muscular/Skeletal
- [ ] Frequent headaches (esp afternoon and evening)
- [ ] Jittery/easily startled
- [ ] Neck and back pain
- [ ] Jaw and temple pain
- [ ] Grinding teeth or clenched jaw
- [ ] Forehead wrinkles or scowls
- [ ] Trembling
- [ ] Tics
- [ ] Easily fatigued
- [ ] Nervous mannerisms (toe tapping, hair pulling, nail biting, etc)

Gastrointestinal
- [ ] Stomach/intestinal pain
- [ ] Nausea
- [ ] Gnawing Hunger
- [ ] Vomiting
- [ ] Diarrhea
- [ ] Constipation
- [ ] Loss of appetite

Feelings
- [ ] Fearful
- [ ] Apprehensive
- [ ] Feeling of loss of control
- [ ] Obsessional or phobic fears
- [ ] Crying or tearful
- [ ] Trouble concentrating
- [ ] Mental confusion
- [ ] Preoccupied
- [ ] Overly shy, timid, fearful of offending an authority figure

Respiratory
- [ ] Rapid shallow breathing
- [ ] Breathlessness
- [ ] Frequent sighing
- [ ] Inability to breathe deeply

Immune System
- [ ] Frequent colds
- [ ] Allergy attacks
- [ ] Asthma attacks
- [ ] Summer colds
- [ ] Inflamation of tissues

Other
- [ ] Frequent urination
- [ ] Excessive perspiration
- [ ] Sleeplessness
- [ ] Sweaty palms

Interpretation

Try to identify your stress pathway (there may be more than one) by looking at the grouping of your checks. If you can identify a pathway then you will know what organ system in your body is responding to stressful life events. This information can then be used to help you develop body awareness necessary for prompt intervention and to identify appropriate interventions for your stress response. Below we will list some of the organ systems and appropriate interventions for these systems.

Cardiovascular

In this organ system thermal or skin conductance biofeedback training are often utilized. Autogenic training meditation and visualization techniques might also be helpful.

Muscular/Skeletal

In this organ system EMG biofeedback training is often utilized. Progressive muscle relaxation techniques and autogenic training are often utilized.

Gastrointestinal

In this organ system thermal or skin conductance biofeedback training might be used. Autogenic training, meditation and visualization techniques might also be helpful.

Skin

In this organ system thermal, skin conductance or skin potential biofeedback training might be utilized. Autogenic training, meditation and visualization techniques might also be helpful.

Respiratory

In this organ system thermal or skin conductance biofeedback training might be used. Autogenic training, meditation and visualization techniques might also be helpful.

Immune System

In this organ system thermal or skin conductance biofeedback training might be used. Autogenic training, meditation and visualization techniques might also be helpful.

Note - Consult your campus directory for a biofeedback lab on campus. You may find it in the departments of Health Education, Psychology, Counseling, or Student Health. You may even have access to biofeedback, relaxation, and stress management training through on of the class taught on campus and get some credits while learning necessary life skills.

These suggestions for interventions are given in with the caveat that the reading find an appropriately trained professional to help them implement their intervention. Every person who has severe and chronic symptoms should have them evaluated by a physician prior to be sure that they do not have a medical condition which would require strict

GUIDELINES FOR EFFECTIVE STRESS MANAGEMENT

Inventory 16

DIRECTIONS: The following skills and behaviors are recommended by stress management experts. Review the list often and attempt to put these skills into practice in your everyday life.

1. Lifestyle Analysis - Analyze aspects of lifestyle for possible stressors. For example, nutritional stressors - caffeine, sedentary lifestyle, time management, noise, etc.
2. Act to alter stressors when it is possible and/or feasible. Eliminate or modify events in your life that are stressful.
3. Analyze your coping styles. Do they help in the long run? Recognize that much of your behavior is learned and, therefore, is subject to modification.
4. Learn to be assertive and how to communicate in an effective manner.
5. Learn to delegate responsibility to others.
6. Learn time management skills.
7. Learn how to say no. Say it assertively, gently and often.
8. Learn to give and accept compliments.
9. Learn and practice a relaxation technique. This is a powerful tool for letting go of stress, preventing further stress responses and feeling in control of your life and body.
10. Exercise regularly in an aerobic manner. This uses stress products and strengthens every part of the body.
11. Avoid sugar, salt, caffeine and saturated fat in your diet. Eat more fruits, vegetables, poultry, fish. Increase your intake of complex carbohydrates.
12. Be patient with yourself. Lasting change is possible, but it takes time.
13. Cultivate friendships and social ties. Social support is one of the main stress buffers.
14. Learn to feel worthy of pleasure. Develop pleasure and fun activities. Do something for fun everyday. It's your right to feel good, but you must pursue it.
15. Develop a sense of humor. Learn to be happy.
16. Read, Read, Read!
17. Enjoy your life!

TYPE A/B BEHAVIOR EVALUATION

Inventory 17

Name ____________________ Date ____________

DIRECTIONS: Please read each item and then select the appropriate response (either 1, 2 or 3). Add the responses to calculate your total score. The scoring box on the bottom of page 250 assigns a Behavior type to the total score.

	Seldom	Sometimes	Often
1. I have the tendency to speak the last sentence far more rapidly than the beginning words.	1	2	3
2. I eat very rapidly, not always fully taking time to adequately chew my food.	1	2	3
3. I get impatient when others are talking and sometimes attempt to finish their sentences.	1	2	3
4. I think people take too long to get to the point of what they are trying to say.	1	2	3
5. I get unduly upset when caught behind a car in traffic that is going at a pace I consider too slow.	1	2	3
6. I find it frustrating to have to wait in line to be seated in a restaurant.	1	2	3
7. I become very impatient with myself when I am obliged to do repetitious tasks (writing checks, washing dishes, vacuuming the floor.)	1	2	3
8. I don't hear what others are saying because I am caught in my own thoughts.	1	2	3
9. While indulging in recreation activities, I think about business or professional problems.	1	2	3
10. I eat meals in the car while driving to an appointment.	1	2	3
11. I don't enjoy conversation unless it centers on those subjects that especially interest me and often just pretend to be listening.	1	2	3
12. I feel guilty when I take time to relax for a few hours.	1	2	3

Type A/B Behavior Evaluation (continued)

	Seldom	Sometimes	Often
13. I no longer notice some of the interesting things about a strange office, store, or home. Furthermore, after leaving these places, I don't remember what was in them.	1	2	3
14. I no longer have time to enjoy many of the pastimes I formerly enjoyed.	1	2	3
15. I find myself trying to schedule more and more activities into less and less time.	1	2	3
16. I think my successes have been largely the result of my ability to get more done in less time than other people.	1	2	3
17. I am aware of or have been told that I have certain nervous gestures (clenching fists, tapping fingers on a table, twitch the corners of my mouth, etc.)	1	2	3
18. I feel somewhat jealous of someone who seems to accomplish more than myself.	1	2	3
19. When playing and relaxing, I still feel the need to display my superiority in that activity.	1	2	3
20. When taking classes in school, I am more concerned about the grade rather than what I have actually learned.	1	2	3

Total Score ______

Behavior Type ______

Scoring

39-60	High Type A
30-38	Moderate Type A
29 & less	Tendency Toward Type B

From *Health and Fitness for Life:Laboratory Manual.* ed. by J.S. Schnendel, Prospect Press, pgs. 63-64, 1983. Adapted from M. Friedman and R.H. Rosenman. *Type A Behavior and Your Heart.* New York:Knopf, 1974. Reprinted by permission of Alfred A. Knopf, Inc. © 1974 by M.Friedman.

HOSTILITY EVALUATION

Inventory **18**

Name ______________________ Date ______________

DIRECTIONS: Hostility basically is an indication of how we feel about the people around us. It is one factor in the Type A behavior profile, and perhaps the most important behavior factor in predicting one's susceptibility to cardiovascular disease. Score each of the following 8 questions. Then add all points to get a total score.

	1 pt.	2 pts.	3 pts.	4 pts.	Score
1. I tend to get agitated too easily.	almost never	seldom	often	almost always	
2. Whenever possible, I try to make my activities competitive.	almost never	seldom	often	almost always	
3. I tend to get upset when I lose.	almost never	seldom	often	almost always	
4. I tend to lose my temper or get irritable when I'm under a lot of pressure.	almost never	seldom	often	almost always	
5. I hate to depend on others.	almost never	seldom	often	almost always	
6. When people make me wait or prevent me from doing things, I think they are selfish and inconsiderate.	almost never	seldom	often	almost always	
7. I feel people around me are incompetent.	almost never	seldom	often	almost always	
8. When angry at someone, I am likely to express my feelings in some way to the other person.	almost never	seldom	often	almost always	
				Total Score	

Scoring

16 & below	Low hostility
17 - 24	Moderate hostility
25 & above	High hostility

BODY FAT ASSESSMENT

Inventory 19

Name ______________________________ Date ______________

DIRECTIONS: The most accurate method of assessing body fat is by hydrostatic weighing with directly measured lung volume (Chapter 9). If possible, an individual should have body fat and optimal weight estimated using hydrostatic weighing. Skinfold measurements can provide a reasonable estimate of body composition if great care is taken to measure at the precise anatomical location and if supervised practice in the use of the skinfold caliper is performed. One of the simplest skinfold techniques for men or women involves the measurement of skinfolds at three sites on the dominant side of the body. These measurements can be made with any skinfold caliper. Proper measurement locations are illustrated below. The sum of the three skinfolds is converted to % fat in the tables. Record the results on the record sheet on page 254.

The amount of body fat necessary for optimal health and fitness is unknown. However, the "average values" for any age group are probably higher than ideal. For Example, an estimate of ideal % fat for a young man and woman would be 10 and 20%, respectively, values which are slightly below the average for the college age group. These "ideal" estimates can be used to age 30 and then higher estimates are probably more appropriate.

The loss of body weight through exercise should be primarily from fat stores. To insure this, the weight loss program must involve routine aerobic activity or circuit resistance training which utilize body fat. Remember, the calculations provide only an estimate of body composition. This procedure can be used only to predict a rough estimate of an appropriate body weight goal.

Female Skinfold Measurements

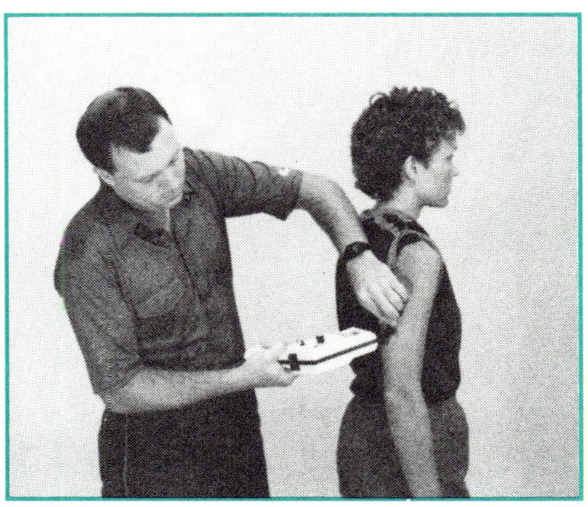

Tricep vertical fold midway between top of the shoulder bone and tip of the elbow.

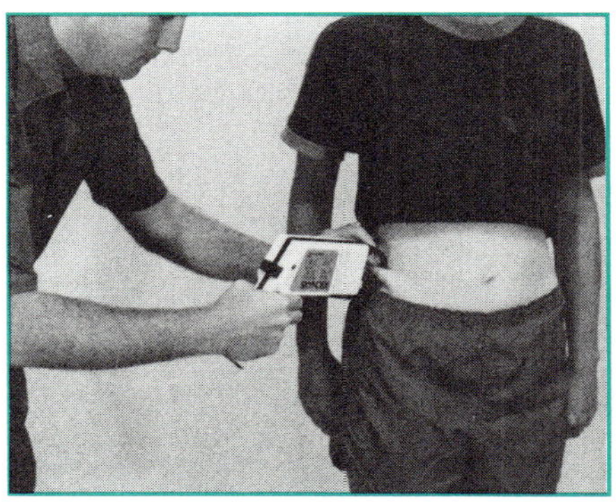

Suprailium diagonal fold over the hip bone.

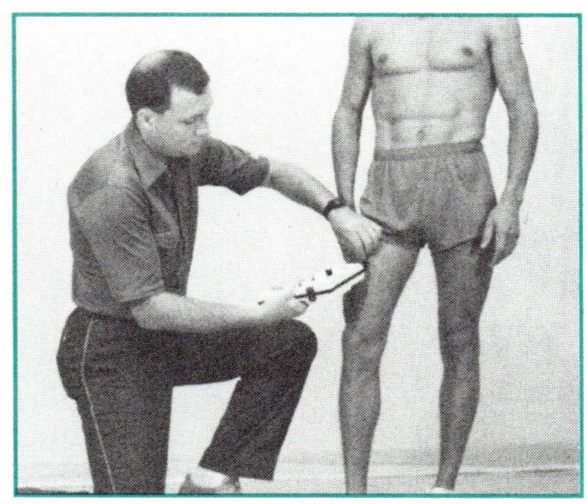

Thigh vertical fold in the middle of the thigh.

Male Skinfold Measurements

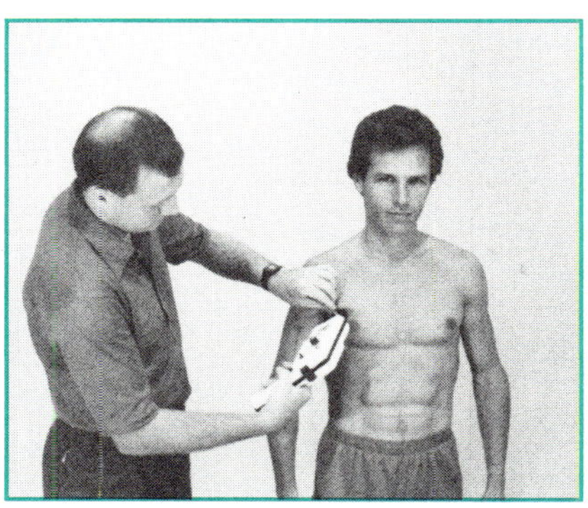

Chest diagonal fold between the nipple and arm pit.

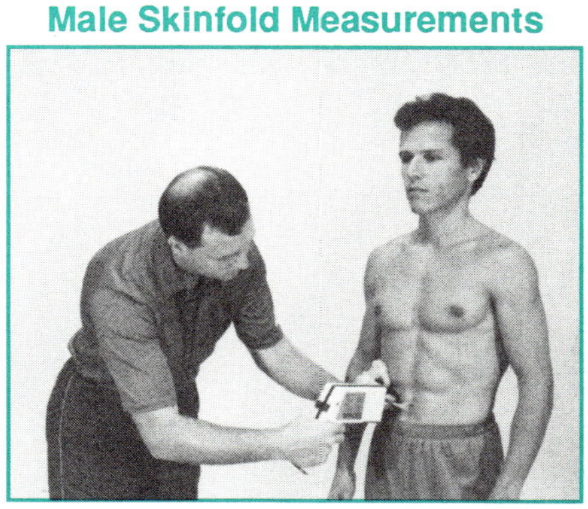

Abdominal horizontal fold just next to the navel.

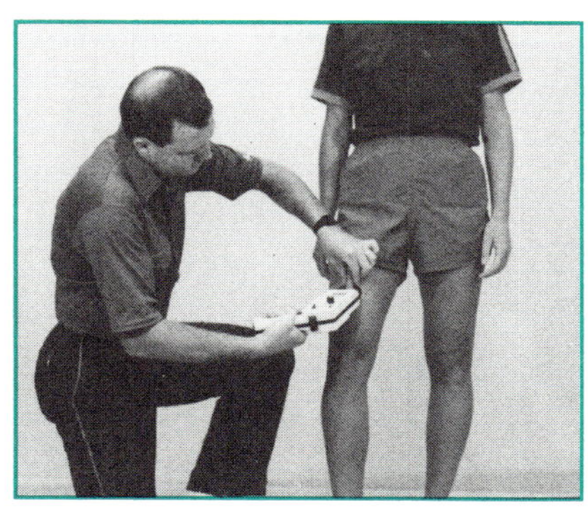

Thigh vertical fold in the middle of the thigh.

Estimation of Percent Body Fat Record Sheet

Jackson and Pollock Technique

Name ______________________ Sex ________ Date ____________

Age in Years ________ Weight in kg. ________ Weight in lbs. ________

Skinfolds Measurement on Dominant Side

Female

1. Triceps	mm
2. Suprailium	mm
3. Thigh	mm
Sum	mm

Male

1. Chest	mm
2. Abdominal	mm
3. Thigh	mm
Sum	mm

Convert sum of the skinfolds to % fat using Tables on following pages.

% Fat	

% Fat Changes

	Evaluation Date	% Fat	Body Weight
1st Test			
2nd Test			
3rd Test			

Female Percent Body Fat Conversion from the Sum of Three Skinfolds

Sum of 3 Skinfolds (mm)	Age in Years 18-22	23-27	28-32	33-37	38-42	43-47	48-52	53-57	58-62
16	7.8	8.1	8.4	8.7	8.9	9.2	9.5	9.8	10.1
18	8.5	8.8	9.1	9.4	9.7	10.0	10.3	10.6	10.9
20	**9.3**	**9.6**	**9.9**	**10.2**	**10.5**	**10.8**	**11.1**	**11.4**	**11.7**
22	10.1	10.4	10.7	11.0	11.3	11.6	11.9	12.2	12.5
24	10.8	11.1	11.4	11.7	12.0	12.3	12.6	12.9	13.2
26	11.6	11.9	12.2	12.5	12.8	13.1	13.4	13.7	14.0
28	12.3	12.6	12.9	13.2	13.5	13.8	14.2	14.5	14.8
30	**13.1**	**13.4**	**13.7**	**14.0**	**14.3**	**14.6**	**14.9**	**15.2**	**15.5**
32	13.8	14.1	14.4	14.7	15.0	15.3	15.6	15.9	16.3
34	14.6	14.9	15.2	15.5	15.8	16.1	16.4	16.7	17.0
36	15.3	15.6	15.9	16.2	16.5	16.8	17.1	17.4	17.7
38	16.0	16.3	16.6	16.9	17.2	17.5	17.8	18.1	18.5
40	**16.7**	**17.0**	**17.3**	**17.6**	**17.9**	**18.3**	**18.6**	**18.9**	**19.2**
42	17.4	17.7	18.0	18.3	18.7	19.0	19.3	19.6	19.9
44	18.1	18.4	18.7	19.1	19.4	19.7	20.0	20.3	20.6
46	18.8	19.1	19.4	19.8	20.1	20.4	20.7	21.0	21.3
48	19.5	19.8	20.1	20.4	20.8	21.1	21.4	21.7	22.0
50	**20.2**	**20.5**	**20.8**	**21.1**	**21.4**	**21.8**	**22.1**	**22.4**	**22.7**
52	20.9	21.2	21.5	21.8	22.1	22.4	22.8	23.1	23.4
54	21.6	21.9	22.2	22.5	22.8	23.1	23.4	23.7	24.1
56	22.2	22.5	22.8	23.2	23.5	23.8	24.1	24.4	24.7
58	22.9	23.2	23.5	23.8	24.1	24.5	24.8	25.1	25.4
60	**23.5**	**23.8**	**24.2**	**24.5**	**24.8**	**25.1**	**26.1**	**26.4**	**26.7**
62	24.2	24.5	24.8	25.1	25.4	25.8	26.1	26.4	26.7
64	24.8	25.1	25.4	25.8	26.1	26.4	26.7	27.0	27.4
66	25.4	25.8	26.1	26.4	26.7	27.0	27.4	27.7	28.0
68	26.1	26.4	26.7	27.0	27.4	27.7	28.0	28.3	28.6
70	**26.7**	**27.0**	**27.3**	**27.7**	**28.0**	**28.3**	**28.6**	**28.9**	**29.3**
72	27.3	27.6	27.9	28.3	28.6	28.9	29.2	29.6	29.9
74	27.9	28.2	28.6	28.9	29.2	29.5	29.8	30.2	30.5
76	28.5	28.8	29.2	29.5	29.8	30.1	30.4	30.8	31.1
78	29.1	29.4	29.7	30.1	30.4	30.7	31.0	31.4	31.7
80	**29.7**	**30.0**	**30.3**	**30.7**	**31.0**	**31.3**	**31.6**	**32.0**	**32.3**
82	30.3	30.6	30.9	31.2	31.6	31.9	32.2	32.5	32.9
84	30.8	31.2	31.5	31.8	32.1	32.5	32.8	33.1	33.4
86	31.4	31.7	32.0	32.4	32.7	33.0	33.4	33.7	34.0
88	32.0	32.3	32.6	32.9	33.3	33.6	33.9	34.2	34.6
90	**32.5**	**32.8**	**33.2**	**33.5**	**33.8**	**34.1**	**34.5**	**34.8**	**35.1**
92	33.0	33.4	33.7	34.0	34.4	34.7	35.0	35.3	35.7
94	33.6	33.9	34.2	34.6	34.9	35.2	35.6	35.9	36.2
96	34.1	34.4	34.8	35.1	35.4	35.8	36.1	36.4	36.8
98	34.6	34.9	35.3	35.6	35.9	36.3	36.6	36.9	37.3
100	**35.1**	**35.5**	**35.8**	**36.1**	**36.5**	**36.8**	**37.1**	**37.5**	**37.8**
102	35.6	36.0	36.3	36.6	37.0	37.3	37.6	38.0	38.3
104	36.1	36.5	36.8	37.1	37.5	37.8	38.1	38.5	38.8
106	36.6	36.9	37.3	37.6	37.9	38.3	38.6	39.0	39.3
108	37.1	37.4	37.8	38.1	38.4	38.8	39.1	39.4	39.8
110	**37.6**	**37.9**	**38.2**	**38.6**	**38.9**	**39.2**	**39.6**	**39.9**	**40.3**
112	38.0	38.4	38.7	39.0	39.4	39.7	40.0	40.4	40.7
114	38.5	38.8	39.2	39.5	39.8	40.2	40.5	40.8	41.2
116	38.9	39.3	39.6	39.9	40.3	40.6	41.0	41.3	41.6
118	39.4	39.7	40.0	40.4	40.7	41.1	41.4	41.7	42.1
120	**39.8**	**40.1**	**40.5**	**40.8**	**41.2**	**41.5**	**41.8**	**42.2**	**42.5**
122	40.2	40.6	40.9	41.2	41.6	41.9	42.3	42.6	42.9
124	40.6	41.0	41.3	41.7	42.0	42.3	42.7	43.0	43.4
126	41.0	41.4	41.7	42.1	42.4	42.7	43.1	43.4	43.8

Example: If a woman's age is 39 years and the sum of three skinfolds equals 58 mm, then her percent fat is 24.1%.

Table was calculated from A.S. Jackson, M.L. Pollock, and A. Ward. Generalized equations for predicting body density of women. *Medicine and Science in Sports and Exercise* 12:175-182, 1980.

Male Percent Body Fat Conversion from the Sum of Three Skinfolds

Sum of 3 Skinfolds (mm)	Age in Years								
	18-22	23-27	28-32	33-37	38-42	43-47	48-52	53-57	58-62
10	1.6	2.2	2.7	3.2	3.8	4.3	4.8	5.4	5.9
12	2.3	2.8	3.4	3.9	4.4	5.0	5.5	6.1	6.6
14	2.9	3.5	4.0	4.6	5.1	5.6	6.2	6.7	7.3
16	3.6	4.1	4.7	5.2	5.7	6.3	6.8	7.4	7.9
18	4.2	4.8	5.3	5.9	6.4	6.9	7.5	8.0	8.6
20	**4.9**	**5.4**	**6.0**	**6.5**	**7.0**	**7.6**	**8.1**	**8.7**	**9.2**
22	5.5	6.1	6.6	7.1	7.7	8.2	8.8	9.3	9.9
24	6.1	6.7	7.2	7.8	8.3	8.9	9.4	10.0	10.5
26	6.8	7.3	7.9	8.4	9.0	9.5	10.1	10.6	11.2
28	7.4	7.9	8.5	9.0	9.6	10.1	10.7	11.2	11.8
30	**8.0**	**8.6**	**9.1**	**9.7**	**10.2**	**10.8**	**11.3**	**11.9**	**12.4**
32	8.6	9.2	9.7	10.3	10.8	11.4	11.9	12.5	13.1
34	9.2	9.8	10.3	10.9	11.5	12.0	12.6	13.1	13.7
36	9.9	10.4	11.0	11.5	12.1	12.6	13.2	13.7	14.3
38	10.5	11.0	11.6	12.1	12.7	13.2	13.8	14.4	14.9
40	**11.1**	**11.6**	**12.2**	**12.7**	**13.3**	**13.8**	**14.4**	**15.0**	**15.5**
42	11.7	12.2	12.8	13.3	13.9	14.5	15.0	15.6	16.1
44	12.3	12.8	13.4	13.9	14.5	15.1	15.6	16.2	16.7
46	12.9	13.4	14.0	14.5	15.1	15.7	16.2	16.8	17.3
48	13.4	14.0	14.6	15.1	15.7	16.2	16.8	17.4	17.9
50	**14.0**	**14.6**	**15.1**	**15.7**	**16.3**	**16.8**	**17.4**	**18.0**	**18.5**
52	14.6	15.2	15.7	16.3	16.9	17.4	18.0	18.6	19.1
54	15.2	15.7	16.3	16.9	17.4	18.0	18.6	19.1	19.7
56	15.7	16.3	16.9	17.4	18.0	18.6	19.1	19.7	20.3
58	16.3	16.9	17.4	18.0	18.6	19.1	19.7	20.3	20.9
60	**16.9**	**17.4**	**18.0**	**18.6**	**19.1**	**19.7**	**20.3**	**20.9**	**21.4**
62	17.4	18.0	18.6	19.1	19.7	20.3	20.9	21.4	22.0
64	18.0	18.5	19.1	19.7	20.3	20.8	21.4	22.0	22.6
66	18.5	19.1	19.7	20.2	20.8	21.4	22.0	22.6	23.1
68	19.1	19.6	20.2	20.8	21.4	21.9	22.5	23.1	23.7
70	**19.6**	**20.2**	**20.8**	**21.3**	**21.9**	**22.5**	**23.1**	**23.7**	**24.2**
72	20.1	20.7	21.3	21.9	22.5	23.1	23.7	24.2	24.8
74	20.7	21.2	21.8	22.4	23.0	23.6	24.2	24.7	25.3
76	21.2	21.8	22.4	22.9	23.5	24.1	24.7	25.3	25.9
78	21.7	22.3	22.9	23.5	24.0	24.6	25.2	25.8	26.4
80	**22.2**	**22.8**	**23.4**	**24.0**	**24.6**	**25.2**	**25.7**	**26.3**	**26.9**
82	22.7	23.3	23.9	24.5	25.1	25.7	26.3	26.8	27.4
84	23.3	23.8	24.4	25.0	25.6	26.2	26.8	27.4	28.0
86	23.8	24.3	24.9	25.5	26.1	26.7	27.3	27.9	28.5
88	24.3	24.8	25.4	26.0	26.6	27.2	27.8	28.4	29.0
90	**24.7**	**25.3**	**25.9**	**26.5**	**27.1**	**27.7**	**28.3**	**28.9**	**29.5**
92	25.2	25.8	26.4	27.0	27.6	28.2	28.8	29.4	30.0
94	25.7	26.3	26.9	27.5	28.1	28.7	29.3	29.9	30.5
96	26.2	26.8	27.4	28.0	28.6	29.2	29.8	30.4	31.0
98	26.7	27.3	27.9	28.4	29.0	29.6	30.2	30.8	31.4
100	**27.1**	**27.7**	**28.3**	**28.9**	**29.5**	**30.1**	**30.7**	**31.3**	**31.9**
102	27.6	28.2	28.8	29.4	30.0	30.6	31.2	31.8	32.4
104	28.1	28.7	29.3	29.9	30.5	31.1	31.7	32.3	32.9
106	28.5	29.1	29.7	30.3	30.9	31.5	32.1	32.7	33.3
108	29.0	29.6	30.2	30.8	31.4	32.0	32.6	33.2	33.8
110	**29.4**	**30.0**	**30.6**	**31.2**	**31.8**	**32.4**	**33.0**	**33.6**	**34.2**
112	29.8	30.4	31.0	31.6	32.3	32.9	33.5	34.1	34.7
114	30.3	30.9	31.5	32.1	32.7	33.3	33.9	34.5	35.1
116	30.7	31.3	31.9	32.5	33.1	33.7	34.3	34.9	35.6

Example: If a man's age is 45 years and the sum of three skinfolds equals 50 mm, then his percent fat is 16.8%.

Table was calculated from A.S. Jackson, M.L. Pollock, and A. Ward. Generalized equations for predicting body density of women. *Medicine and Science in Sports and Exercise* 12:175-182, 1980.

WAIST/HIP RATIO (WHR)

Inventory 20

DIRECTIONS: People with abdominal obesity have been shown to be at higher risk for cardiovascular disease. Scientists believe that fat which is stored in the abdominal region is more easily mobilized into the blood stream where the fat can end up in atherosclerotic plaque.

The WHR requires the measurement of the waist around its narrowest point with an accurate tape measure. The hips are then measured around the broadest point of the buttocks. Each measurement should be taken three times and the two closest values at each site averaged. The ratio can be calculated using either cm or in.

Waist/Hip Ratio Data

Name ______________________ Age ______ Sex ________ Date ____________

Body Weight ______________ kg

Waist Circumference __________ cm (in) Hip Circumference ____________ cm (in)

$$\text{WHR} = \frac{\text{Waist Circumference}}{\text{Hip Circumference}}$$

Classifications

	Men WHR	Women WHR
Excellent	<.70	<.80
Good	~.75	~.85
Poor	>.80	>.90

IDEAL BODY WEIGHT

Inventory 21

Name ______________________ Date ______________

DIRECTIONS: Because of the dangers of excess storage fat, it is vitally important for each person to maintain an ideal body weight. Many people incorrectly gauge this ideal body mass from what they weight on the bathroom scales and never consider the relative proportions of the two major components of body composition. The bathroom-scale approach to determining your weight may be incorrect and also may lead to poor judgments concerning dieting and/or exercise. An individual's ideal body weight should be based on the correct proportion of fat mass present and not on such things as height, weight, or even age.

Complete the Following to Calculate Ideal Body Weight

1. Fat Fraction ____________ = %fat/100
2. Fat Weight ____________ = Body Weight x Fat Fraction
3. Lean Weight ____________ = Body Weight - Fat Weight
4. Ideal Lean Fraction ____________ = 1.00 - Ideal Fat Fraction
   Ideal Fat Fraction is the ideal % fat or the goal % fat (e.g., .10 in men, .20 in women)
5. Ideal Body Weight ____________ = $\frac{\text{Lean Weight}}{\text{Ideal Lean Fraction}}$

The ideal %fat values are often given as 10% for men and 20% for women. These values may seem rather unachievable for many college students and could make the goal of weight control seem out of reach. For example, a college male who weights 220 lbs and has a body fat of 18% would have a fat mass of about 40 lbs. If he attempted to reach the ideal %fat of 10%, he would have to lose 20 lbs of fat. Faced with such a large loss, the individual might consider the task impossible and never attempt to control his weight. Over the next 20 years this uncontrolled fat content might continue to grow until this middle-aged male finds himself at 20% fat and perhaps in serious jeopardy of his health. It might be far more reasonable for this individual to set a short-term goal of 14% fat, which would mean he would have to lose only 10 lbs. Once he has attained this goal, further reductions may become easier to manage.

CALORIC BALANCE

Inventory **22**

DIRECTIONS: The accurate measurement of caloric input of output is very difficult. Many charts are available which estimate the number of calories in a given food, but weights and portions of foods vary so widely that great skill is required to even crudely estimate caloric intake (Appendix B). Likewise, the caloric cost of various activities has been estimated, usually be assessing the oxygen cost (Appendix A). Estimates of energy cost are confounded by differences in body size, metabolism, environmental conditions, etc. Thus, it is very difficult to accurately assess caloric balance.

However, short-term record keeping of the foods eaten and their approximate energy value as well as the approximate number of calories utilized daily can be a valuable experience. Such a record can indicate poor life-style habits and areas where simple changes can make a major difference in caloric balance. In addition, the experience can cause a greater awareness of calorific foods and the best activities of utilizing calories.

Data sheets are provided on which daily caloric intake and output can be recorded. The record should be kept for a minimum of one week and include both weekday and weekend analysis. See Appenix A and B.

Name ______________________ Date ______________ Day ______________

Caloric Intake Data Sheet

Meal	Food	Amount (tsp, cup, oz)	Calories
Breakfast			
Lunch			

Meal	Food	Amount (tsp, cup, oz)	Calories
Dinner			
Snacks			

TOTAL Daily Intake	

Caloric Output Data Sheet

Name ______________________ Date ______________ Day ______________

	Activity	Length of Time	Calories
BMR			
Daily Routine			
		Total Routine	
Exercise Training (e.g. extra walking)			
		Total Training	
		TOTAL Output	

Total Daily Intake		Total Daily Output		Caloric Balance
	-		=	

DIET ANALYSIS SOFTWARE

Inventory 23

The Diet Analysis Software comes in two versions with the (*) showing the primary differences. Both programs are user-friendly, comprehensive, well documented and superb nutrition analysis programs.

1. Nutrition Pro! Nutrition & Fitness Software

$79 plus $5 shipping insurance. (For IBM/compatibles, 384K)

Over 2000 foods analyzed for 18 nutrients
Totals nutrients in foods, menus
Calculate personal RDA based on age, weight, gender, activity
Bar-graphs nutrient excess & deficiency
Use it to plan menus low in key nutrients life fat
Average the daily nutrient intake
Shows % calories from protein, carbs, fat, alcohol
Single Nutrient Detailed Focus: food sources, amounts graph of % contribution to total
Weight loss/weight-gain factor
Tracks up to 10 people
*High/Low Nutrient Search (any 3 nutrients)
*Food Exchanges for diabetic diets & weight-loss
*Food Groups for menu planning
*Ability to Add Your Own foods
*Database with Wider Variety of Foods
*Activity Database of 110 activities/exercises

2. Nutrition Pro! Student Version

$29 plus $5 shipping/insurance. (For IBM/compatibles, 384K)

Similar to the full version except:

Narrowed selection of foods
Food Exchanges not included
Cannot add foods to the program
Cannot do a high/low nutrient search
65 exercises/activities instead of 100.
Food & Activity Diary not included.
2000 foods, more fast foods
16 nutrients - saturated fat & cholesterol not included
Cannot add food to database
High/Low Search - none
Food Exchanges - none
Food Groups - none
65 Exercises/Activities

ONE MILE WALK TEST

Estimation of Aerobic Capacity

Inventory 24

Aerobic capacity usually is assessed by directly measuring or estimating maximal oxygen consumption (VO_2 max). The following test consists of walking one mile as fast as possible on an indoor or outdoor track. The walking pace should be as fast as possible throughout the mile rather than greatly increasing the pace at the end. At the end of the walk, the HR must be measured immediately. This can be accomplished by using a HR monitor watch or by quickly counting the pulses at the wrist (behind the thumb) or on either side of the neck. Count the pulses for exactly six seconds and add a "0" to the six second count. For example, a 6 second count of 14 would yield a HR of 140 bpm. The HR can be used on the chart to estimate VO_2 max. The time of the one-mile walk must be recorded in minutes, e.g. 10:30 = 10.50 min. The person's weight in lbs also must be recorded.

One Mile Walk Data

Name ______________________ Sex ________ Date ______________

Body Weight __________ lbs. Age __________ yr.

Mile Walk Time ______________ (minutes and hundredths of a minute)

Mile Heart Rate ______________ (taken immediately after completion of the mile walk)

Prediction of Aerobic Capacity from One Mile Walk Calculations

Male

+ 154.899

— ____ 0.0947 x Weight

— ____ 0.3709 x Age

— ____ 3.9744 x Mile Time

— ____ 0.1847 x Mile HR

= VO_2 max ml/kg/min

Female

+ 116.579

— ____ 0.0585 x Weight

— ____ 0.3885 x Age

— ____ 2.7961 x Mile Time

— ____ 0.1109 x Mile HR

= VO_2 max ml/kg/min

Calculations are derived from G.M. Kline et al. Estimation of VO_2 max from a one-mile track walk, gender, age, and body weight. *Med. Sci. Sports Exerc.* 19:253-259, 1987.

ADULT FIT-N-DEX

Inventory 25

The software package that brings the speed, flexibility, accuracy and power of computer technology to your adult fitness programs. Apple and IBM compatible, Fit-N-Dex gives health and fitness professionals a low-cost, easy-to-use management and reporting system.

Here's what Fit-N-Dex will do for you:

- Design and organize specific fitness tests.
- Utilize tests to evaluate physical fitness on multiple levels.
- analyze test results
- compare results with national norms.
- Design individualized fitness programs.

Fit-N-Dex evaluates the physcial fitness of men and women between the ages of 18 and 70 for six different parameters:

1) Cardiovascular endurance
2) Flexibility
3) Strength
4) Lung capacity
5) body composition
6) Heredity and life-style factors

Simply collect these test data and enter the scores into your computer. Then select form individualized fitness reports or standard group reports.

Fit-N-Dex will even help you design realistic, individualized fitness goals to help each subject work on his or her particular weaknesses.

The Adult Fitness software Program was written by Dr.Tom Thomas and published by Cramer Products, Inc. It is available for both Apple and IBM - compatible computers for $125. Please specify 5-1/4" or 3-1/2" disk.

For additional information call **eddie bowers publishing, inc.** 1-800-747-2411.

PERSONAL WELLNESS LIFE-STYLE PLAN

Inventory 26

Name ______________________ Date ______________

DIRECTIONS: Complete items 1-10 to establish your Personal Wellness Life-Style Plan (use the sample on page 43 as a guide). You should periodically review these statements as an aid in the assessment of your progress.

1. **Specific** wellness life-style intervention objectives I would be realistically able and willing to work on are as follows:

2. Of the above wellness life-style interventions, the ONE I will select as my PERSONAL HEALTH BEHAVIOR CHANGE is:

3. Specific steps I will take to achieve the objectives in my chosen health behavior changes are:

4. Dates by which I plan to achieve:

5. Rewards (specify LT for long term and ST for short term) I will give myself for completing each step are:

6. Following are some of the benefits (specify LT for long term and ST for short term) I expect to gain from my Personal Wellness Life-Style Plan:

7. Obstacles that might get in the way of my success are:

8. Ways I can avoid or remove these obstacles:

9. I will keep track of my progress by:

10. I will commit myself to this Wellness Life-Style Plan by signing below:

____
("Life-Style Changer")

____
(Date)

____
(Witness)

____
(Date)

STRENGTH ASSESSMENT

Inventory 27

Name ______________________ Date ______________

Push-Ups

DIRECTIONS: Perform the maximum number of push-ups possible, up to 40. The chest must touch the ground and the arm fully extend on each repetition. No rest should be taken between repetitions. Records the results on page 275.

Scoring for the Push-up Test

Strength Category	Number of Push-Ups Men under 35	Men over 35	Women under 35	Women over 35
High	> 35	> 20	> 25	> 15
Average (Adequate)	15-35	10-20	10-25	5-15
Low	5-14	2-9	2-9	1-4

Table B.1.

Sit-Ups

DIRECTIONS: Perform the maximum number of sit-ups possible, up to 75. The feet are not supported. The head should go beyond the upright position in the up phase and touch the floor on the down phase. No rest should be taken between repetitions. Record the results on page 275.

Scoring for the Sit-up Test

Strength Category	Number of Sit-Ups Men under 35	Men over 35	Women under 35	Women over 35
High	> 75	> 50	> 50	> 30
Average (Adequate)	30-75	20-50	25-50	15-30
Low	15-29	10-19	10-24	5-14

Table B.2.

One-Repetition Maximum

DIRECTIONS: A more accurate method of assessing strength requires the use of barbells or a weight machine. Before the test, stretching the muscle to be used is important, and warming-up with light lifting is beneficial. The test requires that the individual progress to lifting as much weight as possible, i.e., a one repetition maximum (1 RM). The maximum lift should be made within three trials to avoid the effects of fatigue. Free-weights or weight machines can be used. Determination of the 1 RM is made on four different lifts: overhead press, chest press, biceps curl, and leg press. These four lifts give an accurate indication of overall body strength. Allow at least two minutes of recovery between each maximal attempt.

Scoring for One Repetition Maximum Strength Tests

Lift	Men's Strength Category			Women Strength Category		
	High	Average	Low	High	Average	Low
Shoulder Press	100*	66	50	66*	45	35
Bench Press	150	100	75	100	70	50
Arm Curl	75	50	40	50	35	25
Leg Press	250	200	150	200	150	100
Total (%)	575	416	315	416	300	210

* All Scores are % of body weight

Reprinted from T.R. Thomas and C.J. Zebas. Scientific Exercise Training. Dubuque, IA: Kendall/Hunt Publishing Co., 1987.

Not all individuals should attempt to achieve a 1 RM. Very sedentary, elderly, very young, or diseased individuals should estimate a 1 RM using the submaximal lift table. In this procedure, the lifter determines the maximal amount of resistance which corresponds to the number of repetitions in the table. For example, an untrained young woman (weight=50 kg) can lift 20 kg 10 times on the bench press (a maximal effort). The 1 RM is estimated by: 20 kg/0.8=25 kg. According to the scoring table, the individual is low in strength for this muscle group. This method provides an estimate only, but does allow the determination of the starting point in the resistance program and a reasonable evaluation of progress made.

Estimation of 1 RM from Submaximal Lifts (# of Reps at 80% load)

Lift	Untrained	Trained*
Shoulder Press	10	10
Bench Press	10	12
Arm Curl	8	10
Leg Press	14	20

* Previous resistance training at least 3 times per week. To estimate 1 RM: Determine the maximal load which can be lifted the designated number of repetition. This load corresponds to 80% maximum. Thus, 1 RM load=80%load/0.8. Table derived from the data of W.K. Hoeger et al. *J. Appl. Sport Sci. Research.* 4(2):47-54, 1990.

Strength Changes Record Sheet

Name ______________________ Sex __________ Date __________

Push-Ups and Sit-Ups

Test	1st test	2nd test	3rd test
Number of Push-Ups			
Strength Category			
Number of Sit-Ups			

One Repetition Maximum

	1st test	2nd test	3rd test
Date			
Body Weight			

Lift	Wt Lifted %BW	Wt Lifted %BW	Wt Lifted %BW
Overhead Press			
Chest Press			
Biceps Curl			
Leg Press			
Total			

$$\% \text{ BW} = \text{Percent of body weight} = \frac{\text{Wt Lifted}}{\text{Body Weight}} \times 100$$

EXERCISE LOG

Inventory 28

Name______________________________ Date ____________________

Target Heart Rate ________________________

Date	Type of Exercise	Distance or Time Involved	Minutes at Target HR	Body Weight

Exercise Log

Name____________________________________ Date ____________________

Target Heart Rate ____________________________

Date	Type of Exercise	Distance or Time Involved	Minutes at Target HR	Body Weight

RESISTANCE TRAINING WORKOUT RECORDS

Inventory 29

Name______________________________ Date ______________

1.) Strength Program

Date	Exercise	Load Lbs.	Load % of 1 RM	Sets	Body Weight	Total Work-out Time

Name____ Date ____________________

2.) Circuit Resistance Training Program (CRT)

Date	Exercise	Load % of 1 RM	Exercise Heart Rate	Aerobic Mode	Body Weight	Total Work-out Time

FAT, FIBER, AND SODIUM LOG

Inventory 30

Name______________________________ Date ____________________

Date	Grams of Fat			Grams of Fiber		Milligrams of Sodium
	Sat.	Polyun.	Monoun.	Soluble	Insoluble	

APPENDIX

A

APPROXIMATE CALORIC EXPENDITURE PER MINUTE FOR VARIOUS PHYSICAL ACTIVITIES

From Melvin H. Williams, *Nutrition for Fitness and Sport,* 3d ed.

Body weight												
Kilograms	45	48	50	52	55	57	59	61	64	66	68	70
Pounds	100	105	110	115	120	125	130	135	140	145	150	155
Sedentary activities												
Lying quietly	99	1.0	1.1	1.1	1.2	1.3	1.3	1.4	1.4	1.5	1.5	1.5
Sitting and writing, card playing, etc.	1.2	1.3	1.4	1.5	1.5	1.6	1.7	1.7	1.8	1.8	1.9	2.0
Standing with light work, cleaning, etc.	2.7	2.9	3.0	3.1	3.3	3.4	3.5	3.7	3.8	3.9	4.1	4.2
Physical activities												
Archery	3.1	3.3	3.5	3.6	3.8	4.0	4.1	4.3	4.5	4.6	4.8	4.9
Badminton												
Recreational singles	3.6	3.8	4.0	4.2	4.4	4.6	4.7	4.9	5.1	5.3	5.4	5.6
Social doubles	2.7	2.9	3.0	3.1	3.3	3.4	3.5	3.7	3.8	3.9	4.1	4.2
Competitive	5.9	6.1	6.4	6.7	7.0	7.3	7.6	7.9	8.2	8.5	8.8	9.1
Baseball												
Player	3.1	3.3	3.4	3.6	3.8	4.0	4.1	4.3	4.4	4.5	4.7	4.8
Pitcher	3.9	4.1	4.3	4.5	4.7	4.9	5.1	5.3	5.5	5.7	5.9	6.0
Basketball												
Half court	3.0	3.1	3.3	3.5	3.6	3.8	3.9	4.1	4.2	4.4	4.5	4.7
Recreational	4.9	5.2	5.5	5.7	6.0	6.2	6.5	6.7	7.0	7.2	7.5	7.7
Vigorous competition	6.5	6.8	7.2	7.5	7.8	8.2	8.5	8.8	9.2	9.5	9.9	10.2
Bicycling, level												
(mph) (min/mile)												
5 12:00	1.9	2.0	2.1	2.2	2.3	2.4	2.5	2.6	2.7	2.8	2.9	3.0
10 6:00	4.2	4.4	4.6	4.8	5.1	5.3	5.5	5.7	5.9	6.1	6.4	6.6
15 4:00	7.3	7.6	8.0	8.4	8.7	9.1	9.5	9.8	10.0	10.5	10.9	11.3
20 3:00	10.7	11.2	11.7	12.3	12.8	13.3	13.9	14.4	14.9	15.5	16.0	16.5
Bowling	2.7	2.8	3.0	3.1	3.3	3.4	3.5	3.7	3.8	3.9	4.1	4.2
Calisthenics												
Light type	3.4	3.6	3.8	4.0	4.1	4.3	4.5	4.7	4.8	5.0	5.2	5.4
Timed vigorous	9.7	10.1	10.6	11.1	11.6	12.1	12.6	13.1	13.6	14.1	14.6	15.1
Canoeing												
(mph) (min/mile)												
2.5 24	1.9	2.0	2.1	2.2	2.3	2.4	2.5	2.6	2.7	2.8	2.9	3.0
4.0 15	4.4	4.6	4.9	5.1	5.3	5.5	5.8	6.0	6.2	6.4	6.7	6.9
5.0 12	5.7	6.0	6.3	6.6	6.9	7.2	7.5	7.8	8.1	8.4	8.7	9.0
Dancing												
Moderately (waltz)	3.1	3.3	3.5	3.6	3.8	4.0	4.1	4.3	4.5	4.6	4.8	4.9
Active (square, disco)	4.5	4.7	5.0	5.2	5.4	5.6	5.9	6.1	6.3	6.6	6.8	7.0
Aerobic (vigorously)	6.0	6.3	6.7	7.0	7.3	7.6	7.9	8.2	8.5	8.8	9.1	9.4

* Note: The energy cost, in Calories, will vary for different physical activities in a given individual depending on several factors. For example, the caloric cost of bicycling will vary depending on the type of bicycle, going uphill or downhill, and wind resistance. Walking with hand weights or ankle weights will increase energy output. Thus, the values expressed here are approximations and may be increased or decreased depending upon factors that influence energy cost.

73 160	75 165	77 170	80 175	82 180	84 185	86 190	89 195	91 200	93 205	95 210	98 215	100 220
1.6	1.6	1.7	1.7	1.8	1.8	1.9	1.9	2.0	2.0	2.1	2.1	2.2
2.0	2.1	2.2	2.2	2.3	2.4	2.4	2.5	2.5	2.6	2.7	2.7	2.8
4.4	4.5	4.6	4.8	4.9	5.0	5.2	5.3	5.4	5.6	5.7	5.9	6.0
5.1	5.3	5.4	5.6	5.7	5.9	6.0	6.2	6.4	6.5	6.7	6.9	7.0
5.8	6.0	6.2	6.4	6.6	6.7	6.9	7.1	7.3	7.4	7.6	7.8	8.0
4.4	4.5	4.6	4.8	4.9	5.0	5.2	5.3	5.4	5.6	5.7	5.9	6.0
9.4	9.7	10.0	10.3	10.6	10.9	11.2	11.5	11.8	12.1	12.4	12.7	13.0
5.0	5.2	5.3	5.5	5.6	5.8	5.9	6.1	6.3	6.4	6.6	6.8	6.9
6.3	6.5	6.7	6.9	7.1	7.3	7.4	7.7	7.9	8.0	8.2	8.5	8.6
4.8	5.0	5.1	5.3	5.4	5.6	5.7	5.9	6.0	6.2	6.4	6.5	6.7
8.0	8.2	8.5	8.7	9.0	9.2	9.5	9.7	10.0	10.2	10.5	10.7	11.0
10.5	10.9	11.2	11.5	11.9	12.2	12.5	12.9	13.2	13.5	13.8	14.2	14.5
3.1	3.2	3.3	3.4	3.5	3.6	3.7	3.8	3.9	4.0	4.1	4.2	4.3
6.8	7.0	7.2	7.4	7.6	7.9	8.1	8.3	8.5	8.7	8.9	9.1	9.4
11.6	12.0	12.4	12.7	13.1	13.4	13.8	14.2	14.5	14.9	15.3	15.6	16.0
17.1	17.6	18.1	18.7	19.2	19.7	20.3	20.8	21.3	21.9	22.4	22.9	23.5
4.4	4.5	4.6	4.8	4.9	5.0	5.2	5.3	5.5	5.6	5.7	5.9	6.0
5.5	5.7	5.9	6.1	6.3	6.4	6.6	6.8	7.0	7.1	7.3	7.5	7.7
15.6	16.1	16.6	17.1	17.6	18.1	18.6	19.1	19.6	20.0	20.5	21.0	21.5
3.1	3.2	3.3	3.4	3.5	3.6	3.7	3.8	3.9	4.0	4.1	4.2	4.3
7.1	7.4	7.6	7.8	8.0	8.2	8.5	8.7	8.9	9.1	9.4	9.6	9.8
9.3	9.5	9.8	10.1	10.4	10.7	11.0	11.3	11.6	11.9	12.2	12.5	12.8
5.1	5.3	5.4	5.6	5.7	5.9	6.0	6.2	6.4	6.5	6.7	6.9	7.0
7.3	7.5	7.7	7.9	8.2	8.4	8.6	8.9	9.1	9.3	9.5	9.8	10.0
9.7	10.0	10.3	10.6	10.9	11.2	11.5	11.8	12.1	12.4	12.7	13.0	13.3

Body weight												
Kilograms	45	48	50	52	55	57	59	61	64	66	68	70
Pounds	100	105	110	115	120	125	130	135	140	145	150	155
Fencing												
Moderately	3.3	3.5	3.6	3.8	4.0	4.1	4.3	4.5	4.6	4.8	5.0	5.2
Vigorously	6.6	7.0	7.3	7.7	8.0	8.3	8.7	9.0	9.4	9.7	10.0	10.4
Football												
Moderate	3.3	3.5	3.6	3.8	4.0	4.1	4.3	4.5	4.6	4.8	5.0	5.2
Touch, vigorous	5.5	5.8	6.1	6.4	6.6	6.9	7.2	7.5	7.8	8.0	8.3	8.6
Golf												
Twosome (carry clubs)	3.6	3.8	4.0	4.2	4.4	4.6	4.7	4.9	5.1	5.3	5.4	5.6
Foursome (carry clubs)	2.7	2.9	3.0	3.1	3.3	3.4	3.5	3.7	3.8	3.9	4.1	4.2
Power-cart	1.9	2.0	2.1	2.2	2.3	2.4	2.5	2.6	2.7	2.8	2.9	3.0
Handball												
Moderate	6.5	6.8	7.2	7.5	7.8	8.2	8.5	8.8	9.2	9.5	9.9	10.2
Competitive	7.7	8.0	8.4	8.8	9.2	9.6	10.0	10.4	10.8	11.1	11.5	11.9
Hiking, pack (3 mph)	4.5	4.7	5.0	5.2	5.4	5.6	5.9	6.1	6.3	6.6	6.8	7.0
Hockey, field	5.0	6.3	6.7	7.0	7.3	7.6	7.9	8.2	8.5	8.8	9.1	9.4
Hockey, ice	6.6	7.0	7.3	7.7	8.0	8.3	8.7	9.0	9.4	9.7	10.0	10.4
Horseback riding												
Walk	1.9	2.0	2.1	2.2	2.3	2.4	2.5	2.6	2.7	2.8	2.9	3.0
Sitting to trot	2.7	2.9	3.0	3.1	3.3	3.4	3.5	3.7	3.8	3.9	4.1	4.2
Posting to trot	4.2	4.4	4.6	4.8	5.1	5.3	5.5	5.7	5.9	6.1	6.4	6.6
Gallop	5.7	6.0	6.3	6.6	6.9	7.2	7.5	7.8	8.1	8.4	8.7	9.0
Horseshoes	2.5	2.6	2.8	2.9	3.0	3.1	3.3	3.4	3.5	3.7	3.8	3.9
Jogging (see Running)												
Judo	8.5	8.9	9.3	9.8	10.2	10.6	11.0	11.5	11.9	12.3	12.8	13.2
Karate	8.5	8.9	9.3	9.8	10.2	10.6	11.0	11.5	11.9	12.3	12.8	13.2
Mountain climbing	6.5	6.8	7.2	7.5	7.8	8.2	8.5	8.8	9.2	9.5	9.8	10.2
Paddle ball	5.7	6.0	6.3	6.6	6.9	7.2	7.5	7.8	8.1	8.4	8.7	9.0
Pool (billiards)	1.5	1.6	1.6	1.7	1.8	1.9	1.9	2.0	2.1	2.2	2.2	2.3
Racketball	6.5	6.8	7.1	7.5	7.8	8.1	8.4	8.8	9.1	9.4	9.8	10.1
Roller skating (9 mph)	4.2	4.4	4.6	4.8	5.1	5.3	5.5	5.7	5.9	6.1	6.4	6.6
Running (steady state)												
(mph) (min/mile)												
5.0 12:00	6.0	6.3	6.6	7.0	7.3	7.6	7.9	8.2	8.5	8.8	9.1	9.4
5.5 10:55	6.7	7.0	7.3	7.7	8.0	8.4	8.7	9.0	9.4	9.7	10.0	10.4
6.0 10:00	7.2	7.6	8.0	8.4	8.7	9.1	9.5	9.8	10.2	10.6	10.9	11.3
7.0 8:35	8.5	8.9	9.3	9.8	10.2	10.6	11.0	11.5	11.9	12.3	12.8	13.2
8.0 7:30	9.7	10.2	10.7	11.2	11.6	12.1	12.6	13.1	13.6	14.1	14.6	15.1
9.0 6:40	10.8	11.3	11.9	12.4	12.9	13.5	14.0	14.6	15.1	15.7	16.2	16.8
10.0 6:00	12.1	12.7	13.3	13.9	14.5	15.1	15.7	16.4	17.0	17.6	18.2	18.8
11.0 5:28	13.3	14.0	14.6	15.3	16.0	16.7	17.3	18.0	18.7	19.4	20.0	20.7
12.0 5:00	14.5	15.2	16.0	16.7	17.4	18.2	18.9	19.7	20.4	21.1	21.9	22.6
Sailing, small boat	2.7	2.9	3.0	3.1	3.3	3.4	3.5	3.7	3.8	3.9	4.1	4.2
Skating, ice (9 mph)	4.2	4.4	4.6	4.8	5.1	5.2	5.5	5.7	5.9	6.1	6.4	6.6
Skiing, cross country												
(mph) (min/mile)												
2.5 24:00	5.0	5.2	5.5	5.7	6.0	6.2	6.5	6.7	7.0	7.2	7.5	7.8
4.0 15:00	6.5	6.8	7.2	7.5	7.8	8.2	8.5	8.8	9.2	9.5	9.9	10.2
5.0 12:00	7.7	8.0	8.4	8.8	9.2	9.6	10.0	10.4	10.8	11.1	11.5	11.9
Skiing, downhill	6.5	6.8	7.2	7.5	7.8	8.2	8.5	8.8	9.2	9.5	9.9	10.2
Soccer	5.9	6.2	6.6	6.9	7.2	7.5	7.8	8.1	8.4	8.7	9.0	9.3

73	75	77	80	82	84	86	89	91	93	95	98	100
160	165	170	175	180	185	190	195	200	205	210	215	220
5.3	5.5	5.7	5.8	6.0	6.2	6.3	6.5	6.7	6.8	7.0	7.1	7.3
10.7	11.0	11.4	11.7	12.1	12.4	12.7	13.1	13.4	13.8	14.1	14.4	14.8
5.3	5.5	5.7	5.8	6.0	6.2	6.3	6.5	6.7	6.8	7.0	7.1	7.3
8.9	9.2	9.4	9.7	10.0	10.3	10.6	10.8	11.1	11.4	11.7	12.0	12.2
5.8	6.0	6.2	6.4	6.6	6.7	6.9	7.1	7.3	7.4	7.6	7.8	8.0
4.4	4.5	4.6	4.8	4.9	5.0	5.2	5.3	5.4	5.6	5.7	5.9	6.0
3.1	3.2	3.3	3.4	3.5	3.6	3.7	3.8	3.9	4.0	4.1	4.2	4.3
10.5	10.9	11.2	11.5	11.9	12.2	12.5	12.9	13.2	13.5	13.8	14.2	14.5
12.3	12.7	13.1	13.5	13.9	14.3	14.7	15.0	15.4	15.8	16.2	16.6	17.0
7.3	7.5	7.7	7.9	8.2	8.4	8.6	8.9	9.1	9.3	9.5	9.8	10.0
9.7	10.0	10.3	10.6	10.9	11.2	11.5	11.8	12.1	12.4	12.7	13.0	13.3
10.7	11.0	11.4	11.7	12.1	12.4	12.7	13.1	13.4	13.8	14.1	14.4	14.8
3.1	3.2	3.3	3.4	3.5	3.6	3.7	3.8	3.9	4.0	4.1	4.2	4.3
4.4	4.5	4.6	4.8	4.9	5.0	5.2	5.3	5.4	5.6	5.7	5.9	6.0
6.8	7.0	7.2	7.4	7.6	7.9	8.1	8.3	8.5	8.7	8.9	9.1	9.4
9.3	9.5	9.8	10.1	10.4	10.7	11.0	11.3	11.6	11.9	12.2	12.5	12.8
4.0	4.2	4.3	4.4	4.5	4.7	4.8	4.9	5.2	5.2	5.3	5.4	5.6
13.6	14.1	14.5	14.9	15.4	15.8	16.2	16.6	17.1	17.5	17.9	18.4	18.8
13.6	14.1	14.5	14.9	15.4	15.8	16.2	16.6	17.1	17.5	17.9	18.4	18.8
10.5	10.8	11.2	11.5	11.8	12.1	12.5	12.8	13.1	13.5	13.8	14.1	14.5
9.3	9.5	9.8	10.1	10.4	10.7	11.0	11.2	11.6	11.9	12.2	12.5	12.8
2.4	2.5	2.6	2.6	2.7	2.8	2.9	2.9	3.0	3.1	3.2	3.2	3.3
10.4	10.7	11.1	11.4	11.7	12.0	12.4	12.7	13.0	13.4	13.7	14.0	14.4
6.8	7.0	7.2	7.4	7.6	7.9	8.1	8.3	8.5	8.7	8.9	9.1	9.4
9.7	10.0	10.3	10.6	10.9	11.2	11.6	11.9	12.2	12.5	12.8	13.1	13.4
10.7	11.1	11.4	11.7	12.1	12.4	12.8	13.1	13.4	13.8	14.1	14.5	14.8
11.7	12.0	12.4	12.8	13.1	13.5	13.8	14.3	14.6	15.0	15.4	15.7	16.1
13.6	14.1	14.5	14.9	15.4	15.8	16.2	16.6	17.1	17.5	17.9	18.4	18.8
15.6	16.1	16.6	17.1	17.6	18.1	18.5	19.0	19.5	20.0	20.5	21.0	21.5
17.3	17.9	18.4	19.0	19.5	20.1	20.6	21.2	21.7	22.2	22.8	23.3	23.9
19.4	20.0	20.7	21.3	21.9	22.5	23.1	23.7	24.2	24.8	25.4	26.0	26.7
21.4	22.1	22.7	23.4	24.1	24.8	25.4	26.1	26.8	27.5	28.1	28.8	29.5
23.3	24.1	24.8	25.6	26.3	27.0	27.8	28.5	29.2	30.0	30.7	31.5	32.2
4.4	4.5	4.6	4.8	4.9	5.0	5.2	5.3	5.4	5.6	5.7	5.9	6.0
6.8	7.0	7.2	7.4	7.6	7.9	8.1	8.3	8.5	8.7	8.9	9.1	9.4
8.0	8.3	8.5	8.8	9.0	9.3	9.5	9.8	10.0	10.3	10.6	10.8	11.1
10.5	10.9	11.2	11.5	11.9	12.2	12.5	12.9	13.2	13.5	13.8	14.2	14.5
12.3	12.7	13.1	13.5	13.9	14.3	14.7	15.0	15.4	15.8	16.2	16.6	17.0
10.5	10.9	11.2	11.5	11.9	12.2	12.5	12.9	13.2	13.5	13.8	14.2	14.5
9.6	9.9	10.2	10.5	10.8	11.1	11.4	11.7	12.0	12.3	12.6	12.9	13.2

Body weight												
Kilograms	45	48	50	52	55	57	59	61	64	66	68	70
Pounds	100	105	110	115	120	125	130	135	140	145	150	155
Squash												
Normal	6.7	7.0	7.3	7.7	8.0	8.4	8.7	9.1	9.5	9.8	10.1	10.5
Competition	7.7	8.0	8.4	8.8	9.2	9.6	10.0	10.4	10.8	11.1	11.5	11.9
Swimming (yards/min)												
Backstroke												
25	2.5	2.6	2.8	2.9	3.0	3.1	3.3	3.4	3.5	3.7	3.8	3.9
30	3.5	3.7	3.9	4.1	4.2	4.4	4.6	4.8	4.9	5.1	5.3	5.5
35	4.5	4.7	5.0	5.2	5.4	5.6	5.9	6.1	6.3	6.6	6.8	7.0
40	5.5	5.8	6.1	6.4	6.6	6.9	7.2	7.5	7.8	8.0	8.3	8.6
Breaststroke												
20	3.1	3.3	3.5	3.6	3.8	4.0	4.1	4.3	4.5	4.6	4.8	4.9
30	4.7	5.0	5.2	5.4	5.7	5.9	6.2	6.4	6.7	6.9	7.1	7.4
40	6.3	6.7	7.0	7.3	7.6	8.0	8.3	8.6	8.9	9.3	9.6	9.9
Front crawl												
20	3.1	3.3	3.5	3.6	3.8	4.0	4.1	4.3	4.5	4.6	4.8	4.9
25	4.0	4.2	4.4	4.6	4.8	5.0	5.2	5.4	5.6	5.8	6.0	6.2
35	4.8	5.1	5.4	5.6	5.9	6.1	6.4	6.6	6.8	7.0	7.3	7.5
45	5.7	6.0	6.3	6.6	6.9	7.2	7.5	7.8	8.1	8.4	8.7	9.0
50	7.0	7.4	7.7	8.1	8.5	8.8	9.2	9.5	9.9	10.3	10.6	11.0
Table tennis	3.4	3.6	3.8	4.0	4.1	4.3	4.5	4.7	4.8	5.0	5.2	5.4
Tennis												
Singles, recreational	5.0	5.2	5.5	5.7	6.0	6.2	6.5	6.7	7.0	7.2	7.5	7.8
Doubles, recreational	3.4	3.6	3.8	4.0	4.1	4.3	4.5	4.7	4.8	5.0	5.2	5.4
Competition	6.4	6.7	7.1	7.4	7.7	8.1	8.4	8.7	9.1	9.4	9.8	10.1
Volleyball												
Moderate, recreational	2.9	3.0	3.2	3.3	3.5	3.6	3.8	3.9	4.1	4.2	4.4	4.5
Vigorous, competition	6.5	6.8	7.1	7.5	7.8	8.1	8.4	8.8	9.1	9.4	9.8	10.1
Walking												
(mph) (min/mile)												
1.0 60:00	1.5	1.6	1.7	1.8	1.8	1.9	2.0	2.1	2.2	2.2	2.3	2.4
2.0 30:00	2.1	2.2	2.3	2.4	2.5	2.6	2.8	2.9	3.0	3.1	3.2	3.3
2.3 26:00	2.3	2.4	2.5	2.7	2.8	2.9	3.0	3.1	3.2	3.4	3.5	3.6
3.0 20.00	2.7	2.9	3.0	3.1	3.3	3.4	3.5	3.7	3.8	3.9	4.1	4.2
3.2 18:45	3.1	3.3	3.4	3.6	3.8	4.0	4.1	4.3	4.4	4.5	4.7	4.8
3.5 17:10	3.3	3.5	3.7	3.9	4.0	4.2	4.4	4.6	4.7	4.9	5.1	5.3
4.0 15:00	4.2	4.4	4.6	4.8	5.1	5.3	5.5	5.7	5.9	6.1	6.4	6.6
4.5 13:20	4.7	5.0	5.2	5.4	5.7	5.9	6.2	6.4	6.7	6.9	7.1	7.4
5.0 12:00	5.4	5.7	6.0	6.3	6.5	6.8	7.1	7.4	7.7	7.9	8.2	8.4
5.4 11:10	6.2	6.6	6.9	7.2	7.5	7.9	8.2	8.5	8.8	9.2	9.5	9.8
5.8 10:20	7.7	8.0	8.4	8.8	9.2	9.6	10.0	10.4	10.8	11.1	11.5	11.9
Water skiing	5.0	5.2	5.5	5.7	6.0	6.2	6.5	6.7	7.0	7.2	7.5	7.8
Weight training	5.2	5.4	5.7	6.0	6.2	6.5	6.8	7.0	7.3	7.6	7.8	8.1
Wrestling	8.5	8.9	9.3	9.8	10.2	10.6	11.0	11.5	11.9	12.3	12.8	13.2

73	75	77	80	82	84	86	89	91	93	95	98	100
160	165	170	175	180	185	190	195	200	205	210	215	220
10.8	11.2	11.5	11.8	12.2	12.5	12.9	13.2	13.5	13.9	14.2	14.6	14.9
12.3	12.7	13.1	13.5	13.9	14.3	14.7	15.0	15.4	15.8	16.2	16.6	17.0
4.0	4.2	4.3	4.4	4.5	4.7	4.8	4.9	5.1	5.2	5.3	5.4	5.6
5.6	5.8	6.0	6.2	6.4	6.5	6.7	6.9	7.1	7.2	7.4	7.6	7.8
7.3	7.5	7.7	7.9	8.2	8.4	8.6	8.9	9.1	9.3	9.5	9.8	10.0
8.9	9.2	9.4	9.7	10.0	10.3	10.6	10.8	11.1	11.4	11.7	12.0	12.2
5.1	5.3	5.4	5.6	5.7	5.9	6.0	6.2	6.4	6.5	6.7	6.9	7.0
7.6	7.9	8.1	8.3	8.6	8.8	9.1	9.3	9.5	9.8	10.0	10.3	10.5
10.2	10.5	10.9	11.2	11.5	11.9	12.2	12.5	12.8	13.1	13.5	13.8	14.1
5.1	5.3	5.4	5.6	5.7	5.9	6.0	6.2	6.4	6.5	6.7	6.9	7.0
6.4	6.6	6.8	7.0	7.2	7.4	7.6	7.8	8.0	8.2	8.4	8.6	8.8
7.8	8.0	8.3	8.5	8.8	9.0	9.2	9.4	9.7	9.9	10.2	10.4	10.7
9.3	9.5	9.8	10.1	10.4	10.7	11.0	11.3	11.6	11.9	12.2	12.5	12.8
11.3	11.7	12.0	12.4	12.8	13.1	13.5	13.8	14.2	14.5	14.9	15.2	15.6
5.5	5.7	5.9	6.1	6.3	6.4	6.6	6.8	7.0	7.1	7.3	7.5	7.7
8.0	8.3	8.5	8.8	9.0	9.3	9.5	9.8	10.0	10.3	10.6	10.8	11.1
5.5	5.7	5.9	6.1	6.3	6.4	6.6	6.8	7.0	7.1	7.3	7.5	7.7
10.4	10.8	11.1	11.4	11.8	12.1	12.4	12.8	13.1	13.4	13.7	14.1	14.4
4.7	4.8	5.0	5.1	5.3	5.4	5.6	5.7	5.9	6.0	6.1	6.3	6.4
10.4	10.7	11.1	11.4	11.7	12.0	12.4	12.7	13.0	13.4	13.7	14.0	14.4
2.4	2.5	2.6	2.7	2.8	2.9	2.9	3.0	3.1	3.2	3.2	3.3	3.4
3.4	3.5	3.6	3.7	3.9	4.0	4.1	4.2	4.3	4.4	4.5	4.6	4.7
3.7	3.8	4.0	4.1	4.2	4.3	4.4	4.5	4.7	4.8	4.9	5.0	5.1
4.4	4.5	4.6	4.8	4.9	5.0	5.2	5.3	5.4	5.6	5.7	5.9	6.0
5.0	5.2	5.3	5.5	5.6	5.8	5.9	6.1	6.3	6.4	6.6	6.8	6.9
5.4	5.6	5.8	6.0	6.2	6.3	6.5	6.7	6.9	7.0	7.2	7.4	7.6
6.8	7.0	7.2	7.4	7.6	7.9	8.1	8.3	8.5	8.7	8.9	9.1	9.4
7.6	7.9	8.1	8.3	8.6	8.8	9.1	9.3	9.5	9.8	10.0	10.3	10.5
8.7	9.0	9.2	9.5	9.8	10.1	10.4	10.6	10.9	11.2	11.5	11.8	12.0
10.1	10.4	10.8	11.1	11.4	11.8	12.1	12.4	12.7	13.0	13.4	13.7	14.0
12.3	12.7	13.1	13.5	13.9	14.3	14.7	15.0	15.4	15.8	16.2	16.6	17.0
8.0	8.3	8.5	8.8	9.0	9.3	9.5	9.8	10.0	10.3	10.6	10.8	11.1
8.3	8.6	8.9	9.1	9.4	9.7	9.9	10.2	10.5	10.7	11.0	11.2	11.5
13.6	14.1	14.5	14.9	15.4	15.8	16.2	16.6	17.1	17.5	17.9	18.4	18.8

APPENDIX

B

NUTRITIVE VALUE OF FOODS

United States Department of Agriculture, *Home and Garden Bulletin #72*, Washington, DC: U.S. Government Printing Office, 1991.

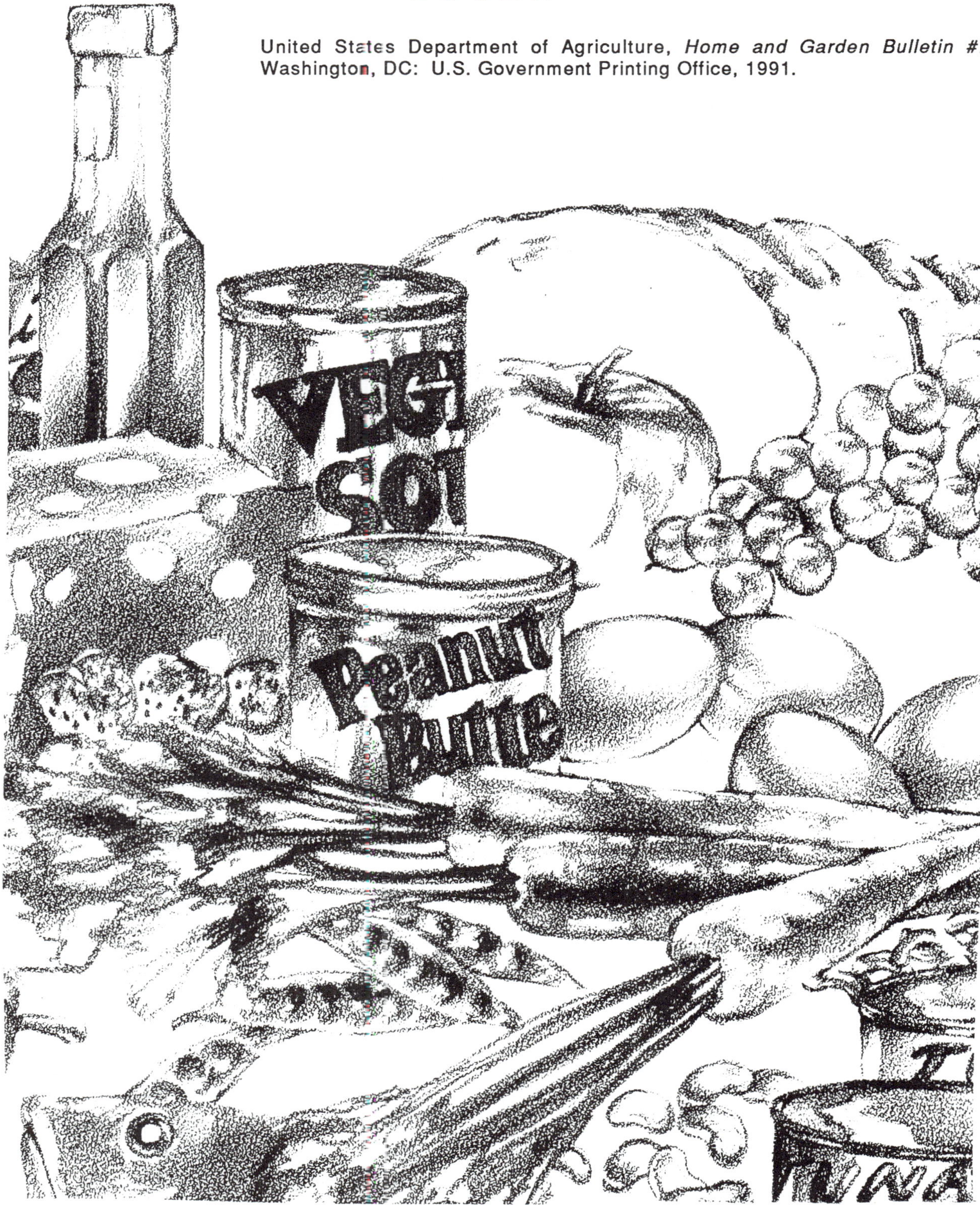

Contents

Explanation of the Tables 290
Further Information 293

Table
1) Equivalents by Volume and Weight 290

2) Nutritive Value of the Edible Part of Food: 294
  Beverages (Item 1-29) 294
  Dairy proudcts (Item 30-120) 296
  Eggs (Item 121-127) 300
  Fats and Oils (Item 128-173) 302
  Fish and shellfish (Item 174-197) 304
  Fruits and fruit juices (Item 198-310) 304
  Grain products (Item 311-524) 312
  Legumes, nuts, and seeds (Item 525-574) 326
  Meat and meat products (Item 575-628) 328
  Mixed dishes and fast foods (Item 629-655) 332
  Poultry and poultry products (Item 656-676) 334
  Soups, sauces, and gravies (Item 677-709) 334
  Sugars and sweets (Item 710-749) 336
  Vegetables and vegetable products (Item 750-880) 338
  Miscellaneous items (Item 881-908) 348

3) Yield of Cooked Meat per Pound of Raw Meat as Purchased 350

4) Recommended Daily Dietary Allowances (RDA) 351

5) Food Sources of Additional Nutrients 352

6) Amount of Fat that Provides 30 and 35 Percent of Calories at Specified Calorie Levels 352

Explanation of the Tables

Some helpful volume and weight equivalents are shown in table 1.

Table 1.—Equivalents by Volume and Weight

Volume

Level measure	Equivalent
1 gallon (3.786 liters; 3,786 milliliters)	4 quarts
1 quart (0.946 liter; 946 milliliters)	4 cups 2 pints
1 cup (237 milliliters)	8 fluid ounces 1/2 pint 16 tablespoons
2 tablespoons (30 milliliters)	1 fluid ounce
1 tablespoon (15 milliliters)	3 teaspoons

Weight

Avoirdupois weight	Equivalent
1 pound (16 ounces)	453.6 grams
1 ounce	28.35 grams
3-1/2 ounces	100 grams

Nutritive Value of Foods (Table 2)

Table 2 shows the nutritive values of 908 common foods.

Foods listed.—Foods are grouped under the following main headings:

- Beverages
- Dairy products
- Eggs
- Fats and oils
- Fish and shellfish
- Fruits and fruit juices
- Grain products
- Legumes, nuts, and seeds
- Meat and meat products
- Mixed dishes and fast foods
- Poultry and poultry products
- Soups, sauces, and gravies
- Sugars and sweets
- Vegetables and vegetable products
- Miscellaneous items

Most of the foods listed are in ready-to-eat form. Some are basic products widely used in food preparation, such as flour, fat, and cornmeal.

The approximate measure shown for each food is in cups, ounces, pounds, some other well-known unit, or a piece of a certain size. The measures shown do not necessarily represent a serving, but the unit given may be used to calculate a variety of serving sizes. For example, values are given for 1 cup of applesauce. If a serving is 1/2 cup, divide the values by 2 or multiply by 0.5; for a 2/3 cup serving multiply values by 0.67. The cup measure refers to the standard measuring cup of 8 fluid ounces. The ounce is one-sixteenth of a pound avoirdupois, unless "fluid ounce" is indicated. The weight of a fluid ounce varies according to the food measured. If the household measure of a food is listed as 1 ounce, the nutrients are based on a weight of 28.35 grams, although only 28 grams is shown in the table. All other measures are based on the actual weight shown.

The weight in grams for an approximate measure of each food is shown. The weight applies to only the edible portion of the food, such as the banana pulp without the peel. For fruits and vegetables, whenever possible a market unit and its weight are given in the food description to indicate the weight of an item as purchased including the inedible parts that will be removed.

Food values.—Table 2 also shows values for water; food energy; protein; fat; total saturated, monounsaturated, and polyunsaturated fatty acids; cholesterol; carbohydrate; five minerals (calcium, phosphorus, iron, potassium, and sodium); and five vitamins (vitamin A, thiamin, riboflavin, niacin, and ascorbic acid or vitamin C). Water content is included because the percentage of moisture present is needed for identification and comparison of many food items. Values are in grams or milligrams except for food energy and vitamin A.

Food energy is reported in calories. The calorie is the unit of measurement of the energy furnished the body by protein, fat, and carbohydrate. Alcohol also contributes to the calorie content of alcoholic beverages. Calorie values have been rounded to the nearest 5 calories. Vitamin A is reported in two different units: International Units (IU), used in the past for expressing vitamin A activity, and Retinol Equivalents (RE), the units currently used by the Food and Nutrition Board for expressing the Recommended Daily Dietary Allowances for vitamin A. International Units are rounded to the nearest 10 IU.

Nutrient data are from revised sections 1 through 12 of Agriculture Handbook No. 8. Values for foods not in the published AH-8 sections have been reviewed and updated as necessary using information currently available in the National Nutrient Data Bank. Most differences in this bulletin from values in the published sections of AH-8 are due to rounding.

Values for food energy (calories) and nutrients shown in table 2 are the amounts present in the part of the item that is customarily eaten—corn without cob, meat without bone, peaches without skin, European-type grapes without seeds. If additional parts are eaten—the peach skin, for example—amounts of some nutrients obtained will be somewhat greater than those shown.

Thiamin, riboflavin, niacin, and iron values in enriched white flours, white bread and rolls, cornmeals, pastas, farina, and rice are based on the current enrichment levels established for those products by the Food and Drug Administration. (Enrichment levels for riboflavin in rice have not been put into effect and are not used in table 2.) Enriched flour is used in most home-prepared and commercially prepared baked goods.

Niacin values are for preformed niacin occurring naturally in foods. The values do not include additional niacin that may be formed in the body from tryptophan, an essential amino acid in the protein of most foods. Among the better sources of tryptophan are milk, meats, eggs, legumes, and nuts.

Values for many prepared items have been calculated from the ingredients in typical recipes. Examples are biscuits, corn muffins, macaroni and cheese, custard, and many dessert-type items. Adjustments were made for nutrient losses during cooking.

Values for toast and cooked vegetables are without fat added, either during preparation or at the table. Values for cooked vegetables, dry beans, pasta, noodles, rice, meat, poultry, and fish are without salt added. Cutting or shredding vegetables may destroy a portion of some vitamins, especially ascorbic acid. Since such losses are variable, no deduction has been made.

The mineral contribution of water was not considered for coffee, tea, soups, sauces, or concentrated fruit juices prepared with water. Sweetened items contain sugar unless identified as artifically sweetened.

Several manufactured items—including some milk products, ready-to-eat breakfast cereals, imitation cream products, fruit drinks, and various mixes—are included in table 2. Such foods may be fortified with one or more nutrients; the label will describe any fortification. Values shown here for these foods may be based on products from several manufacturers and, therefore, may differ somewhat from the values provided by any one source.

For meat, values describe it after it has been cooked and drained of the drippings. For many cuts, two sets of values are shown: meat including lean and fat parts, and lean meat from which the fat has been removed either before or after cooking.

Yield of Cooked Meat (Table 3)

Meat undergoes certain losses from the time it is purchased to the time it is eaten. Among these are losses during cooking from evaporation of moisture, loss of fat in the drippings, and removal of parts such as bone, gristle, and fat before or after cooking.

Table 3 shows, for several retail cuts, the yield of cooked meat from 1 pound of raw meat. Yield is given as ounces of:

Cooked meat with bone and fat

Cooked lean and fat

Cooked lean only

Among the factors influencing the yield of meat is the proportion of fat and lean. Many cuts have an outside layer of fat extending all or part way around. The thickness of this fat layer varies depending on the cutting and trimming practices in the market. The information on yield in table 3 and on nutritive value in table 2 applies to retail cuts trimmed according to typical market practices. Deposits of fat within a cut (marbling) may be extensive. They usually are not affected by retail trimming but may be discarded at the table.

Recommended Daily Dietary Allowances (Table 4)

Table 4 shows Recommended Daily Dietary Allowances (RDA) for calories and for several nutrients essential for maintenance of good nutrition in healthy, normally active persons. This table is adapted from a more extensive table published by the Food and Nutrition Board of the National Academy of Sciences, National Research Council, in 1980.

Nutrients not shown in tables 2 and 4 but for which the Food and Nutrition Board published RDA in 1980 are vitamin B_6, vitamin B_{12}, folacin, vitamin D, vitamin E, magnesium, iodine, and zinc. More detailed information about RDA's may be obtained from the publication from which table 4 is adapted.

Food Sources of Additional Nutrients (Table 5)

Table 5 lists foods that are of special value in supplying the eight nutrients not shown in tables 2 and 4. Foods are considered to be of special value as a source of a nutrient if a serving of the food is relatively high in the nutrient.

The RDA for one nutrient shown in tables 2 and 4 is notably difficult to achieve by some individuals. Iron allowances are not met in diets for many preschool-age children and females of childbearing age. Choosing foods rich in iron—lean meats, shellfish, liver, heart, kidney, dry beans and peas, dark-green vegetables, dried fruit, and cereals with added iron—can help in meeting iron allowances. Iron supplements, in addition to a varied diet, are recommended for pregnant and lactating women.

Fat That Provides 30 and 35 Percent of Calories (Table 6)

Several scientific groups suggest that Americans moderate the amount of fat in their diets. Some recommend that fat be limited to amounts that will provide no more than 30 to 35 percent of calories. Table 6 shows the amount of fat that provides 30 and 35 percent of calories for diets of several total daily calorie intakes. For example, a woman wishing to moderate her fat intake to 35 percent of her 2,000-calorie diet should select foods that total no more than 78 grams of fat per day. She can estimate the grams of fat in the foods she eats from table 2.

Further Information

A number of other publications of the Human Nutrition Information Service, U.S. Department of Agriculture, give helpful information about nutrients and which foods they are found in.

Agriculture Handbook No. 8, "Composition of Foods. . . Raw, Processed, Prepared," is a more technical publication with data for a much more extensive list of foods. It is being revised in sections. The revised sections now available are:

No. 8-1 Dairy and Egg Products
8-2 Spices and Herbs
8-3 Baby Foods
8-4 Fats and Oils
8-5 Poultry Products
8-6 Soups, Sauces, and Gravies
8-7 Sausages and Luncheon Meats
8-8 Breakfast Cereals
8-9 Fruits and Fruit Juices
8-10 Pork Products
8-11 Vegetables and Vegetable Products
8-12 Nut and Seed Products

Other publications containing information on a specific nutrient are "The Sodium Content of Your Food," Home and Garden Bulletin No. 233, and "Calories and Weight," Agriculture Information Bulletin No. 364. Additional information on evaluating and planning diets is available from "The Hassle Free Guide to a Better Diet," L-567, and "Nutrition and Your Health: Dietary Guidelines for Americans," Home and Garden Bulletin No. 232.

These publications may be purchased from the Superintendent of Documents, U.S. Government Printing Office, Washington, DC 20401, or any U.S. Government Printing Office bookstore.

Table 2. Nutritive Value of the Edible Part of Food

(Tr indicates nutrient present in trace amount.)

Item No.	Foods, approximate measures, units and weight (weight of edible portion only)			Water	Food energy	Protein	Fat	Fatty acids: Saturated	Fatty acids: Monounsaturated	Fatty acids: Polyunsaturated
			Grams	Percent	Calories	Grams	Grams	Grams	Grams	Grams
	Beverages									
	Alcoholic:									
	Beer:									
1	Regular	12 fl oz	360	92	150	1	0	0.0	0.0	0.0
2	Light	12 fl oz	355	95	95	1	0	0.0	0.0	0.0
	Gin, rum, vodka, whiskey:									
3	80-proof	1-1/2 fl oz	42	67	95	0	0	0.0	0.0	0.0
4	86-proof	1-1/2 fl oz	42	64	105	0	0	0.0	0.0	0.0
5	90-proof	1-1/2 fl oz	42	62	110	0	0	0.0	0.0	0.0
	Wines:									
6	Dessert	3-1/2 fl oz	103	77	140	Tr	0	0.0	0.0	0.0
	Table:									
7	Red	3-1/2 fl oz	102	88	75	Tr	0	0.0	0.0	0.0
8	White	3-1/2 fl oz	102	87	80	Tr	0	0.0	0.0	0.0
	Carbonated:[2]									
9	Club soda	12 fl oz	355	100	0	0	0	0.0	0.0	0.0
	Cola type:									
10	Regular	12 fl oz	369	89	160	0	0	0.0	0.0	0.0
11	Diet, artificially sweetened	12 fl oz	355	100	Tr	0	0	0.0	0.0	0.0
12	Ginger ale	12 fl oz	366	91	125	0	0	0.0	0.0	0.0
13	Grape	12 fl oz	372	88	180	0	0	0.0	0.0	0.0
14	Lemon-lime	12 fl oz	372	89	155	0	0	0.0	0.0	0.0
15	Orange	12 fl oz	372	88	180	0	0	0.0	0.0	0.0
16	Pepper type	12 fl oz	369	89	160	0	0	0.0	0.0	0.0
17	Root beer	12 fl oz	370	89	165	0	0	0.0	0.0	0.0
	Cocoa and chocolate-flavored beverages. See Dairy Products (items 95-98).									
	Coffee:									
18	Brewed	6 fl oz	180	100	Tr	Tr	Tr	Tr	Tr	Tr
19	Instant, prepared (2 tsp powder plus 6 fl oz water)	6 fl oz	182	99	Tr	Tr	Tr	Tr	Tr	Tr
	Fruit drinks, noncarbonated:									
	Canned:									
20	Fruit punch drink	6 fl oz	190	88	85	Tr	0	0.0	0.0	0.0
21	Grape drink	6 fl oz	187	86	100	Tr	0	0.0	0.0	0.0
22	Pineapple-grapefruit juice drink	6 fl oz	187	87	90	Tr	Tr	Tr	Tr	Tr
	Frozen:									
	Lemonade concentrate:									
23	Undiluted	6-fl-oz can	219	49	425	Tr	Tr	Tr	Tr	Tr
24	Diluted with 4-1/3 parts water by volume	6 fl oz	185	89	80	Tr	Tr	Tr	Tr	Tr
	Limeade concentrate:									
25	Undiluted	6-fl-oz can	218	50	410	Tr	Tr	Tr	Tr	Tr
26	Diluted with 4-1/3 parts water by volume	6 fl oz	185	89	75	Tr	Tr	Tr	Tr	Tr
	Fruit juices. See type under Fruits and Fruit Juices.									
	Milk beverages. See Dairy Products (items 92-105).									
	Tea:									
27	Brewed	8 fl oz	240	100	Tr	Tr	Tr	Tr	Tr	Tr
	Instant, powder, prepared:									
28	Unsweetened (1 tsp powder plus 8 fl oz water)	8 fl oz	241	100	Tr	Tr	Tr	Tr	Tr	Tr
29	Sweetened (3 tsp powder plus 8 fl oz water)	8 fl oz	262	91	85	Tr	Tr	Tr	Tr	Tr

[1]Value not determined.
[2]Mineral content varies depending on water source.

Nutrients in Indicated Quantity													
Cho-les-terol	Carbo-hydrate	Calcium	Phos-phorus	Iron	Potas-sium	Sodium	Vitamin A value (IU)	Vitamin A value (RE)	Thiamin	Ribo-flavin	Niacin	Ascorbic acid	Item No.
Milli-grams	Grams	Milli-grams	Milli-grams	Milli-grams	Milli-grams	Milli-grams	Inter-national units	Retinol equiva-lents	Milli-grams	Milli-grams	Milli-grams	Milli-grams	
0	13	14	50	0.1	115	18	0	0	0.02	0.09	1.8	0	1
0	5	14	43	0.1	64	11	0	0	0.03	0.11	1.4	0	2
0	Tr	Tr	Tr	Tr	1	Tr	0	0	Tr	Tr	Tr	0	3
0	Tr	Tr	Tr	Tr	1	Tr	0	0	Tr	Tr	Tr	0	4
0	Tr	Tr	Tr	Tr	1	Tr	0	0	Tr	Tr	Tr	0	5
0	3	8	9	0.2	95	9	([1])	([1])	0.01	0.02	0.2	0	6
0	3	8	18	0.4	113	5	([1])	([1])	0.00	0.03	0.1	0	7
0	3	9	14	0.3	83	5	([1])	([1])	0.00	0.01	0.1	0	8
0	0	18	0	Tr	0	78	0	0	0.00	0.00	0.0	0	9
0	41	11	52	0.2	7	18	0	0	0.00	0.00	0.0	0	10
0	Tr	14	39	0.2	7	[3]32	0	0	0.00	0.00	0.0	0	11
0	32	11	0	0.1	4	29	0	0	0.00	0.00	0.0	0	12
0	45	15	0	0.4	4	48	0	0	0.00	0.00	0.0	0	13
0	39	7	0	0.4	4	33	0	0	0.00	0.00	0.0	0	14
0	45	15	4	0.3	7	52	0	0	0.00	0.00	0.0	0	15
0	41	11	41	0.1	4	37	0	0	0.00	0.00	0.0	0	16
0	42	15	0	0.2	4	48	0	0	0.00	0.00	0.0	0	17
0	Tr	4	2	Tr	124	2	0	0	0.00	0.02	0.4	0	18
0	1	2	6	0.1	71	Tr	0	0	0.00	0.03	0.6	0	19
0	22	15	2	0.4	48	15	20	2	0.03	0.04	Tr	[4]61	20
0	26	2	2	0.3	9	11	Tr	Tr	0.01	0.01	Tr	[4]64	21
0	23	13	7	0.9	97	24	60	6	0.06	0.04	0.5	[4]110	22
0	112	9	13	0.4	153	4	40	4	0.04	0.07	0.7	66	23
0	21	2	2	0.1	30	1	10	1	0.01	0.02	0.2	13	24
0	108	11	13	0.2	129	Tr	Tr	Tr	0.02	0.02	0.2	26	25
0	20	2	2	Tr	24	Tr	Tr	Tr	Tr	Tr	Tr	4	26
0	Tr	0	2	Tr	36	1	0	0	0.00	0.03	Tr	0	27
0	1	1	4	Tr	61	1	0	0	0.00	0.02	0.1	0	28
0	22	1	3	Tr	49	Tr	0	0	0.00	0.04	0.1	0	29

[3]Blend of aspartame and saccharin; if only sodium saccharin is used, sodium is 75 mg; if only aspartame is used, sodium is 23 mg.

[4]With added ascorbic acid.

Table 2. Nutritive Value of the Edible Part of Food (Continued)

(Tr indicates nutrient present in trace amount.)

Item No.	Foods, approximate measures, units, and weight (weight of edible portion only)			Water	Food energy	Protein	Fat	Fatty acids: Saturated	Fatty acids: Monounsaturated	Fatty acids: Polyunsaturated
	Dairy Products		Grams	Percent	Calories	Grams	Grams	Grams	Grams	Grams
	Butter. See Fats and Oils (items 128-130).									
	Cheese:									
	Natural:									
30	Blue	1 oz	28	42	100	6	8	5.3	2.2	0.2
31	Camembert (3 wedges per 4-oz container)	1 wedge	38	52	115	8	9	5.8	2.7	0.3
	Cheddar:									
32	Cut pieces	1 oz	28	37	115	7	9	6.0	2.7	0.3
33		1 in³	17	37	70	4	6	3.6	1.6	0.2
34	Shredded	1 cup	113	37	455	28	37	23.8	10.6	1.1
	Cottage (curd not pressed down):									
	Creamed (cottage cheese, 4% fat):									
35	Large curd	1 cup	225	79	235	28	10	6.4	2.9	0.3
36	Small curd	1 cup	210	79	215	26	9	6.0	2.7	0.3
37	With fruit	1 cup	226	72	280	22	8	4.9	2.2	0.2
38	Lowfat (2%)	1 cup	226	79	205	31	4	2.8	1.2	0.1
39	Uncreamed (cottage cheese dry curd, less than 1/2% fat)	1 cup	145	80	125	25	1	0.4	0.2	Tr
40	Cream	1 oz	28	54	100	2	10	6.2	2.8	0.4
41	Feta	1 oz	28	55	75	4	6	4.2	1.3	0.2
	Mozzarella, made with:									
42	Whole milk	1 oz	28	54	80	6	6	3.7	1.9	0.2
43	Part skim milk (low moisture)	1 oz	28	49	80	8	5	3.1	1.4	0.1
44	Muenster	1 oz	28	42	105	7	9	5.4	2.5	0.2
	Parmesan, grated:									
45	Cup, not pressed down	1 cup	100	18	455	42	30	19.1	8.7	0.7
46	Tablespoon	1 tbsp	5	18	25	2	2	1.0	0.4	Tr
47	Ounce	1 oz	28	18	130	12	9	5.4	2.5	0.2
48	Provolone	1 oz	28	41	100	7	8	4.8	2.1	0.2
	Ricotta, made with:									
49	Whole milk	1 cup	246	72	430	28	32	20.4	8.9	0.9
50	Part skim milk	1 cup	246	74	340	28	19	12.1	5.7	0.6
51	Swiss	1 oz	28	37	105	8	8	5.0	2.1	0.3
	Pasteurized process cheese:									
52	American	1 oz	28	39	105	6	9	5.6	2.5	0.3
53	Swiss	1 oz	28	42	95	7	7	4.5	2.0	0.2
54	Pasteurized process cheese food, American	1 oz	28	43	95	6	7	4.4	2.0	0.2
55	Pasteurized process cheese spread, American	1 oz	28	48	80	5	6	3.8	1.8	0.2
	Cream, sweet:									
56	Half-and-half (cream and milk)	1 cup	242	81	315	7	28	17.3	8.0	1.0
57		1 tbsp	15	81	20	Tr	2	1.1	0.5	0.1
58	Light, coffee, or table	1 cup	240	74	470	6	46	28.8	13.4	1.7
59		1 tbsp	15	74	30	Tr	3	1.8	0.8	0.1
	Whipping, unwhipped (volume about double when whipped):									
60	Light	1 cup	239	64	700	5	74	46.2	21.7	2.1
61		1 tbsp	15	64	45	Tr	5	2.9	1.4	0.1
62	Heavy	1 cup	238	58	820	5	88	54.8	25.4	3.3
63		1 tbsp	15	58	50	Tr	6	3.5	1.6	0.2
64	Whipped topping, (pressurized)	1 cup	60	61	155	2	13	8.3	3.9	0.5
65		1 tbsp	3	61	10	Tr	1	0.4	0.2	Tr
66	Cream, sour	1 cup	230	71	495	7	48	30.0	13.9	1.8
67		1 tbsp	12	71	25	Tr	3	1.6	0.7	0.1

Nutrients in Indicated Quantity

Cholesterol	Carbohydrate	Calcium	Phosphorus	Iron	Potassium	Sodium	Vitamin A value (IU)	Vitamin A value (RE)	Thiamin	Riboflavin	Niacin	Ascorbic acid	Item No.
Milligrams	Grams	Milligrams	Milligrams	Milligrams	Milligrams	Milligrams	International units	Retinol equivalents	Milligrams	Milligrams	Milligrams	Milligrams	
21	1	150	110	0.1	73	396	200	65	0.01	0.11	0.3	0	30
27	Tr	147	132	0.1	71	320	350	96	0.01	0.19	0.2	0	31
30	Tr	204	145	0.2	28	176	300	86	0.01	0.11	Tr	0	32
18	Tr	123	87	0.1	17	105	180	52	Tr	0.06	Tr	0	33
119	1	815	579	0.8	111	701	1,200	342	0.03	0.42	0.1	0	34
34	6	135	297	0.3	190	911	370	108	0.05	0.37	0.3	Tr	35
31	6	126	277	0.3	177	850	340	101	0.04	0.34	0.3	Tr	36
25	30	108	236	0.2	151	915	280	81	0.04	0.29	0.2	Tr	37
19	8	155	340	0.4	217	918	160	45	0.05	0.42	0.3	Tr	38
10	3	46	151	0.3	47	19	40	12	0.04	0.21	0.2	0	39
31	1	23	30	0.3	34	84	400	124	Tr	0.06	Tr	0	40
25	1	140	96	0.2	18	316	130	36	0.04	0.24	0.3	0	41
22	1	147	105	0.1	19	106	220	68	Tr	0.07	Tr	0	42
15	1	207	149	0.1	27	150	180	54	0.01	0.10	Tr	0	43
27	Tr	203	133	0.1	38	178	320	90	Tr	0.09	Tr	0	44
79	4	1,376	807	1.0	107	1,861	700	173	0.05	0.39	0.3	0	45
4	Tr	69	40	Tr	5	93	40	9	Tr	0.02	Tr	0	46
22	1	390	229	0.3	30	528	200	49	0.01	0.11	0.1	0	47
20	1	214	141	0.1	39	248	230	75	0.01	0.09	Tr	0	48
124	7	509	389	0.9	257	207	1,210	330	0.03	0.48	0.3	0	49
76	13	669	449	1.1	307	307	1,060	278	0.05	0.46	0.2	0	50
26	1	272	171	Tr	31	74	240	72	0.01	0.10	Tr	0	51
27	Tr	174	211	0.1	46	406	340	82	0.01	0.10	Tr	0	52
24	1	219	216	0.2	61	388	230	65	Tr	0.08	Tr	0	53
18	2	163	130	0.2	79	337	260	62	0.01	0.13	Tr	0	54
16	2	159	202	0.1	69	381	220	54	0.01	0.12	Tr	0	55
89	10	254	230	0.2	314	98	1,050	259	0.08	0.36	0.2	2	56
6	1	16	14	Tr	19	6	70	16	0.01	0.02	Tr	Tr	57
159	9	231	192	0.1	292	95	1,730	437	0.08	0.36	0.1	2	58
10	1	14	12	Tr	18	6	110	27	Tr	0.02	Tr	Tr	59
265	7	166	146	0.1	231	82	2,690	705	0.06	0.30	0.1	1	60
17	Tr	10	9	Tr	15	5	170	44	Tr	0.02	Tr	Tr	61
326	7	154	149	0.1	179	89	3,500	1,002	0.05	0.26	0.1	1	62
21	Tr	10	9	Tr	11	6	220	63	Tr	0.02	Tr	Tr	63
46	7	61	54	Tr	88	78	550	124	0.02	0.04	Tr	0	64
2	Tr	3	3	Tr	4	4	30	6	Tr	Tr	Tr	0	65
102	10	268	195	0.1	331	123	1,820	448	0.08	0.34	0.2	2	66
5	1	14	10	Tr	17	6	90	23	Tr	0.02	Tr	Tr	67

Table 2. Nutritive Value of the Edible Part of Food (Continued)
(Tr indicates nutrient present in trace amount.)

Item No.	Foods, approximate measures, units, and weight (weight of edible portion only)			Water	Food energy	Protein	Fat	Fatty acids: Saturated	Fatty acids: Monounsaturated	Fatty acids: Polyunsaturated
	Dairy Products—Con.		Grams	Percent	Calories	Grams	Grams	Grams	Grams	Grams
	Cream products, imitation (made with vegetable fat):									
	Sweet:									
	Creamers:									
68	Liquid (frozen)	1 tbsp	15	77	20	Tr	1	1.4	Tr	Tr
69	Powdered	1 tsp	2	2	10	Tr	1	0.7	Tr	Tr
	Whipped topping:									
70	Frozen	1 cup	75	50	240	1	19	16.3	1.2	0.4
71		1 tbsp	4	50	15	Tr	1	0.9	0.1	Tr
	Powdered, made with whole									
72	milk	1 cup	80	67	150	3	10	8.5	0.7	0.2
73		1 tbsp	4	67	10	Tr	Tr	0.4	Tr	Tr
74	Pressurized	1 cup	70	60	185	1	16	13.2	1.3	0.2
75		1 tbsp	4	60	10	Tr	1	0.8	0.1	Tr
76	Sour dressing (filled cream type product, nonbutterfat)	1 cup	235	75	415	8	39	31.2	4.6	1.1
77		1 tbsp	12	75	20	Tr	2	1.6	0.2	0.1
	Ice cream. See Milk desserts, frozen (items 106-111).									
	Ice milk. See Milk desserts, frozen (items 112-114).									
	Milk:									
	Fluid:									
78	Whole (3.3% fat)	1 cup	244	88	150	8	8	5.1	2.4	0.3
	Lowfat (2%):									
79	No milk solids added	1 cup	244	89	120	8	5	2.9	1.4	0.2
80	Milk solids added, label claim less than 10 g of protein per cup	1 cup	245	89	125	9	5	2.9	1.4	0.2
	Lowfat (1%):									
81	No milk solids added	1 cup	244	90	100	8	3	1.6	0.7	0.1
82	Milk solids added, label claim less than 10 g of protein per cup	1 cup	245	90	105	9	2	1.5	0.7	0.1
	Nonfat (skim):									
83	No milk solids added	1 cup	245	91	85	8	Tr	0.3	0.1	Tr
84	Milk solids added, label claim less than 10 g of protein per cup	1 cup	245	90	90	9	1	0.4	0.2	Tr
85	Buttermilk	1 cup	245	90	100	8	2	1.3	0.6	0.1
	Canned:									
86	Condensed, sweetened	1 cup	306	27	980	24	27	16.8	7.4	1.0
	Evaporated:									
87	Whole milk	1 cup	252	74	340	17	19	11.6	5.9	0.6
88	Skim milk	1 cup	255	79	200	19	1	0.3	0.2	Tr
	Dried:									
89	Buttermilk	1 cup	120	3	465	41	7	4.3	2.0	0.3
	Nonfat, instantized:									
90	Envelope, 3.2 oz, net wt.[6]	1 envelope	91	4	325	32	1	0.4	0.2	Tr
91	Cup	1 cup	68	4	245	24	Tr	0.3	0.1	Tr
	Milk beverages:									
	Chocolate milk (commercial):									
92	Regular	1 cup	250	82	210	8	8	5.3	2.5	0.3
93	Lowfat (2%)	1 cup	250	84	180	8	5	3.1	1.5	0.2
94	Lowfat (1%)	1 cup	250	85	160	8	3	1.5	0.8	0.1

[5] Vitamin A value is largely from beta-carotene used for coloring.
[6] Yields 1 qt of fluid milk when reconstituted according to package directions.

Nutrients in Indicated Quantity													
Cholesterol	Carbohydrate	Calcium	Phosphorus	Iron	Potassium	Sodium	Vitamin A value (IU)	Vitamin A value (RE)	Thiamin	Riboflavin	Niacin	Ascorbic acid	Item No.
Milligrams	Grams	Milligrams	Milligrams	Milligrams	Milligrams	Milligrams	International units	Retinol equivalents	Milligrams	Milligrams	Milligrams	Milligrams	
0	2	1	10	Tr	29	12	[5]10	[5]1	0.00	0.00	0.0	0	68
0	1	Tr	8	Tr	16	4	Tr	Tr	0.00	Tr	0.0	0	69
0	17	5	6	0.1	14	19	[5]650	[5]65	0.00	0.00	0.0	0	70
0	1	Tr	Tr	Tr	1	1	[5]30	[5]3	0.00	0.00	0.0	0	71
8	13	72	69	Tr	121	53	[5]290	[5]39	0.02	0.09	Tr	1	72
Tr	1	4	3	Tr	6	3	[5]10	[5]2	Tr	Tr	Tr	Tr	73
0	11	4	13	Tr	13	43	[5]330	[5]33	0.00	0.00	0.0	0	74
0	1	Tr	1	Tr	1	2	[5]20	[5]2	0.00	0.00	0.0	0	75
13	11	266	205	0.1	380	113	20	5	0.09	0.38	0.2	2	76
1	1	14	10	Tr	19	6	Tr	Tr	Tr	0.02	Tr	Tr	77
33	11	291	228	0.1	370	120	310	76	0.09	0.40	0.2	2	78
18	12	297	232	0.1	377	122	500	139	0.10	0.40	0.2	2	79
18	12	313	245	0.1	397	128	500	140	0.10	0.42	0.2	2	80
10	12	300	235	0.1	381	123	500	144	0.10	0.41	0.2	2	81
10	12	313	245	0.1	397	128	500	145	0.10	0.42	0.2	2	82
4	12	302	247	0.1	406	126	500	149	0.09	0.34	0.2	2	83
5	12	316	255	0.1	418	130	500	149	0.10	0.43	0.2	2	84
9	12	285	219	0.1	371	257	80	20	0.08	0.38	0.1	2	85
104	166	868	775	0.6	1,136	389	1,000	248	0.28	1.27	0.6	8	86
74	25	657	510	0.5	764	267	610	136	0.12	0.80	0.5	5	87
9	29	738	497	0.7	845	293	1,000	298	0.11	0.79	0.4	3	88
83	59	1,421	1,119	0.4	1,910	621	260	65	0.47	1.89	1.1	7	89
17	47	1,120	896	0.3	1,552	499	[7]2,160	[7]646	0.38	1.59	0.8	5	90
12	35	837	670	0.2	1,160	373	[7]1,610	[7]483	0.28	1.19	0.6	4	91
31	26	280	251	0.6	417	149	300	73	0.09	0.41	0.3	2	92
17	26	284	254	0.6	422	151	500	143	0.09	0.41	0.3	2	93
7	26	287	256	0.6	425	152	500	148	0.10	0.42	0.3	2	94

[7]With added vitamin A.

Table 2. Nutritive Value of the Edible Part of Food (Continued)

(Tr indicates nutrient present in trace amount.)

Item No.	Foods, approximate measures, units, and weight (weight of edible portion only)			Water	Food energy	Protein	Fat	Fatty acids: Saturated	Fatty acids: Monounsaturated	Fatty acids: Polyunsaturated
	Dairy Products—Con.		Grams	Percent	Calories	Grams	Grams	Grams	Grams	Grams
	Milk beverages:									
	Cocoa and chocolate-flavored beverages:									
95	Powder containing nonfat dry milk	1 oz	28	1	100	3	1	0.6	0.3	Tr
96	Prepared (6 oz water plus 1 oz powder)	1 serving	206	86	100	3	1	0.6	0.3	Tr
97	Powder without nonfat dry milk	3/4 oz	21	1	75	1	1	0.3	0.2	Tr
98	Prepared (8 oz whole milk plus 3/4 oz powder)	1 serving	265	81	225	9	9	5.4	2.5	0.3
99	Eggnog (commercial)	1 cup	254	74	340	10	19	11.3	5.7	0.9
	Malted milk:									
	Chocolate:									
100	Powder	3/4 oz	21	2	85	1	1	0.5	0.3	0.1
101	Prepared (8 oz whole milk plus 3/4 oz powder)	1 serving	265	81	235	9	9	5.5	2.7	0.4
	Natural:									
102	Powder	3/4 oz	21	3	85	3	2	0.9	0.5	0.3
103	Prepared (8 oz whole milk plus 3/4 oz powder)	1 serving	265	81	235	11	10	6.0	2.9	0.6
	Shakes, thick:									
104	Chocolate	10-oz container	283	72	335	9	8	4.8	2.2	0.3
105	Vanilla	10-oz container	283	74	315	11	9	5.3	2.5	0.3
	Milk desserts, frozen:									
	Ice cream, vanilla:									
	Regular (about 11% fat):									
106	Hardened	1/2 gal	1,064	61	2,155	38	115	71.3	33.1	4.3
107		1 cup	133	61	270	5	14	8.9	4.1	0.5
108		3 fl oz	50	61	100	2	5	3.4	1.6	0.2
109	Soft serve (frozen custard)	1 cup	173	60	375	7	23	13.5	6.7	1.0
110	Rich (about 16% fat), hardened	1/2 gal	1,188	59	2,805	33	190	118.3	54.9	7.1
111		1 cup	148	59	350	4	24	14.7	6.8	0.9
	Ice milk, vanilla:									
112	Hardened (about 4% fat)	1/2 gal	1,048	69	1,470	41	45	28.1	13.0	1.7
113		1 cup	131	69	185	5	6	3.5	1.6	0.2
114	Soft serve (about 3% fat)	1 cup	175	70	225	8	5	2.9	1.3	0.2
115	Sherbet (about 2% fat)	1/2 gal	1,542	66	2,160	17	31	19.0	8.8	1.1
116		1 cup	193	66	270	2	4	2.4	1.1	0.1
	Yogurt:									
	With added milk solids:									
	Made with lowfat milk:									
117	Fruit-flavored[8]	8-oz container	227	74	230	10	2	1.6	0.7	0.1
118	Plain	8-oz container	227	85	145	12	4	2.3	1.0	0.1
119	Made with nonfat milk	8-oz container	227	85	125	13	Tr	0.3	0.1	Tr
	Without added milk solids:									
120	Made with whole milk	8-oz container	227	88	140	8	7	4.8	2.0	0.2
	Eggs									
	Eggs, large (24 oz per dozen):									
	Raw:									
121	Whole, without shell	1 egg	50	75	75	6	5	1.6	1.9	0.7
122	White	1 white	33	88	15	4	0	0.0	0.0	0.0
123	Yolk	1 yolk	17	49	60	3	5	1.6	1.9	0.7
	Cooked:									
124	Fried in margarine	1 egg	46	69	90	6	7	1.9	2.7	1.3
125	Hard-cooked, shell removed	1 egg	50	75	75	6	5	1.6	2.0	0.7
126	Poached	1 egg	50	75	75	6	5	1.5	1.9	0.7
127	Scrambled (milk added) in margarine	1 egg	61	73	100	7	7	2.2	2.9	1.3

[8]Carbohydrate content varies widely because of amount of sugar added and amount and solids content of added flavoring. Consult the label if more precise values for carbohydrate and calories are needed.

Nutrients in Indicated Quantity

Cholesterol	Carbohydrate	Calcium	Phosphorus	Iron	Potassium	Sodium	Vitamin A value (IU)	Vitamin A value (RE)	Thiamin	Riboflavin	Niacin	Ascorbic acid	Item No.
Milligrams	Grams	Milligrams	Milligrams	Milligrams	Milligrams	Milligrams	International units	Retinol equivalents	Milligrams	Milligrams	Milligrams	Milligrams	
1	22	90	88	0.3	223	139	Tr	Tr	0.03	0.17	0.2	Tr	95
1	22	90	88	0.3	223	139	Tr	Tr	0.03	0.17	0.2	Tr	96
0	19	7	26	0.7	136	56	Tr	Tr	Tr	0.03	0.1	Tr	97
33	30	298	254	0.9	508	176	310	76	0.10	0.43	0.3	3	98
149	34	330	278	0.5	420	138	890	203	0.09	0.48	0.3	4	99
1	18	13	37	0.4	130	49	20	5	0.04	0.04	0.4	0	100
34	29	304	265	0.5	500	168	330	80	0.14	0.43	0.7	2	101
4	15	56	79	0.2	159	96	70	17	0.11	0.14	1.1	0	102
37	27	347	307	0.3	529	215	380	93	0.20	0.54	1.3	2	103
30	60	374	357	0.9	634	314	240	59	0.13	0.63	0.4	0	104
33	50	413	326	0.3	517	270	320	79	0.08	0.55	0.4	0	105
476	254	1,406	1,075	1.0	2,052	929	4,340	1,064	0.42	2.63	1.1	6	106
59	32	176	134	0.1	257	116	540	133	0.05	0.33	0.1	1	107
22	12	66	51	Tr	96	44	200	50	0.02	0.12	0.1	Tr	108
153	38	236	199	0.4	338	153	790	199	0.08	0.45	0.2	1	109
703	256	1,213	927	0.8	1,771	868	7,200	1,758	0.36	2.27	0.9	5	110
88	32	151	115	0.1	221	108	900	219	0.04	0.28	0.1	1	111
146	232	1,409	1,035	1.5	2,117	836	1,710	419	0.61	2.78	0.9	6	112
18	29	176	129	0.2	265	105	210	52	0.08	0.35	0.1	1	113
13	38	274	202	0.3	412	163	175	44	0.12	0.54	0.2	1	114
113	469	827	594	2.5	1,585	706	1,480	308	0.26	0.71	1.0	31	115
14	59	103	74	0.3	198	88	190	39	0.03	0.09	0.1	4	116
10	43	345	271	0.2	442	133	100	25	0.08	0.40	0.2	1	117
14	16	415	326	0.2	531	159	150	36	0.10	0.49	0.3	2	118
4	17	452	355	0.2	579	174	20	5	0.11	0.53	0.3	2	119
29	11	274	215	0.1	351	105	280	68	0.07	0.32	0.2	1	120
213	1	25	89	0.7	60	63	320	95	0.03	0.25	Tr	0	121
0	Tr	2	4	Tr	48	55	0	0	Tr	0.15	Tr	0	122
213	Tr	23	81	0.6	16	7	320	97	0.03	0.11	Tr	0	123
211	1	25	89	0.7	61	162	390	114	0.03	0.24	Tr	0	124
213	1	25	86	0.6	63	62	280	84	0.03	0.26	Tr	0	125
212	1	25	89	0.7	60	140	320	95	0.02	0.22	Tr	0	126
215	1	44	104	0.7	84	171	420	119	0.03	0.27	Tr	Tr	127

Table 2. Nutritive Value of the Edible Part of Food (Continued)

(Tr indicates nutrient present in trace amount.)

Item No.	Foods, approximate measures, units, and weight (weight of edible portion only)			Water	Food energy	Protein	Fat	Fatty acids: Saturated	Fatty acids: Monounsaturated	Fatty acids: Polyunsaturated
	Fats and Oils		Grams	Percent	Calories	Grams	Grams	Grams	Grams	Grams
	Butter (4 sticks per lb):									
128	Stick	1/2 cup	113	16	810	1	92	57.1	26.4	3.4
129	Tablespoon (1/8 stick)	1 tbsp	14	16	100	Tr	11	7.1	3.3	0.4
130	Pat (1 in square, 1/3 in high; 90 per lb)	1 pat	5	16	35	Tr	4	2.5	1.2	0.2
131	Fats, cooking (vegetable shortenings)	1 cup	205	0	1,810	0	205	51.3	91.2	53.5
132		1 tbsp	13	0	115	0	13	3.3	5.8	3.4
133	Lard	1 cup	205	0	1,850	0	205	80.4	92.5	23.0
134		1 tbsp	13	0	115	0	13	5.1	5.9	1.5
	Margarine:									
135	Imitation (about 40% fat), soft	8-oz container	227	58	785	1	88	17.5	35.6	31.3
136		1 tbsp	14	58	50	Tr	5	1.1	2.2	1.9
	Regular (about 80% fat):									
	Hard (4 sticks per lb):									
137	Stick	1/2 cup	113	16	810	1	91	17.9	40.5	28.7
138	Tablespoon (1/8 stick)	1 tbsp	14	16	100	Tr	11	2.2	5.0	3.6
139	Pat (1 in square, 1/3 in high; 90 per lb)	1 pat	5	16	35	Tr	4	0.8	1.8	1.3
140	Soft	8-oz container	227	16	1,625	2	183	31.3	64.7	78.5
141		1 tbsp	14	16	100	Tr	11	1.9	4.0	4.8
	Spread (about 60% fat):									
	Hard (4 sticks per lb):									
142	Stick	1/2 cup	113	37	610	1	69	15.9	29.4	20.5
143	Tablespoon (1/8 stick)	1 tbsp	14	37	75	Tr	9	2.0	3.6	2.5
144	Pat (1 in square, 1/3 in high; 90 per lb)	1 pat	5	37	25	Tr	3	0.7	1.3	0.9
145	Soft	8-oz container	227	37	1,225	1	138	29.1	71.5	31.3
146		1 tbsp	14	37	75	Tr	9	1.8	4.4	1.9
	Oils, salad or cooking:									
147	Corn	1 cup	218	0	1,925	0	218	27.7	52.8	128.0
148		1 tbsp	14	0	125	0	14	1.8	3.4	8.2
149	Olive	1 cup	216	0	1,910	0	216	29.2	159.2	18.1
150		1 tbsp	14	0	125	0	14	1.9	10.3	1.2
151	Peanut	1 cup	216	0	1,910	0	216	36.5	99.8	69.1
152		1 tbsp	14	0	125	0	14	2.4	6.5	4.5
153	Safflower	1 cup	218	0	1,925	0	218	19.8	26.4	162.4
154		1 tbsp	14	0	125	0	14	1.3	1.7	10.4
155	Soybean oil, hydrogenated (partially hardened)	1 cup	218	0	1,925	0	218	32.5	93.7	82.0
156		1 tbsp	14	0	125	0	14	2.1	6.0	5.3
157	Soybean-cottonseed oil blend, hydrogenated	1 cup	218	0	1,925	0	218	39.2	64.3	104.9
158		1 tbsp	14	0	125	0	14	2.5	4.1	6.7
159	Sunflower	1 cup	218	0	1,925	0	218	22.5	42.5	143.2
160		1 tbsp	14	0	125	0	14	1.4	2.7	9.2
	Salad dressings:									
	Commercial:									
161	Blue cheese	1 tbsp	15	32	75	1	8	1.5	1.8	4.2
	French:									
162	Regular	1 tbsp	16	35	85	Tr	9	1.4	4.0	3.5
163	Low calorie	1 tbsp	16	75	25	Tr	2	0.2	0.3	1.0
	Italian:									
164	Regular	1 tbsp	15	34	80	Tr	9	1.3	3.7	3.2
165	Low calorie	1 tbsp	15	86	5	Tr	Tr	Tr	Tr	Tr
	Mayonnaise:									
166	Regular	1 tbsp	14	15	100	Tr	11	1.7	3.2	5.8
167	Imitation	1 tbsp	15	63	35	Tr	3	0.5	0.7	1.6
168	Mayonnaise type	1 tbsp	15	40	60	Tr	5	0.7	1.4	2.7
169	Tartar sauce	1 tbsp	14	34	75	Tr	8	1.2	2.6	3.9
	Thousand island:									
170	Regular	1 tbsp	16	46	60	Tr	6	1.0	1.3	3.2
171	Low calorie	1 tbsp	15	69	25	Tr	2	0.2	0.4	0.9

[9] For salted butter; unsalted butter contains 12 mg sodium per stick, 2 mg per tbsp, or 1 mg per pat.
[10] Values for vitamin A are year-round average.

Nutrients in Indicated Quantity													
Cho-les-terol	Carbo-hydrate	Calcium	Phos-phorus	Iron	Potas-sium	Sodium	Vitamin A value (IU)	Vitamin A value (RE)	Thiamin	Ribo-flavin	Niacin	Ascorbic acid	Item No.
Milli-grams	Grams	Milli-grams	Milli-grams	Milli-grams	Milli-grams	Milli-grams	Inter-national units	Retinol equiva-lents	Milli-grams	Milli-grams	Milli-grams	Milli-grams	
247	Tr	27	26	0.2	29	[9]933	[10]3,460	[10]852	0.01	0.04	Tr	0	128
31	Tr	3	3	Tr	4	[9]116	[10]430	[10]106	Tr	Tr	Tr	0	129
11	Tr	1	1	Tr	1	[9]41	[10]150	[10]38	Tr	Tr	Tr	0	130
0	0	0	0	0.0	0	0	0	0	0.00	0.00	0.0	0	131
0	0	0	0	0.0	0	0	0	0	0.00	0.00	0.0	0	132
195	0	0	0	0.0	0	0	0	0	0.00	0.00	0.0	0	133
12	0	0	0	0.0	0	0	0	0	0.00	0.00	0.0	0	134
0	1	40	31	0.0	57	[11]2,178	[12]7,510	[12]2,254	0.01	0.05	Tr	Tr	135
0	Tr	2	2	0.0	4	[11]134	[12]460	[12]139	Tr	Tr	Tr	Tr	136
0	1	34	26	0.1	48	[11]1,066	[12]3,740	[12]1,122	0.01	0.04	Tr	Tr	137
0	Tr	4	3	Tr	6	[11]132	[12]460	[12]139	Tr	0.01	Tr	Tr	138
0	Tr	1	1	Tr	2	[11]47	[12]170	[12]50	Tr	Tr	Tr	Tr	139
0	1	60	46	0.0	86	[11]2,449	[12]7,510	[12]2,254	0.02	0.07	Tr	Tr	140
0	Tr	4	3	0.0	5	[11]151	[12]460	[12]139	Tr	Tr	Tr	Tr	141
0	0	24	18	0.0	34	[11]1,123	[12]3,740	[12]1,122	0.01	0.03	Tr	Tr	142
0	0	3	2	0.0	4	[11]139	[12]460	[12]139	Tr	Tr	Tr	Tr	143
0	0	1	1	0.0	1	[11]50	[12]170	[12]50	Tr	Tr	Tr	Tr	144
0	0	47	37	0.0	68	[11]2,256	[12]7,510	[12]2,254	0.02	0.06	Tr	Tr	145
0	0	3	2	0.0	4	[11]139	[12]460	[12]139	Tr	Tr	Tr	Tr	146
0	0	0	0	0.0	0	0	0	0	0.00	0.00	0.0	0	147
0	0	0	0	0.0	0	0	0	0	0.00	0.00	0.0	0	148
0	0	0	0	0.0	0	0	0	0	0.00	0.00	0.0	0	149
0	0	0	0	0.0	0	0	0	0	0.00	0.00	0.0	0	150
0	0	0	0	0.0	0	0	0	0	0.00	0.00	0.0	0	151
0	0	0	0	0.0	0	0	0	0	0.00	0.00	0.0	0	152
0	0	0	0	0.0	0	0	0	0	0.00	0.00	0.0	0	153
0	0	0	0	0.0	0	0	0	0	0.00	0.00	0.0	0	154
0	0	0	0	0.0	0	0	0	0	0.00	0.00	0.0	0	155
0	0	0	0	0.0	0	0	0	0	0.00	0.00	0.0	0	156
0	0	0	0	0.0	0	0	0	0	0.00	0.00	0.0	0	157
0	0	0	0	0.0	0	0	0	0	0.00	0.00	0.0	0	158
0	0	0	0	0.0	0	0	0	0	0.00	0.00	0.0	0	159
0	0	0	0	0.0	0	0	0	0	0.00	0.00	0.0	0	160
3	1	12	11	Tr	6	164	30	10	Tr	0.02	Tr	Tr	161
0	1	2	1	Tr	2	188	Tr	Tr	Tr	Tr	Tr	Tr	162
0	2	6	5	Tr	3	306	Tr	Tr	Tr	Tr	Tr	Tr	163
0	1	1	1	Tr	5	162	30	3	Tr	Tr	Tr	Tr	164
0	2	1	1	Tr	4	136	Tr	Tr	Tr	Tr	Tr	Tr	165
8	Tr	3	4	0.1	5	80	40	12	0.00	0.00	Tr	0	166
4	2	Tr	Tr	0.0	2	75	0	0	0.00	0.00	0.0	0	167
4	4	2	4	Tr	1	107	30	13	Tr	Tr	Tr	0	168
4	1	3	4	0.1	11	182	30	9	Tr	Tr	0.0	Tr	169
4	2	2	3	0.1	18	112	50	15	Tr	Tr	Tr	0	170
2	2	2	3	0.1	17	150	50	14	Tr	Tr	Tr	0	171

[11]For salted margarine.

[12]Based on average vitamin A content of fortified margarine. Federal specifications for fortified margarine require a minimum of 15,000 IU per pound.

Table 2. Nutritive Value of the Edible Part of Food (Continued)

(Tr indicates nutrient present in trace amount.)

Item No.	Foods, approximate measures, units, and weight (weight of edible portion only)			Water	Food energy	Protein	Fat	Fatty acids: Saturated	Fatty acids: Monounsaturated	Fatty acids: Polyunsaturated
			Grams	Percent	Calories	Grams	Grams	Grams	Grams	Grams
	Fats and Oils—Con.									
	Salad dressings:									
	Prepared from home recipe:									
172	Cooked type[13]	1 tbsp	16	69	25	1	2	0.5	0.6	0.3
173	Vinegar and oil	1 tbsp	16	47	70	0	8	1.5	2.4	3.9
	Fish and Shellfish									
	Clams:									
174	Raw, meat only	3 oz	85	82	65	11	1	0.3	0.3	0.3
175	Canned, drained solids	3 oz	85	77	85	13	2	0.5	0.5	0.4
176	Crabmeat, canned	1 cup	135	77	135	23	3	0.5	0.8	1.4
177	Fish sticks, frozen, reheated, (stick, 4 by 1 by 1/2 in)	1 fish stick	28	52	70	6	3	0.8	1.4	0.8
	Flounder or Sole, baked, with lemon juice:									
178	With butter	3 oz	85	73	120	16	6	3.2	1.5	0.5
179	With margarine	3 oz	85	73	120	16	6	1.2	2.3	1.9
180	Without added fat	3 oz	85	78	80	17	1	0.3	0.2	0.4
181	Haddock, breaded, fried[14]	3 oz	85	61	175	17	9	2.4	3.9	2.4
182	Halibut, broiled, with butter and lemon juice	3 oz	85	67	140	20	6	3.3	1.6	0.7
183	Herring, pickled	3 oz	85	59	190	17	13	4.3	4.6	3.1
184	Ocean perch, breaded, fried[14]	1 fillet	85	59	185	16	11	2.6	4.6	2.8
	Oysters:									
185	Raw, meat only (13-19 medium Selects)	1 cup	240	85	160	20	4	1.4	0.5	1.4
186	Breaded, fried[14]	1 oyster	45	65	90	5	5	1.4	2.1	1.4
	Salmon:									
187	Canned (pink), solids and liquid	3 oz	85	71	120	17	5	0.9	1.5	2.1
188	Baked (red)	3 oz	85	67	140	21	5	1.2	2.4	1.4
189	Smoked	3 oz	85	59	150	18	8	2.6	3.9	0.7
190	Sardines, Atlantic, canned in oil, drained solids	3 oz	85	62	175	20	9	2.1	3.7	2.9
191	Scallops, breaded, frozen, reheated	6 scallops	90	59	195	15	10	2.5	4.1	2.5
	Shrimp:									
192	Canned, drained solids	3 oz	85	70	100	21	1	0.2	0.2	0.4
193	French fried (7 medium)[16]	3 oz	85	55	200	16	10	2.5	4.1	2.6
194	Trout, broiled, with butter and lemon juice	3 oz	85	63	175	21	9	4.1	2.9	1.6
	Tuna, canned, drained solids:									
195	Oil pack, chunk light	3 oz	85	61	165	24	7	1.4	1.9	3.1
196	Water pack, solid white	3 oz	85	63	135	30	1	0.3	0.2	0.3
197	Tuna salad[17]	1 cup	205	63	375	33	19	3.3	4.9	9.2
	Fruits and Fruit Juices									
	Apples:									
	Raw:									
	Unpeeled, without cores:									
198	2-3/4-in diam. (about 3 per lb with cores)	1 apple	138	84	80	Tr	Tr	0.1	Tr	0.1
199	3-1/4-in diam. (about 2 per lb with cores)	1 apple	212	84	125	Tr	1	0.1	Tr	0.2
200	Peeled, sliced	1 cup	110	84	65	Tr	Tr	0.1	Tr	0.1
201	Dried, sulfured	10 rings	64	32	155	1	Tr	Tr	Tr	0.1
202	Apple juice, bottled or canned[19]	1 cup	248	88	115	Tr	Tr	Tr	Tr	0.1
	Applesauce, canned:									
203	Sweetened	1 cup	255	80	195	Tr	Tr	0.1	Tr	0.1
204	Unsweetened	1 cup	244	88	105	Tr	Tr	Tr	Tr	Tr

[13] Fatty acid values apply to product made with regular margarine.
[14] Dipped in egg, milk, and breadcrumbs; fried in vegetable shortening.
[15] If bones are discarded, value for calcium will be greatly reduced.
[16] Dipped in egg, breadcrumbs, and flour; fried in vegetable shortening.

Nutrients in Indicated Quantity													
Cholesterol	Carbohydrate	Calcium	Phosphorus	Iron	Potassium	Sodium	Vitamin A value (IU)	Vitamin A value (RE)	Thiamin	Riboflavin	Niacin	Ascorbic acid	Item No.
Milligrams	Grams	Milligrams	Milligrams	Milligrams	Milligrams	Milligrams	International units	Retinol equivalents	Milligrams	Milligrams	Milligrams	Milligrams	
9	2	13	14	0.1	19	117	70	20	0.01	0.02	Tr	Tr	172
0	Tr	0	0	0.0	1	Tr	0	0	0.00	0.00	0.0	0	173
43	2	59	138	2.6	154	102	90	26	0.09	0.15	1.1	9	174
54	2	47	116	3.5	119	102	90	26	0.01	0.09	0.9	3	175
135	1	61	246	1.1	149	1,350	50	14	0.11	0.11	2.6	0	176
26	4	11	58	0.3	94	53	20	5	0.03	0.05	0.6	0	177
68	Tr	13	187	0.3	272	145	210	54	0.05	0.08	1.6	1	178
55	Tr	14	187	0.3	273	151	230	69	0.05	0.08	1.6	1	179
59	Tr	13	197	0.3	286	101	30	10	0.05	0.08	1.7	1	180
75	7	34	183	1.0	270	123	70	20	0.06	0.10	2.9	0	181
62	Tr	14	206	0.7	441	103	610	174	0.06	0.07	7.7	1	182
85	0	29	128	0.9	85	850	110	33	0.04	0.18	2.8	0	183
66	7	31	191	1.2	241	138	70	20	0.10	0.11	2.0	0	184
120	8	226	343	15.6	290	175	740	223	0.34	0.43	6.0	24	185
35	5	49	73	3.0	64	70	150	44	0.07	0.10	1.3	4	186
34	0	[15]167	243	0.7	307	443	60	18	0.03	0.15	6.8	0	187
60	0	26	269	0.5	305	55	290	87	0.18	0.14	5.5	0	188
51	0	12	208	0.8	327	1,700	260	77	0.17	0.17	6.8	0	189
85	0	[15]371	424	2.6	349	425	190	56	0.03	0.17	4.6	0	190
70	10	39	203	2.0	369	298	70	21	0.11	0.11	1.6	0	191
128	1	98	224	1.4	104	1,955	50	15	0.01	0.03	1.5	0	192
168	11	61	154	2.0	189	384	90	26	0.06	0.09	2.8	0	193
71	Tr	26	259	1.0	297	122	230	60	0.07	0.07	2.3	1	194
55	0	7	199	1.6	298	303	70	20	0.04	0.09	10.1	0	195
48	0	17	202	0.6	255	468	110	32	0.03	0.10	13.4	0	196
80	19	31	281	2.5	531	877	230	53	0.06	0.14	13.3	6	197
0	21	10	10	0.2	159	Tr	70	7	0.02	0.02	0.1	8	198
0	32	15	15	0.4	244	Tr	110	11	0.04	0.03	0.2	12	199
0	16	4	8	0.1	124	Tr	50	5	0.02	0.01	0.1	4	200
0	42	9	24	0.9	288	[18]56	0	0	0.00	0.10	0.6	2	201
0	29	17	17	0.9	295	7	Tr	Tr	0.05	0.04	0.2	[20]2	202
0	51	10	18	0.9	156	8	30	3	0.03	0.07	0.5	[20]4	203
0	28	7	17	0.3	183	5	70	7	0.03	0.06	0.5	[20]3	204

[17] Made with drained chunk light tuna, celery, onion, pickle relish, and mayonnaise-type salad dressing.
[18] Sodium bisulfite used to preserve color; unsulfited product would contain less sodium.
[19] Also applies to pasteurized apple cider.
[20] Without added ascorbic acid. For value with added ascorbic acid, refer to label.

Table 2. Nutritive Value of the Edible Part of Food (Continued)

(Tr indicates nutrient present in trace amount.)

Item No.	Foods, approximate measures, units, and weight (weight of edible portion only)			Water	Food energy	Protein	Fat	Fatty acids		
								Saturated	Monounsaturated	Polyunsaturated
	Fruits and Fruit Juices—Con.		Grams	Percent	Calories	Grams	Grams	Grams	Grams	Grams
	Apricots:									
205	Raw, without pits (about 12 per lb with pits)	3 apricots	106	86	50	1	Tr	Tr	0.2	0.1
	Canned (fruit and liquid):									
206	Heavy syrup pack	1 cup	258	78	215	1	Tr	Tr	0.1	Tr
207		3 halves	85	78	70	Tr	Tr	Tr	Tr	Tr
208	Juice pack	1 cup	248	87	120	2	Tr	Tr	Tr	Tr
209		3 halves	84	87	40	1	Tr	Tr	Tr	Tr
	Dried:									
210	Uncooked (28 large or 37 medium halves per cup)	1 cup	130	31	310	5	1	Tr	0.3	0.1
211	Cooked, unsweetened, fruit and liquid	1 cup	250	76	210	3	Tr	Tr	0.2	0.1
212	Apricot nectar, canned	1 cup	251	85	140	1	Tr	Tr	0.1	Tr
	Avocados, raw, whole, without skin and seed:									
213	California (about 2 per lb with skin and seed)	1 avocado	173	73	305	4	30	4.5	19.4	3.5
214	Florida (about 1 per lb with skin and seed)	1 avocado	304	80	340	5	27	5.3	14.8	4.5
	Bananas, raw, without peel:									
215	Whole (about 2-1/2 per lb with peel)	1 banana	114	74	105	1	1	0.2	Tr	0.1
216	Sliced	1 cup	150	74	140	2	1	0.3	0.1	0.1
217	Blackberries, raw	1 cup	144	86	75	1	1	0.2	0.1	0.1
	Blueberries:									
218	Raw	1 cup	145	85	80	1	1	Tr	0.1	0.3
219	Frozen, sweetened	10-oz container	284	77	230	1	Tr	Tr	0.1	0.2
220		1 cup	230	77	185	1	Tr	Tr	Tr	0.1
	Cantaloup. See Melons (item 251).									
	Cherries:									
221	Sour, red, pitted, canned, water pack	1 cup	244	90	90	2	Tr	0.1	0.1	0.1
222	Sweet, raw, without pits and stems	10 cherries	68	81	50	1	1	0.1	0.2	0.2
223	Cranberry juice cocktail, bottled, sweetened	1 cup	253	85	145	Tr	Tr	Tr	Tr	0.1
224	Cranberry sauce, sweetened, canned, strained	1 cup	277	61	420	1	Tr	Tr	0.1	0.2
	Dates:									
225	Whole, without pits	10 dates	83	23	230	2	Tr	0.1	0.1	Tr
226	Chopped	1 cup	178	23	490	4	1	0.3	0.2	Tr
227	Figs, dried	10 figs	187	28	475	6	2	0.4	0.5	1.0
	Fruit cocktail, canned, fruit and liquid:									
228	Heavy syrup pack	1 cup	255	80	185	1	Tr	Tr	Tr	0.1
229	Juice pack	1 cup	248	87	115	1	Tr	Tr	Tr	Tr
	Grapefruit:									
230	Raw, without peel, membrane and seeds (3-3/4-in diam., 1 lb 1 oz, whole, with refuse)	1/2 grapefruit	120	91	40	1	Tr	Tr	Tr	Tr
231	Canned, sections with syrup	1 cup	254	84	150	1	Tr	Tr	Tr	0.1
	Grapefruit juice:									
232	Raw	1 cup	247	90	95	1	Tr	Tr	Tr	0.1
	Canned:									
233	Unsweetened	1 cup	247	90	95	1	Tr	Tr	Tr	0.1
234	Sweetened	1 cup	250	87	115	1	Tr	Tr	Tr	0.1
	Frozen concentrate, unsweetened									
235	Undiluted	6-fl-oz can	207	62	300	4	1	0.1	0.1	0.2
236	Diluted with 3 parts water by volume	1 cup	247	89	100	1	Tr	Tr	Tr	0.1

[20] Without added ascorbic acid. For value with added ascorbic acid, refer to label.
[21] With added ascorbic acid.

Nutrients in Indicated Quantity

Cholesterol	Carbohydrate	Calcium	Phosphorus	Iron	Potassium	Sodium	Vitamin A value (IU)	Vitamin A value (RE)	Thiamin	Riboflavin	Niacin	Ascorbic acid	Item No.
Milligrams	Grams	Milligrams	Milligrams	Milligrams	Milligrams	Milligrams	International units	Retinol equivalents	Milligrams	Milligrams	Milligrams	Milligrams	
0	12	15	20	0.6	314	1	2,770	277	0.03	0.04	0.6	11	205
0	55	23	31	0.8	361	10	3,170	317	0.05	0.06	1.0	8	206
0	18	8	10	0.3	119	3	1,050	105	0.02	0.02	0.3	3	207
0	31	30	50	0.7	409	10	4,190	419	0.04	0.05	0.9	12	208
0	10	10	17	0.3	139	3	1,420	142	0.02	0.02	0.3	4	209
0	80	59	152	6.1	1,791	13	9,410	941	0.01	0.20	3.9	3	210
0	55	40	103	4.2	1,222	8	5,910	591	0.02	0.08	2.4	4	211
0	36	18	23	1.0	286	8	3,300	330	0.02	0.04	0.7	[20]2	212
0	12	19	73	2.0	1,097	21	1,060	106	0.19	0.21	3.3	14	213
0	27	33	119	1.6	1,484	15	1,860	186	0.33	0.37	5.8	24	214
0	27	7	23	0.4	451	1	90	9	0.05	0.11	0.6	10	215
0	35	9	30	0.5	594	2	120	12	0.07	0.15	0.8	14	216
0	18	46	30	0.8	282	Tr	240	24	0.04	0.06	0.6	30	217
0	20	9	15	0.2	129	9	150	15	0.07	0.07	0.5	19	218
0	62	17	20	1.1	170	3	120	12	0.06	0.15	0.7	3	219
0	50	14	16	0.9	138	2	100	10	0.05	0.12	0.6	2	220
0	22	27	24	3.3	239	17	1,840	184	0.04	0.10	0.4	5	221
0	11	10	13	0.3	152	Tr	150	15	0.03	0.04	0.3	5	222
0	38	8	3	0.4	61	10	10	1	0.01	0.04	0.1	[21]108	223
0	108	11	17	0.6	72	80	60	6	0.04	0.06	0.3	6	224
0	61	27	33	1.0	541	2	40	4	0.07	0.08	1.8	0	225
0	131	57	71	2.0	1,161	5	90	9	0.16	0.18	3.9	0	226
0	122	269	127	4.2	1,331	21	250	25	0.13	0.16	1.3	1	227
0	48	15	28	0.7	224	15	520	52	0.05	0.05	1.0	5	228
0	29	20	35	0.5	236	10	760	76	0.03	0.04	1.0	7	229
0	10	14	10	0.1	167	Tr	[22]10	[22]1	0.04	0.02	0.3	41	230
0	39	36	25	1.0	328	5	Tr	Tr	0.10	0.05	0.6	54	231
0	23	22	37	0.5	400	2	20	2	0.10	0.05	0.5	94	232
0	22	17	27	0.5	378	2	20	2	0.10	0.05	0.6	72	233
0	28	20	28	0.9	405	5	20	2	0.10	0.06	0.8	67	234
0	72	56	101	1.0	1,002	6	60	6	0.30	0.16	1.6	248	235
0	24	20	35	0.3	336	2	20	2	0.10	0.05	0.5	83	236

[22]For white grapefruit; pink grapefruit have about 310 IU or 31 RE.

Table 2. Nutritive Value of the Edible Part of Food (Continued)

(Tr indicates nutrient present in trace amount.)

Item No.	Foods, approximate measures, units, and weight (weight of edible portion only)			Water	Food energy	Protein	Fat	Fatty acids: Saturated	Fatty acids: Monounsaturated	Fatty acids: Polyunsaturated
	Fruits and Fruit Juices—Con.		Grams	Percent	Calories	Grams	Grams	Grams	Grams	Grams
	Grapes, European type (adherent skin), raw:									
237	Thompson Seedless	10 grapes	50	81	35	Tr	Tr	0.1	Tr	0.1
238	Tokay and Emperor, seeded types	10 grapes	57	81	40	Tr	Tr	0.1	Tr	0.1
	Grape juice:									
239	Canned or bottled	1 cup	253	84	155	1	Tr	0.1	Tr	0.1
	Frozen concentrate, sweetened:									
240	Undiluted	6-fl-oz can	216	54	385	1	1	0.2	Tr	0.2
241	Diluted with 3 parts water by volume	1 cup	250	87	125	Tr	Tr	0.1	Tr	0.1
242	Kiwifruit, raw, without skin (about 5 per lb with skin)	1 kiwifruit	76	83	45	1	Tr	Tr	0.1	0.1
243	Lemons, raw, without peel and seeds (about 4 per lb with peel and seeds)	1 lemon	58	89	15	1	Tr	Tr	Tr	0.1
	Lemon juice:									
244	Raw	1 cup	244	91	60	1	Tr	Tr	Tr	Tr
245	Canned or bottled, unsweetened	1 cup	244	92	50	1	1	0.1	Tr	0.2
246		1 tbsp	15	92	5	Tr	Tr	Tr	Tr	Tr
247	Frozen, single-strength, unsweetened	6-fl-oz can	244	92	55	1	1	0.1	Tr	0.2
	Lime juice:									
248	Raw	1 cup	246	90	65	1	Tr	Tr	Tr	0.1
249	Canned, unsweetened	1 cup	246	93	50	1	1	0.1	0.1	0.2
250	Mangos, raw, without skin and seed (about 1-1/2 per lb with skin and seed)	1 mango	207	82	135	1	1	0.1	0.2	0.1
	Melons, raw, without rind and cavity contents:									
251	Cantaloup, orange-fleshed (5-in diam., 2-1/3 lb, whole, with rind and cavity contents)	1/2 melon	267	90	95	2	1	0.1	0.1	0.3
252	Honeydew (6-1/2-in diam., 5-1/4 lb, whole, with rind and cavity contents)	1/10 melon	129	90	45	1	Tr	Tr	Tr	0.1
253	Nectarines, raw, without pits (about 3 per lb with pits)	1 nectarine	136	86	65	1	1	0.1	0.2	0.3
	Oranges, raw:									
254	Whole, without peel and seeds (2-5/8-in diam., about 2-1/2 per lb, with peel and seeds)	1 orange	131	87	60	1	Tr	Tr	Tr	Tr
255	Sections without membranes	1 cup	180	87	85	2	Tr	Tr	Tr	Tr
	Orange juice:									
256	Raw, all varieties	1 cup	248	88	110	2	Tr	0.1	0.1	0.1
257	Canned, unsweetened	1 cup	249	89	105	1	Tr	Tr	0.1	0.1
258	Chilled	1 cup	249	88	110	2	1	0.1	0.1	0.2
	Frozen concentrate:									
259	Undiluted	6-fl-oz can	213	58	340	5	Tr	0.1	0.1	0.1
260	Diluted with 3 parts water by volume	1 cup	249	88	110	2	Tr	Tr	Tr	Tr
261	Orange and grapefruit juice, canned	1 cup	247	89	105	1	Tr	Tr	Tr	Tr
262	Papayas, raw, 1/2-in cubes	1 cup	140	86	65	1	Tr	0.1	0.1	Tr
	Peaches:									
	Raw:									
263	Whole, 2-1/2-in diam., peeled, pitted (about 4 per lb with peels and pits)	1 peach	87	88	35	1	Tr	Tr	Tr	Tr
264	Sliced	1 cup	170	88	75	1	Tr	Tr	0.1	0.1
	Canned, fruit and liquid:									
265	Heavy syrup pack	1 cup	256	79	190	1	Tr	Tr	0.1	0.1
266		1 half	81	79	60	Tr	Tr	Tr	Tr	Tr
267	Juice pack	1 cup	248	87	110	2	Tr	Tr	Tr	Tr
268		1 half	77	87	35	Tr	Tr	Tr	Tr	Tr

[20]Without added ascorbic acid. For value with added ascorbic acid, refer to label.
[21]With added ascorbic acid.

Nutrients in Indicated Quantity

Cholesterol	Carbohydrate	Calcium	Phosphorus	Iron	Potassium	Sodium	Vitamin A value (IU)	Vitamin A value (RE)	Thiamin	Riboflavin	Niacin	Ascorbic acid	Item No.
Milligrams	Grams	Milligrams	Milligrams	Milligrams	Milligrams	Milligrams	International units	Retinol equivalents	Milligrams	Milligrams	Milligrams	Milligrams	
0	9	6	7	0.1	93	1	40	4	0.05	0.03	0.2	5	237
0	10	6	7	0.1	105	1	40	4	0.05	0.03	0.2	6	238
0	38	23	28	0.6	334	8	20	2	0.07	0.09	0.7	[20]Tr	239
0	96	28	32	0.8	160	15	60	6	0.11	0.20	0.9	[21]179	240
0	32	10	10	0.3	53	5	20	2	0.04	0.07	0.3	[21]60	241
0	11	20	30	0.3	252	4	130	13	0.02	0.04	0.4	74	242
0	5	15	9	0.3	80	1	20	2	0.02	0.01	0.1	31	243
0	21	17	15	0.1	303	2	50	5	0.07	0.02	0.2	112	244
0	16	27	22	0.3	249	[23]51	40	4	0.10	0.02	0.5	61	245
0	1	2	1	Tr	15	[23]3	Tr	Tr	0.01	Tr	Tr	4	246
0	16	20	20	0.3	217	2	30	3	0.14	0.03	0.3	77	247
0	22	22	17	0.1	268	2	20	2	0.05	0.02	0.2	72	248
0	16	30	25	0.6	185	[23]39	40	4	0.08	0.01	0.4	16	249
0	35	21	23	0.3	323	4	8,060	806	0.12	0.12	1.2	57	250
0	22	29	45	0.6	825	24	8,610	861	0.10	0.06	1.5	113	251
0	12	8	13	0.1	350	13	50	5	0.10	0.02	0.8	32	252
0	16	7	22	0.2	288	Tr	1,000	100	0.02	0.06	1.3	7	253
0	15	52	18	0.1	237	Tr	270	27	0.11	0.05	0.4	70	254
0	21	72	25	0.2	326	Tr	370	37	0.16	0.07	0.5	96	255
0	26	27	42	0.5	496	2	500	50	0.22	0.07	1.0	124	256
0	25	20	35	1.1	436	5	440	44	0.15	0.07	0.8	86	257
0	25	25	27	0.4	473	2	190	19	0.28	0.05	0.7	82	258
0	81	68	121	0.7	1,436	6	590	59	0.60	0.14	1.5	294	259
0	27	22	40	0.2	473	2	190	19	0.20	0.04	0.5	97	260
0	25	20	35	1.1	390	7	290	29	0.14	0.07	0.8	72	261
0	17	35	12	0.3	247	9	400	40	0.04	0.04	0.5	92	262
0	10	4	10	0.1	171	Tr	470	47	0.01	0.04	0.9	6	263
0	19	9	20	0.2	335	Tr	910	91	0.03	0.07	1.7	11	264
0	51	8	28	0.7	236	15	850	85	0.03	0.06	1.6	7	265
0	16	2	9	0.2	75	5	270	27	0.01	0.02	0.5	2	266
0	29	15	42	0.7	317	10	940	94	0.02	0.04	1.4	9	267
0	9	5	13	0.2	99	3	290	29	0.01	0.01	0.4	3	268

[23]Sodium benzoate and sodium bisulfite added as preservatives.

Table 2. Nutritive Value of the Edible Part of Food (Continued)

(Tr indicates nutrient present in trace amount.)

Item No.	Foods, approximate measures, units, and weight (weight of edible portion only)			Water	Food energy	Protein	Fat	Fatty acids: Saturated	Fatty acids: Monounsaturated	Fatty acids: Polyunsaturated
	Fruits and Fruit Juices—Con.		Grams	Percent	Calories	Grams	Grams	Grams	Grams	Grams
	Peaches:									
	Dried:									
269	Uncooked	1 cup	160	32	380	6	1	0.1	0.4	0.6
270	Cooked, unsweetened, fruit and liquid	1 cup	258	78	200	3	1	0.1	0.2	0.3
271	Frozen, sliced, sweetened	10-oz container	284	75	265	2	Tr	Tr	0.1	0.2
272		1 cup	250	75	235	2	Tr	Tr	0.1	0.2
	Pears:									
	Raw, with skin, cored:									
273	Bartlett, 2-1/2-in diam. (about 2-1/2 per lb with cores and stems)	1 pear	166	84	100	1	1	Tr	0.1	0.2
274	Bosc, 2-1/2-in diam. (about 3 per lb with cores and stems)	1 pear	141	84	85	1	1	Tr	0.1	0.1
275	D'Anjou, 3-in diam. (about 2 per lb with cores and stems)	1 pear	200	84	120	1	1	Tr	0.2	0.2
	Canned, fruit and liquid:									
276	Heavy syrup pack	1 cup	255	80	190	1	Tr	Tr	0.1	0.1
277		1 half	79	80	60	Tr	Tr	Tr	Tr	Tr
278	Juice pack	1 cup	248	86	125	1	Tr	Tr	Tr	Tr
279		1 half	77	86	40	Tr	Tr	Tr	Tr	Tr
	Pineapple:									
280	Raw, diced	1 cup	155	87	75	1	1	Tr	0.1	0.2
	Canned, fruit and liquid:									
	Heavy syrup pack:									
281	Crushed, chunks, tidbits	1 cup	255	79	200	1	Tr	Tr	Tr	0.1
282	Slices	1 slice	58	79	45	Tr	Tr	Tr	Tr	Tr
	Juice pack:									
283	Chunks or tidbits	1 cup	250	84	150	1	Tr	Tr	Tr	0.1
284	Slices	1 slice	58	84	35	Tr	Tr	Tr	Tr	Tr
285	Pineapple juice, unsweetened, canned	1 cup	250	86	140	1	Tr	Tr	Tr	0.1
	Plantains, without peel:									
286	Raw	1 plantain	179	65	220	2	1	0.3	0.1	0.1
287	Cooked, boiled, sliced	1 cup	154	67	180	1	Tr	0.1	Tr	0.1
	Plums, without pits:									
	Raw:									
288	2-1/8-in diam. (about 6-1/2 per lb with pits)	1 plum	66	85	35	1	Tr	Tr	0.3	0.1
289	1-1/2-in diam. (about 15 per lb with pits)	1 plum	28	85	15	Tr	Tr	Tr	0.1	Tr
	Canned, purple, fruit and liquid:									
290	Heavy syrup pack	1 cup	258	76	230	1	Tr	Tr	0.2	0.1
291		3 plums	133	76	120	Tr	Tr	Tr	0.1	Tr
292	Juice pack	1 cup	252	84	145	1	Tr	Tr	Tr	Tr
293		3 plums	95	84	55	Tr	Tr	Tr	Tr	Tr
	Prunes, dried:									
294	Uncooked	4 extra large or 5 large prunes	49	32	115	1	Tr	Tr	0.2	0.1
295	Cooked, unsweetened, fruit and liquid	1 cup	212	70	225	2	Tr	Tr	0.3	0.1
296	Prune juice, canned or bottled	1 cup	256	81	180	2	Tr	Tr	0.1	Tr
	Raisins, seedless:									
297	Cup, not pressed down	1 cup	145	15	435	5	1	0.2	Tr	0.2
298	Packet, 1/2 oz (1-1/2 tbsp)	1 packet	14	15	40	Tr	Tr	Tr	Tr	Tr
	Raspberries:									
299	Raw	1 cup	123	87	60	1	1	Tr	0.1	0.4
300	Frozen, sweetened	10-oz container	284	73	295	2	Tr	Tr	Tr	0.3
301		1 cup	250	73	255	2	Tr	Tr	Tr	0.2

[21] With added ascorbic acid.

Nutrients in Indicated Quantity													
Cho-les-terol	Carbo-hydrate	Calcium	Phos-phorus	Iron	Potas-sium	Sodium	Vitamin A value (IU)	Vitamin A value (RE)	Thiamin	Ribo-flavin	Niacin	Ascorbic acid	Item No.
Milli-grams	Grams	Milli-grams	Milli-grams	Milli-grams	Milli-grams	Milli-grams	Inter-national units	Retinol equiva-lents	Milli-grams	Milli-grams	Milli-grams	Milli-grams	
0	98	45	190	6.5	1,594	11	3,460	346	Tr	0.34	7.0	8	269
0	51	23	98	3.4	826	5	510	51	0.01	0.05	3.9	10	270
0	68	9	31	1.1	369	17	810	81	0.04	0.10	1.9	[21]268	271
0	60	8	28	0.9	325	15	710	71	0.03	0.09	1.6	[21]236	272
0	25	18	18	0.4	208	Tr	30	3	0.03	0.07	0.2	7	273
0	21	16	16	0.4	176	Tr	30	3	0.03	0.06	0.1	6	274
0	30	22	22	0.5	250	Tr	40	4	0.04	0.08	0.2	8	275
0	49	13	18	0.6	166	13	10	1	0.03	0.06	0.6	3	276
0	15	4	6	0.2	51	4	Tr	Tr	0.01	0.02	0.2	1	277
0	32	22	30	0.7	238	10	10	1	0.03	0.03	0.5	4	278
0	10	7	9	0.2	74	3	Tr	Tr	0.01	0.01	0.2	1	279
0	19	11	11	0.6	175	2	40	4	0.14	0.06	0.7	24	280
0	52	36	18	1.0	265	3	40	4	0.23	0.06	0.7	19	281
0	12	8	4	0.2	60	1	10	1	0.05	0.01	0.2	4	282
0	39	35	15	0.7	305	3	100	10	0.24	0.05	0.7	24	283
0	9	8	3	0.2	71	1	20	2	0.06	0.01	0.2	6	284
0	34	43	20	0.7	335	3	10	1	0.14	0.06	0.6	27	285
0	57	5	61	1.1	893	7	2,020	202	0.09	0.10	1.2	33	286
0	48	3	43	0.9	716	8	1,400	140	0.07	0.08	1.2	17	287
0	9	3	7	0.1	114	Tr	210	21	0.03	0.06	0.3	6	288
0	4	1	3	Tr	48	Tr	90	9	0.01	0.03	0.1	3	289
0	60	23	34	2.2	235	49	670	67	0.04	0.10	0.8	1	290
0	31	12	17	1.1	121	25	340	34	0.02	0.05	0.4	1	291
0	38	25	38	0.9	388	3	2,540	254	0.06	0.15	1.2	7	292
0	14	10	14	0.3	146	1	960	96	0.02	0.06	0.4	3	293
0	31	25	39	1.2	365	2	970	97	0.04	0.08	1.0	2	294
0	60	49	74	2.4	708	4	650	65	0.05	0.21	1.5	6	295
0	45	31	64	3.0	707	10	10	1	0.04	0.18	2.0	10	296
0	115	71	141	3.0	1,089	17	10	1	0.23	0.13	1.2	5	297
0	11	7	14	0.3	105	2	Tr	Tr	0.02	0.01	0.1	Tr	298
0	14	27	15	0.7	187	Tr	160	16	0.04	0.11	1.1	31	299
0	74	43	48	1.8	324	3	170	17	0.05	0.13	0.7	47	300
0	65	38	43	1.6	285	3	150	15	0.05	0.11	0.6	41	301

Table 2. Nutritive Value of the Edible Part of Food (Continued)

(Tr indicates nutrient present in trace amount.)

Item No.	Foods, approximate measures, units, and weight (weight of edible portion only)			Water	Food energy	Protein	Fat	Fatty acids: Saturated	Fatty acids: Monounsaturated	Fatty acids: Polyunsaturated
	Fruits and Fruit Juices—Con.		Grams	Percent	Calories	Grams	Grams	Grams	Grams	Grams
302	Rhubarb, cooked, added sugar	1 cup	240	68	280	1	Tr	Tr	Tr	0.1
	Strawberries:									
303	Raw, capped, whole	1 cup	149	92	45	1	1	Tr	0.1	0.3
304	Frozen, sweetened, sliced	10-oz container	284	73	275	2	Tr	Tr	0.1	0.2
305		1 cup	255	73	245	1	Tr	Tr	Tr	0.2
	Tangerines:									
306	Raw, without peel and seeds (2-3/8-in diam., about 4 per lb, with peel and seeds)	1 tangerine	84	88	35	1	Tr	Tr	Tr	Tr
307	Canned, light syrup, fruit and liquid	1 cup	252	83	155	1	Tr	Tr	Tr	0.1
308	Tangerine juice, canned, sweetened	1 cup	249	87	125	1	Tr	Tr	Tr	0.1
	Watermelon, raw, without rind and seeds:									
309	Piece (4 by 8 in wedge with rind and seeds; 1/16 of 32-2/3-lb melon, 10 by 16 in)	1 piece	482	92	155	3	2	0.3	0.2	1.0
310	Diced	1 cup	160	92	50	1	1	0.1	0.1	0.3
	Grain Products									
311	Bagels, plain or water, enriched, 3-1/2-in diam.[24]	1 bagel	68	29	200	7	2	0.3	0.5	0.7
312	Barley, pearled, light, uncooked	1 cup	200	11	700	16	2	0.3	0.2	0.9
	Biscuits, baking powder, 2-in diam. (enriched flour, vegetable shortening):									
313	From home recipe	1 biscuit	28	28	100	2	5	1.2	2.0	1.3
314	From mix	1 biscuit	28	29	95	2	3	0.8	1.4	0.9
315	From refrigerated dough	1 biscuit	20	30	65	1	2	0.6	0.9	0.6
	Breadcrumbs, enriched:									
316	Dry, grated	1 cup	100	7	390	13	5	1.5	1.6	1.0
	Soft. See White bread (item 351).									
	Breads:									
317	Boston brown bread, canned, slice, 3-1/4 in by 1/2 in[25]	1 slice	45	45	95	2	1	0.3	0.1	0.1
	Cracked-wheat bread (3/4 enriched wheat flour, 1/4 cracked wheat flour):[25]									
318	Loaf, 1 lb	1 loaf	454	35	1,190	42	16	3.1	4.3	5.7
319	Slice (18 per loaf)	1 slice	25	35	65	2	1	0.2	0.2	0.3
320	Toasted	1 slice	21	26	65	2	1	0.2	0.2	0.3
	French or vienna bread, enriched:[25]									
321	Loaf, 1 lb	1 loaf	454	34	1,270	43	18	3.8	5.7	5.9
	Slice:									
322	French, 5 by 2-1/2 by 1 in	1 slice	35	34	100	3	1	0.3	0.4	0.5
323	Vienna, 4-3/4 by 4 by 1/2 in	1 slice	25	34	70	2	1	0.2	0.3	0.3
	Italian bread, enriched:									
324	Loaf, 1 lb	1 loaf	454	32	1,255	41	4	0.6	0.3	1.6
325	Slice, 4-1/2 by 3-1/4 by 3/4 in	1 slice	30	32	85	3	Tr	Tr	Tr	0.1
	Mixed grain bread, enriched:[25]									
326	Loaf, 1 lb	1 loaf	454	37	1,165	45	17	3.2	4.1	6.5
327	Slice (18 per loaf)	1 slice	25	37	65	2	1	0.2	0.2	0.4
328	Toasted	1 slice	23	27	65	2	1	0.2	0.2	0.4

[24] Egg bagels have 44 mg cholesterol and 22 IU or 7 RE vitamin A per bagel.
[25] Made with vegetable shortening.

Nutrients in Indicated Quantity														
Cholesterol	Carbohydrate	Calcium	Phosphorus	Iron	Potassium	Sodium	Vitamin A value (IU)	Vitamin A value (RE)	Thiamin	Riboflavin	Niacin	Ascorbic acid	Item No.
Milligrams	Grams	Milligrams	Milligrams	Milligrams	Milligrams	Milligrams	International units	Retinol equivalents	Milligrams	Milligrams	Milligrams	Milligrams	
0	75	348	19	0.5	230	2	170	17	0.04	0.06	0.5	8	302
0	10	21	28	0.6	247	1	40	4	0.03	0.10	0.3	84	303
0	74	31	37	1.7	278	9	70	7	0.05	0.14	1.1	118	304
0	66	28	33	1.5	250	8	60	6	0.04	0.13	1.0	106	305
0	9	12	8	0.1	132	1	770	77	0.09	0.02	0.1	26	306
0	41	18	25	0.9	197	15	2,120	212	0.13	0.11	1.1	50	307
0	30	45	35	0.5	443	2	1,050	105	0.15	0.05	0.2	55	308
0	35	39	43	0.8	559	10	1,760	176	0.39	0.10	1.0	46	309
0	11	13	14	0.3	186	3	590	59	0.13	0.03	0.3	15	310
0	38	29	46	1.8	50	245	0	0	0.26	0.20	2.4	0	311
0	158	32	378	4.2	320	6	0	0	0.24	0.10	6.2	0	312
Tr	13	47	36	0.7	32	195	10	3	0.08	0.08	0.8	Tr	313
Tr	14	53	128	0.7	56	262	20	4	0.12	0.11	0.8	Tr	314
1	10	4	79	0.5	18	249	0	0	0.08	0.05	0.7	0	315
5	73	122	141	4.1	152	736	0	0	0.35	0.35	4.8	0	316
3	21	41	72	0.9	131	113	[26] 0	[26] 0	0.06	0.04	0.7	0	317
0	227	295	581	12.1	608	1,966	Tr	Tr	1.73	1.73	15.3	Tr	318
0	12	16	32	0.7	34	106	Tr	Tr	0.10	0.09	0.8	Tr	319
0	12	16	32	0.7	34	106	Tr	Tr	0.07	0.09	0.8	Tr	320
0	230	499	386	14.0	409	2,633	Tr	Tr	2.09	1.59	18.2	Tr	321
0	18	39	30	1.1	32	203	Tr	Tr	0.16	0.12	1.4	Tr	322
0	13	28	21	0.8	23	145	Tr	Tr	0.12	0.09	1.0	Tr	323
0	256	77	350	12.7	336	2,656	0	0	1.80	1.10	15.0	0	324
0	17	5	23	0.8	22	176	0	0	0.12	0.07	1.0	0	325
0	212	472	962	14.8	990	1,870	Tr	Tr	1.77	1.73	18.9	Tr	326
0	12	27	55	0.8	56	106	Tr	Tr	0.10	0.10	1.1	Tr	327
0	12	27	55	0.8	56	106	Tr	Tr	0.08	0.10	1.1	Tr	328

[26] Made with white cornmeal. If made with yellow cornmeal, value is 32 IU or 3 RE.

Table 2. Nutritive Value of the Edible Part of Food (Continued)

(Tr indicates nutrient present in trace amount.)

Item No.	Foods, approximate measures, units, and weight (weight of edible portion only)			Water	Food energy	Protein	Fat	Fatty acids: Saturated	Fatty acids: Monounsaturated	Fatty acids: Polyunsaturated
	Grain Products—Con.		Grams	Percent	Calories	Grams	Grams	Grams	Grams	Grams
	Breads:									
	Oatmeal bread, enriched:[25]									
329	Loaf, 1 lb	1 loaf	454	37	1,145	38	20	3.7	7.1	8.2
330	Slice (18 per loaf)	1 slice	25	37	65	2	1	0.2	0.4	0.5
331	Toasted	1 slice	23	30	65	2	1	0.2	0.4	0.5
332	Pita bread, enriched, white, 6-1/2-in diam.	1 pita	60	31	165	6	1	0.1	0.1	0.4
	Pumpernickel (2/3 rye flour, 1/3 enriched wheat flour):[25]									
333	Loaf, 1 lb	1 loaf	454	37	1,160	42	16	2.6	3.6	6.4
334	Slice, 5 by 4 by 3/8 in	1 slice	32	37	80	3	1	0.2	0.3	0.5
335	Toasted	1 slice	29	28	80	3	1	0.2	0.3	0.5
	Raisin bread, enriched:[25]									
336	Loaf, 1 lb	1 loaf	454	33	1,260	37	18	4.1	6.5	6.7
337	Slice (18 per loaf)	1 slice	25	33	65	2	1	0.2	0.3	0.4
338	Toasted	1 slice	21	24	65	2	1	0.2	0.3	0.4
	Rye bread, light (2/3 enriched wheat flour, 1/3 rye flour):[25]									
339	Loaf, 1 lb	1 loaf	454	37	1,190	38	17	3.3	5.2	5.5
340	Slice, 4-3/4 by 3-3/4 by 7/16 in	1 slice	25	37	65	2	1	0.2	0.3	0.3
341	Toasted	1 slice	22	28	65	2	1	0.2	0.3	0.3
	Wheat bread, enriched:[25]									
342	Loaf, 1 lb	1 loaf	454	37	1,160	43	19	3.9	7.3	4.5
343	Slice (18 per loaf)	1 slice	25	37	65	2	1	0.2	0.4	0.3
344	Toasted	1 slice	23	28	65	3	1	0.2	0.4	0.3
	White bread, enriched:[25]									
345	Loaf, 1 lb	1 loaf	454	37	1,210	38	18	5.6	6.5	4.2
346	Slice (18 per loaf)	1 slice	25	37	65	2	1	0.3	0.4	0.2
347	Toasted	1 slice	22	28	65	2	1	0.3	0.4	0.2
348	Slice (22 per loaf)	1 slice	20	37	55	2	1	0.2	0.3	0.2
349	Toasted	1 slice	17	28	55	2	1	0.2	0.3	0.2
350	Cubes	1 cup	30	37	80	2	1	0.4	0.4	0.3
351	Crumbs, soft	1 cup	45	37	120	4	2	0.6	0.6	0.4
	Whole-wheat bread:[25]									
352	Loaf, 1 lb	1 loaf	454	38	1,110	44	20	5.8	6.8	5.2
353	Slice (16 per loaf)	1 slice	28	38	70	3	1	0.4	0.4	0.3
354	Toasted	1 slice	25	29	70	3	1	0.4	0.4	0.3
	Bread stuffing (from enriched bread), prepared from mix:									
355	Dry type	1 cup	140	33	500	9	31	6.1	13.3	9.6
356	Moist type	1 cup	203	61	420	9	26	5.3	11.3	8.0
	Breakfast cereals:									
	Hot type, cooked:									
	Corn (hominy) grits:									
357	Regular and quick, enriched	1 cup	242	85	145	3	Tr	Tr	0.1	0.2
358	Instant, plain	1 pkt	137	85	80	2	Tr	Tr	Tr	0.1
	Cream of Wheat®:									
359	Regular, quick, instant	1 cup	244	86	140	4	Tr	0.1	Tr	0.2
360	Mix'n Eat, plain	1 pkt	142	82	100	3	Tr	Tr	Tr	0.1
361	Malt-O-Meal®	1 cup	240	88	120	4	Tr	Tr	Tr	0.1
	Oatmeal or rolled oats:									
362	Regular, quick, instant, nonfortified	1 cup	234	85	145	6	2	0.4	0.8	1.0
	Instant, fortified:									
363	Plain	1 pkt	177	86	105	4	2	0.3	0.6	0.7
364	Flavored	1 pkt	164	76	160	5	2	0.3	0.7	0.8

[25] Made with vegetable shortening.
[27] Nutrient added.
[28] Cooked without salt. If salt is added according to label recommendations, sodium content is 540 mg.
[29] For white corn grits. Cooked yellow grits contain 145 IU or 14 RE.
[30] Value based on label declaration for added nutrients.

Nutrients in Indicated Quantity

Cholesterol	Carbohydrate	Calcium	Phosphorus	Iron	Potassium	Sodium	Vitamin A value (IU)	Vitamin A value (RE)	Thiamin	Riboflavin	Niacin	Ascorbic acid	Item No.
Milligrams	Grams	Milligrams	Milligrams	Milligrams	Milligrams	Milligrams	International units	Retinol equivalents	Milligrams	Milligrams	Milligrams	Milligrams	
0	212	267	563	12.0	707	2,231	0	0	2.09	1.20	15.4	0	329
0	12	15	31	0.7	39	124	0	0	0.12	0.07	0.9	0	330
0	12	15	31	0.7	39	124	0	0	0.09	0.07	0.9	0	331
0	33	49	60	1.4	71	339	0	0	0.27	0.12	2.2	0	332
0	218	322	990	12.4	1,966	2,461	0	0	1.54	2.36	15.0	0	333
0	16	23	71	0.9	141	177	0	0	0.11	0.17	1.1	0	334
0	16	23	71	0.9	141	177	0	0	0.09	0.17	1.1	0	335
0	239	463	395	14.1	1,058	1,657	Tr	Tr	1.50	2.81	18.6	Tr	336
0	13	25	22	0.8	59	92	Tr	Tr	0.08	0.15	1.0	Tr	337
0	13	25	22	0.8	59	92	Tr	Tr	0.06	0.15	1.0	Tr	338
0	218	363	658	12.3	926	3,164	0	0	1.86	1.45	15.0	0	339
0	12	20	36	0.7	51	175	0	0	0.10	0.08	0.8	0	340
0	12	20	36	0.7	51	175	0	0	0.08	0.08	0.8	0	341
0	213	572	835	15.8	627	2,447	Tr	Tr	2.09	1.45	20.5	Tr	342
0	12	32	47	0.9	35	138	Tr	Tr	0.12	0.08	1.2	Tr	343
0	12	32	47	0.9	35	138	Tr	Tr	0.10	0.08	1.2	Tr	344
0	222	572	490	12.9	508	2,334	Tr	Tr	2.13	1.41	17.0	Tr	345
0	12	32	27	0.7	28	129	Tr	Tr	0.12	0.08	0.9	Tr	346
0	12	32	27	0.7	28	129	Tr	Tr	0.09	0.08	0.9	Tr	347
0	10	25	21	0.6	22	101	Tr	Tr	0.09	0.06	0.7	Tr	348
0	10	25	21	0.6	22	101	Tr	Tr	0.07	0.06	0.7	Tr	349
0	15	38	32	0.9	34	154	Tr	Tr	0.14	0.09	1.1	Tr	350
0	22	57	49	1.3	50	231	Tr	Tr	0.21	0.14	1.7	Tr	351
0	206	327	1,180	15.5	799	2,887	Tr	Tr	1.59	0.95	17.4	Tr	352
0	13	20	74	1.0	50	180	Tr	Tr	0.10	0.06	1.1	Tr	353
0	13	20	74	1.0	50	180	Tr	Tr	0.08	0.06	1.1	Tr	354
0	50	92	136	2.2	126	1,254	910	273	0.17	0.20	2.5	0	355
67	40	81	134	2.0	118	1,023	850	256	0.10	0.18	1.6	0	356
0	31	0	29	[27]1.5	53	[28]0	[29]0	[29]0	[27]0.24	[27]0.15	[27]2.0	0	357
0	18	7	16	[27]1.0	29	343	0	0	[27]0.18	[27]0.08	[27]1.3	0	358
0	29	[30]54	[31]43	[30]10.9	46	[31,32]5	0	0	[30]0.24	[30]0.07	[30]1.5	0	359
0	21	[30]20	[30]20	[30]8.1	38	241	[30]1,250	[30]376	[30]0.43	[30]0.28	[30]5.0	0	360
0	26	5	[30]24	[30]9.6	31	[33]2	0	0	[30]0.48	[30]0.24	[30]5.8	0	361
0	25	19	178	1.6	131	[34]2	40	4	0.26	0.05	0.3	0	362
0	18	[27]163	133	[27]6.3	99	[27]285	[27]1,510	[27]453	[27]0.53	[27]0.28	[27]5.5	0	363
0	31	[27]168	148	[27]6.7	137	[27]254	[27]1,530	[27]460	[27]0.53	[27]0.38	[27]5.9	Tr	364

[31] For regular and instant cereal. For quick cereal, phosphorus is 102 mg and sodium is 142 mg.
[32] Cooked without salt. If salt is added according to label recommendations, sodium content is 390 mg.
[33] Cooked without salt. If salt is added according to label recommendations, sodium content is 324 mg.
[34] Cooked without salt. If salt is added according to label recommendations, sodium content is 374 mg.

Table 2. Nutritive Value of the Edible Part of Food (Continued)
(Tr indicates nutrient present in trace amount.)

Item No.	Foods, approximate measures, units, and weight (weight of edible portion only)			Water	Food energy	Protein	Fat	Fatty acids: Saturated	Fatty acids: Monounsaturated	Fatty acids: Polyunsaturated
	Grain Products—Con.		Grams	Percent	Calories	Grams	Grams	Grams	Grams	Grams
	Breakfast cereals:									
	Ready to eat:									
365	All-Bran® (about 1/3 cup)	1 oz	28	3	70	4	1	0.1	0.1	0.3
366	Cap'n Crunch® (about 3/4 cup)	1 oz	28	3	120	1	3	1.7	0.3	0.4
367	Cheerios® (about 1-1/4 cup)	1 oz	28	5	110	4	2	0.3	0.6	0.7
	Corn Flakes (about 1-1/4 cup):									
368	Kellogg's®	1 oz	28	3	110	2	Tr	Tr	Tr	Tr
369	Toasties®	1 oz	28	3	110	2	Tr	Tr	Tr	Tr
	40% Bran Flakes:									
370	Kellogg's® (about 3/4 cup)	1 oz	28	3	90	4	1	0.1	0.1	0.3
371	Post® (about 2/3 cup)	1 oz	28	3	90	3	Tr	0.1	0.1	0.2
372	Froot Loops® (about 1 cup)	1 oz	28	3	110	2	1	0.2	0.1	0.1
373	Golden Grahams® (about 3/4 cup)	1 oz	28	2	110	2	1	0.7	0.1	0.2
374	Grape-Nuts® (about 1/4 cup)	1 oz	28	3	100	3	Tr	Tr	Tr	0.1
375	Honey Nut Cheerios® (about 3/4 cup)	1 oz	28	3	105	3	1	0.1	0.3	0.3
376	Lucky Charms® (about 1 cup)	1 oz	28	3	110	3	1	0.2	0.4	0.4
377	Nature Valley® Granola (about 1/3 cup)	1 oz	28	4	125	3	5	3.3	0.7	0.7
378	100% Natural Cereal (about 1/4 cup)	1 oz	28	2	135	3	6	4.1	1.2	0.5
379	Product 19® (about 3/4 cup)	1 oz	28	3	110	3	Tr	Tr	Tr	0.1
	Raisin Bran:									
380	Kellogg's® (about 3/4 cup)	1 oz	28	8	90	3	1	0.1	0.1	0.3
381	Post® (about 1/2 cup)	1 oz	28	9	85	3	1	0.1	0.1	0.3
382	Rice Krispies® (about 1 cup)	1 oz	28	2	110	2	Tr	Tr	Tr	0.1
383	Shredded Wheat (about 2/3 cup)	1 oz	28	5	100	3	1	0.1	0.1	0.3
384	Special K® (about 1-1/3 cup)	1 oz	28	2	110	6	Tr	Tr	Tr	Tr
385	Super Sugar Crisp® (about 7/8 cup)	1 oz	28	2	105	2	Tr	Tr	Tr	0.1
386	Sugar Frosted Flakes, Kellogg's® (about 3/4 cup)	1 oz	28	3	110	1	Tr	Tr	Tr	Tr
387	Sugar Smacks® (about 3/4 cup)	1 oz	28	3	105	2	1	0.1	0.1	0.2
388	Total® (about 1 cup)	1 oz	28	4	100	3	1	0.1	0.1	0.3
389	Trix® (about 1 cup)	1 oz	28	3	110	2	Tr	0.2	0.1	0.1
390	Wheaties® (about 1 cup)	1 oz	28	5	100	3	Tr	0.1	Tr	0.2
391	Buckwheat flour, light, sifted	1 cup	98	12	340	6	1	0.2	0.4	0.4
392	Bulgur, uncooked	1 cup	170	10	600	19	3	1.2	0.3	1.2
	Cakes prepared from cake mixes with enriched flour:[35]									
	Angelfood:									
393	Whole cake, 9-3/4-in diam. tube cake	1 cake	635	38	1,510	38	2	0.4	0.2	1.0
394	Piece, 1/12 of cake	1 piece	53	38	125	3	Tr	Tr	Tr	0.1
	Coffeecake, crumb:									
395	Whole cake, 7-3/4 by 5-5/8 by 1-1/4 in	1 cake	430	30	1,385	27	41	11.8	16.7	9.6
396	Piece, 1/6 of cake	1 piece	72	30	230	5	7	2.0	2.8	1.6
	Devil's food with chocolate frosting:									
397	Whole, 2-layer cake, 8- or 9-in diam.	1 cake	1,107	24	3,755	49	136	55.6	51.4	19.7
398	Piece, 1/16 of cake	1 piece	69	24	235	3	8	3.5	3.2	1.2
399	Cupcake, 2-1/2-in diam.	1 cupcake	35	24	120	2	4	1.8	1.6	0.6
	Gingerbread:									
400	Whole cake, 8 in square	1 cake	570	37	1,575	18	39	9.6	16.4	10.5
401	Piece, 1/9 of cake	1 piece	63	37	175	2	4	1.1	1.8	1.2

[27] Nutrient added.
[30] Value based on label declaration for added nutrients.

Nutrients in Indicated Quantity													
Cho-les-terol	Carbo-hydrate	Calcium	Phos-phorus	Iron	Potas-sium	Sodium	Vitamin A value (IU)	Vitamin A value (RE)	Thiamin	Ribo-flavin	Niacin	Ascorbic acid	Item No.
Milli-grams	Grams	Milli-grams	Milli-grams	Milli-grams	Milli-grams	Milli-grams	Inter-national units	Retinol equiva-lents	Milli-grams	Milli-grams	Milli-grams	Milli-grams	
0	21	23	264	[30]4.5	350	320	[30]1,250	[30]375	[30]0.37	[30]0.43	[30]5.0	[30]15	365
0	23	5	36	[27]7.5	37	213	40	4	[27]0.50	[27]0.55	[27]6.6	0	366
0	20	48	134	[30]4.5	101	307	[30]1,250	[30]375	[30]0.37	[30]0.43	[30]5.0	[30]15	367
0	24	1	18	[30]1.8	26	351	[30]1,250	[30]375	[30]0.37	[30]0.43	[30]5.0	[30]15	368
0	24	1	12	[27]0.7	33	297	[30]1,250	[30]375	[30]0.37	[30]0.43	[30]5.0	0	369
0	22	14	139	[30]8.1	180	264	[30]1,250	[30]375	[30]0.37	[30]0.43	[30]5.0	0	370
0	22	12	179	[30]4.5	151	260	[30]1,250	[30]375	[30]0.37	[30]0.43	[30]5.0	0	371
0	25	3	24	[30]4.5	26	145	[30]1,250	[30]375	[30]0.37	[30]0.43	[30]5.0	[30]15	372
Tr	24	17	41	[30]4.5	63	346	[30]1,250	[30]375	[30]0.37	[30]0.43	[30]5.0	[30]15	373
0	23	11	71	1.2	95	197	[30]1,250	[30]375	[30]0.37	[30]0.43	[30]5.0	0	374
0	23	20	105	[30]4.5	99	257	[30]1,250	[30]375	[30]0.37	[30]0.43	[30]5.0	[30]15	375
0	23	32	79	[30]4.5	59	201	[30]1,250	[30]375	[30]0.37	[30]0.43	[30]5.0	[30]15	376
0	19	18	89	0.9	98	58	20	2	0.10	0.05	0.2	0	377
Tr	18	49	104	0.8	140	12	20	2	0.09	0.15	0.6	0	378
0	24	3	40	[30]18.0	44	325	[30]5,000	[30]1,501	[30]1.50	[30]1.70	[30]20.0	[30]60	379
0	21	10	105	[30]3.5	147	207	[30]960	[30]288	[30]0.28	[30]0.34	[30]3.9	0	380
0	21	13	119	[30]4.5	175	185	[30]1,250	[30]375	[30]0.37	[30]0.43	[30]5.0	0	381
0	25	4	34	[30]1.8	29	340	[30]1,250	[30]375	[30]0.37	[30]0.43	[30]5.0	[30]15	382
0	23	11	100	1.2	102	3	0	0	0.07	0.08	1.5	0	383
Tr	21	8	55	[30]4.5	49	265	[30]1,250	[30]375	[30]0.37	[30]0.43	[30]5.0	[30]15	384
0	26	6	52	[30]1.8	105	25	[30]1,250	[30]375	[30]0.37	[30]0.43	[30]5.0	0	385
0	26	1	21	[30]1.8	18	230	[30]1,250	[30]375	[30]0.37	[30]0.43	[30]5.0	[30]15	386
0	25	3	31	[30]1.8	42	75	[30]1,250	[30]375	[30]0.37	[30]0.43	[30]5.0	[30]15	387
0	22	48	118	[30]18.0	106	352	[30]5,000	[30]1,501	[30]1.50	[30]1.70	[30]20.0	[30]60	388
0	25	6	19	[30]4.5	27	181	[30]1,250	[30]375	[30]0.37	[30]0.43	[30]5.0	[30]15	389
0	23	43	98	[30]4.5	106	354	[30]1,250	[30]375	[30]0.37	[30]0.43	[30]5.0	[30]15	390
0	78	11	86	1.0	314	2	0	0	0.08	0.04	0.4	0	391
0	129	49	575	9.5	389	7	0	0	0.48	0.24	7.7	0	392
0	342	527	1,086	2.7	845	3,226	0	0	0.32	1.27	1.6	0	393
0	29	44	91	0.2	71	269	0	0	0.03	0.11	0.1	0	394
279	225	262	748	7.3	469	1,853	690	194	0.82	0.90	7.7	1	395
47	38	44	125	1.2	78	310	120	32	0.14	0.15	1.3	Tr	396
598	645	653	1,162	22.1	1,439	2,900	1,660	498	1.11	1.66	10.0	1	397
37	40	41	72	1.4	90	181	100	31	0.07	0.10	0.6	Tr	398
19	20	21	37	0.7	46	92	50	16	0.04	0.05	0.3	Tr	399
6	291	513	570	10.8	1,562	1,733	0	0	0.86	1.03	7.4	1	400
1	32	57	63	1.2	173	192	0	0	0.09	0.11	0.8	Tr	401

[35] Excepting angelfood cake, cakes were made from mixes containing vegetable shortening and frostings were made with margarine.

Table 2. Nutritive Value of the Edible Part of Food (Continued)

(Tr indicates nutrient present in trace amount.)

Item No.	Foods, approximate measures, units, and weight (weight of edible portion only)			Water	Food energy	Protein	Fat	Fatty acids: Saturated	Fatty acids: Monounsaturated	Fatty acids: Polyunsaturated
	Grain Products—Con.		Grams	Percent	Calories	Grams	Grams	Grams	Grams	Grams
	Cakes prepared from cake mixes with enriched flour:[35]									
	Yellow with chocolate frosting:									
402	Whole, 2-layer cake, 8- or 9-in diam.	1 cake	1,108	26	3,735	45	125	47.8	48.8	21.8
403	Piece, 1/16 of cake	1 piece	69	26	235	3	8	3.0	3.0	1.4
	Cakes prepared from home recipes using enriched flour:									
	Carrot, with cream cheese frosting:[36]									
404	Whole cake, 10-in diam. tube cake	1 cake	1,536	23	6,175	63	328	66.0	135.2	107.5
405	Piece, 1/16 of cake	1 piece	96	23	385	4	21	4.1	8.4	6.7
	Fruitcake, dark:[36]									
406	Whole cake, 7-1/2-in diam., 2-1/4-in high tube cake	1 cake	1,361	18	5,185	74	228	47.6	113.0	51.7
407	Piece, 1/32 of cake, 2/3-in arc	1 piece	43	18	165	2	7	1.5	3.6	1.6
	Plain sheet cake:[37]									
	Without frosting:									
408	Whole cake, 9-in square	1 cake	777	25	2,830	35	108	29.5	45.1	25.6
409	Piece, 1/9 of cake	1 piece	86	25	315	4	12	3.3	5.0	2.8
	With uncooked white frosting:									
410	Whole cake, 9-in square	1 cake	1,096	21	4,020	37	129	41.6	50.4	26.3
411	Piece, 1/9 of cake	1 piece	121	21	445	4	14	4.6	5.6	2.9
	Pound:[38]									
412	Loaf, 8-1/2 by 3-1/2 by 3-1/4 in	1 loaf	514	22	2,025	33	94	21.1	40.9	26.7
413	Slice, 1/17 of loaf	1 slice	30	22	120	2	5	1.2	2.4	1.6
	Cakes, commercial, made with enriched flour:									
	Pound:									
414	Loaf, 8-1/2 by 3-1/2 by 3 in	1 loaf	500	24	1,935	26	94	52.0	30.0	4.0
415	Slice, 1/17 of loaf	1 slice	29	24	110	2	5	3.0	1.7	0.2
	Snack cakes:									
416	Devil's food with creme filling (2 small cakes per pkg)	1 small cake	28	20	105	1	4	1.7	1.5	0.6
417	Sponge with creme filling (2 small cakes per pkg)	1 small cake	42	19	155	1	5	2.3	2.1	0.5
	White with white frosting:									
418	Whole, 2-layer cake, 8- or 9-in diam.	1 cake	1,140	24	4,170	43	148	33.1	61.6	42.2
419	Piece, 1/16 of cake	1 piece	71	24	260	3	9	2.1	3.8	2.6
	Yellow with chocolate frosting:									
420	Whole, 2-layer cake, 8- or 9-in diam.	1 cake	1,108	23	3,895	40	175	92.0	58.7	10.0
421	Piece, 1/16 of cake	1 piece	69	23	245	2	11	5.7	3.7	0.6
	Cheesecake:									
422	Whole cake, 9-in diam.	1 cake	1,110	46	3,350	60	213	119.9	65.5	14.4
423	Piece, 1/12 of cake	1 piece	92	46	280	5	18	9.9	5.4	1.2
	Cookies made with enriched flour:									
	Brownies with nuts:									
424	Commercial, with frosting, 1-1/2 by 1-3/4 by 7/8 in	1 brownie	25	13	100	1	4	1.6	2.0	0.6
425	From home recipe, 1-3/4 by 1-3/4 by 7/8 in[36]	1 brownie	20	10	95	1	6	1.4	2.8	1.2
	Chocolate chip:									
426	Commercial, 2-1/4-in diam., 3/8 in thick	4 cookies	42	4	180	2	9	2.9	3.1	2.6

[35] Excepting angelfood cake, cakes were made from mixes containing vegetable shortening and frostings were made with margarine.

[36] Made with vegetable oil.

Nutrients in Indicated Quantity														
Cho-les-terol	Carbo-hydrate	Calcium	Phos-phorus	Iron	Potas-sium	Sodium	Vitamin A value (IU)	Vitamin A value (RE)	Thiamin	Ribo-flavin	Niacin	Ascorbic acid	Item No.
Milli-grams	Grams	Milli-grams	Milli-grams	Milli-grams	Milli-grams	Milli-grams	Inter-national units	Retinol equiva-lents	Milli-grams	Milli-grams	Milli-grams	Milli-grams	
576	638	1,008	2,017	15.5	1,208	2,515	1,550	465	1.22	1.66	11.1	1	402
36	40	63	126	1.0	75	157	100	29	0.08	0.10	0.7	Tr	403
1183	775	707	998	21.0	1,720	4,470	2,240	246	1.83	1.97	14.7	23	404
74	48	44	62	1.3	108	279	140	15	0.11	0.12	0.9	1	405
640	783	1,293	1,592	37.6	6,138	2,123	1,720	422	2.41	2.55	17.0	504	406
20	25	41	50	1.2	194	67	50	13	0.08	0.08	0.5	16	407
552	434	497	793	11.7	614	2,331	1,320	373	1.24	1.40	10.1	2	408
61	48	55	88	1.3	68	258	150	41	0.14	0.15	1.1	Tr	409
636	694	548	822	11.0	669	2,488	2,190	647	1.21	1.42	9.9	2	410
70	77	61	91	1.2	74	275	240	71	0.13	0.16	1.1	Tr	411
555	265	339	473	9.3	483	1,645	3,470	1,033	0.93	1.08	7.8	1	412
32	15	20	28	0.5	28	96	200	60	0.05	0.06	0.5	Tr	413
1100	257	146	517	8.0	443	1,857	2,820	715	0.96	1.12	8.1	0	414
64	15	8	30	0.5	26	108	160	41	0.06	0.06	0.5	0	415
15	17	21	26	1.0	34	105	20	4	0.06	0.09	0.7	0	416
7	27	14	44	0.6	37	155	30	9	0.07	0.06	0.6	0	417
46	670	536	1,585	15.5	832	2,827	640	194	3.19	2.05	27.6	0	418
3	42	33	99	1.0	52	176	40	12	0.20	0.13	1.7	0	419
609	620	366	1,884	19.9	1,972	3,080	1,850	488	0.78	2.22	10.0	0	420
38	39	23	117	1.2	123	192	120	30	0.05	0.14	0.6	0	421
2053	317	622	977	5.3	1,088	2,464	2,820	833	0.33	1.44	5.1	56	422
170	26	52	81	0.4	90	204	230	69	0.03	0.12	0.4	5	423
14	16	13	26	0.6	50	59	70	18	0.08	0.07	0.3	Tr	424
18	11	9	26	0.4	35	51	20	6	0.05	0.05	0.3	Tr	425
5	28	13	41	0.8	68	140	50	15	0.10	0.23	1.0	Tr	426

[37]Cake made with vegetable shortening; frosting with margarine.
[38]Made with margarine.

Table 2. Nutritive Value of the Edible Part of Food (Continued)

(Tr indicates nutrient present in trace amount.)

Item No.	Foods, approximate measures, units, and weight (weight of edible portion only)			Water	Food energy	Protein	Fat	Fatty acids: Saturated	Fatty acids: Monounsaturated	Fatty acids: Polyunsaturated
	Grain Products—Con.		Grams	Percent	Calories	Grams	Grams	Grams	Grams	Grams
	Cookies made with enriched flour:									
	Chocolate chip:									
427	From home recipe, 2-1/3-in diam.[25]	4 cookies	40	3	185	2	11	3.9	4.3	2.0
428	From refrigerated dough, 2-1/4-in diam., 3/8 in thick	4 cookies	48	5	225	2	11	4.0	4.4	2.0
429	Fig bars, square, 1-5/8 by 1-5/8 by 3/8 in or rectangular, 1-1/2 by 1-3/4 by 1/2 in	4 cookies	56	12	210	2	4	1.0	1.5	1.0
430	Oatmeal with raisins, 2-5/8-in diam., 1/4 in thick	4 cookies	52	4	245	3	10	2.5	4.5	2.8
431	Peanut butter cookie, from home recipe, 2-5/8-in diam.[25]	4 cookies	48	3	245	4	14	4.0	5.8	2.8
432	Sandwich type (chocolate or vanilla), 1-3/4-in diam., 3/8 in thick	4 cookies	40	2	195	2	8	2.0	3.6	2.2
	Shortbread:									
433	Commercial	4 small cookies	32	6	155	2	8	2.9	3.0	1.1
434	From home recipe[38]	2 large cookies	28	3	145	2	8	1.3	2.7	3.4
435	Sugar cookie, from refrigerated dough, 2-1/2-in diam., 1/4 in thick	4 cookies	48	4	235	2	12	2.3	5.0	3.6
436	Vanilla wafers, 1-3/4-in diam., 1/4 in thick	10 cookies	40	4	185	2	7	1.8	3.0	1.8
437	Corn chips	1-oz package	28	1	155	2	9	1.4	2.4	3.7
	Cornmeal:									
438	Whole-ground, unbolted, dry form	1 cup	122	12	435	11	5	0.5	1.1	2.5
439	Bolted (nearly whole-grain), dry form	1 cup	122	12	440	11	4	0.5	0.9	2.2
	Degermed, enriched:									
440	Dry form	1 cup	138	12	500	11	2	0.2	0.4	0.9
441	Cooked	1 cup	240	88	120	3	Tr	Tr	0.1	0.2
	Crackers:[39]									
	Cheese:									
442	Plain, 1 in square	10 crackers	10	4	50	1	3	0.9	1.2	0.3
443	Sandwich type (peanut butter)	1 sandwich	8	3	40	1	2	0.4	0.8	0.3
444	Graham, plain, 2-1/2 in square	2 crackers	14	5	60	1	1	0.4	0.6	0.4
445	Melba toast, plain	1 piece	5	4	20	1	Tr	0.1	0.1	0.1
446	Rye wafers, whole-grain, 1-7/8 by 3-1/2 in	2 wafers	14	5	55	1	1	0.3	0.4	0.3
447	Saltines[40]	4 crackers	12	4	50	1	1	0.5	0.4	0.2
448	Snack-type, standard	1 round cracker	3	3	15	Tr	1	0.2	0.4	0.1
449	Wheat, thin	4 crackers	8	3	35	1	1	0.5	0.5	0.4
450	Whole-wheat wafers	2 crackers	8	4	35	1	2	0.5	0.6	0.4
451	Croissants, made with enriched flour, 4-1/2 by 4 by 1-3/4 in	1 croissant	57	22	235	5	12	3.5	6.7	1.4
	Danish pastry, made with enriched flour:									
	Plain without fruit or nuts:									
452	Packaged ring, 12 oz	1 ring	340	27	1,305	21	71	21.8	28.6	15.6
453	Round piece, about 4-1/4-in diam., 1 in high	1 pastry	57	27	220	4	12	3.6	4.8	2.6
454	Ounce	1 oz	28	27	110	2	6	1.8	2.4	1.3
455	Fruit, round piece	1 pastry	65	30	235	4	13	3.9	5.2	2.9
	Doughnuts, made with enriched flour:									
456	Cake type, plain, 3-1/4-in diam., 1 in high	1 doughnut	50	21	210	3	12	2.8	5.0	3.0
457	Yeast-leavened, glazed, 3-3/4-in diam., 1-1/4 in high	1 doughnut	60	27	235	4	13	5.2	5.5	0.9
458	English muffins, plain, enriched	1 muffin	57	42	140	5	1	0.3	0.2	0.3
459	Toasted	1 muffin	50	29	140	5	1	0.3	0.2	0.3

[25]Made with vegetable shortening.
[38]Made with margarine.

Nutrients in Indicated Quantity

Cholesterol	Carbohydrate	Calcium	Phosphorus	Iron	Potassium	Sodium	Vitamin A value (IU)	Vitamin A value (RE)	Thiamin	Riboflavin	Niacin	Ascorbic acid	Item No.
Milligrams	Grams	Milligrams	Milligrams	Milligrams	Milligrams	Milligrams	International units	Retinol equivalents	Milligrams	Milligrams	Milligrams	Milligrams	
18	26	13	34	1.0	82	82	20	5	0.06	0.06	0.6	0	427
22	32	13	34	1.0	62	173	30	8	0.06	0.10	0.9	0	428
27	42	40	34	1.4	162	180	60	6	0.08	0.07	0.7	Tr	429
2	36	18	58	1.1	90	148	40	12	0.09	0.08	1.0	0	430
22	28	21	60	1.1	110	142	20	5	0.07	0.07	1.9	0	431
0	29	12	40	1.4	66	189	0	0	0.09	0.07	0.8	0	432
27	20	13	39	0.8	38	123	30	8	0.10	0.09	0.9	0	433
0	17	6	31	0.6	18	125	300	89	0.08	0.06	0.7	Tr	434
29	31	50	91	0.9	33	261	40	11	0.09	0.06	1.1	0	435
25	29	16	36	0.8	50	150	50	14	0.07	0.10	1.0	0	436
0	16	35	52	0.5	52	233	110	11	0.04	0.05	0.4	1	437
0	90	24	312	2.2	346	1	620	62	0.46	0.13	2.4	0	438
0	91	21	272	2.2	303	1	590	59	0.37	0.10	2.3	0	439
0	108	8	137	5.9	166	1	610	61	0.61	0.36	4.8	0	440
0	26	2	34	1.4	38	0	140	14	0.14	0.10	1.2	0	441
6	6	11	17	0.3	17	112	20	5	0.05	0.04	0.4	0	442
1	5	7	25	0.3	17	90	Tr	Tr	0.04	0.03	0.6	0	443
0	11	6	20	0.4	36	86	0	0	0.02	0.03	0.6	0	444
0	4	6	10	0.1	11	44	0	0	0.01	0.01	0.1	0	445
0	10	7	44	0.5	65	115	0	0	0.06	0.03	0.5	0	446
4	9	3	12	0.5	17	165	0	0	0.06	0.05	0.6	0	447
0	2	3	6	0.1	4	30	Tr	Tr	0.01	0.01	0.1	0	448
0	5	3	15	0.3	17	69	Tr	Tr	0.04	0.03	0.4	0	449
0	5	3	22	0.2	31	59	0	0	0.02	0.03	0.4	0	450
13	27	20	64	2.1	68	452	50	13	0.17	0.13	1.3	0	451
292	152	360	347	6.5	316	1,302	360	99	0.95	1.02	8.5	Tr	452
49	26	60	58	1.1	53	218	60	17	0.16	0.17	1.4	Tr	453
24	13	30	29	0.5	26	109	30	8	0.08	0.09	0.7	Tr	454
56	28	17	80	1.3	57	233	40	11	0.16	0.14	1.4	Tr	455
20	24	22	111	1.0	58	192	20	5	0.12	0.12	1.1	Tr	456
21	26	17	55	1.4	64	222	Tr	Tr	0.28	0.12	1.8	0	457
0	27	96	67	1.7	331	378	0	0	0.26	0.19	2.2	0	458
0	27	96	67	1.7	331	378	0	0	0.23	0.19	2.2	0	459

[39] Crackers made with enriched flour except for rye wafers and whole-wheat wafers.
[40] Made with lard.

Table 2. Nutritive Value of the Edible Part of Food (Continued)

(Tr indicates nutrient present in trace amount.)

Item No.	Foods, approximate measures, units, and weight (weight of edible portion only)			Water	Food energy	Protein	Fat	Fatty acids: Saturated	Fatty acids: Monounsaturated	Fatty acids: Polyunsaturated
	Grain Products—Con.		Grams	Percent	Calories	Grams	Grams	Grams	Grams	Grams
460	French toast, from home recipe	1 slice	65	53	155	6	7	1.6	2.0	1.6
	Macaroni, enriched, cooked (cut lengths, elbows, shells):									
461	Firm stage (hot)	1 cup	130	64	190	7	1	0.1	0.1	0.3
	Tender stage:									
462	Cold	1 cup	105	72	115	4	Tr	0.1	0.1	0.2
463	Hot	1 cup	140	72	155	5	1	0.1	0.1	0.2
	Muffins made with enriched flour, 2-1/2-in diam., 1-1/2 in high:									
	From home recipe:									
464	Blueberry[25]	1 muffin	45	37	135	3	5	1.5	2.1	1.2
465	Bran[36]	1 muffin	45	35	125	3	6	1.4	1.6	2.3
466	Corn (enriched, degermed cornmeal and flour)[25]	1 muffin	45	33	145	3	5	1.5	2.2	1.4
	From commercial mix (egg and water added):									
467	Blueberry	1 muffin	45	33	140	3	5	1.4	2.0	1.2
468	Bran	1 muffin	45	28	140	3	4	1.3	1.6	1.0
469	Corn	1 muffin	45	30	145	3	6	1.7	2.3	1.4
470	Noodles (egg noodles), enriched, cooked	1 cup	160	70	200	7	2	0.5	0.6	0.6
471	Noodles, chow mein, canned	1 cup	45	11	220	6	11	2.1	7.3	0.4
	Pancakes, 4-in diam.:									
472	Buckwheat, from mix (with buckwheat and enriched flours), egg and milk added	1 pancake	27	58	55	2	2	0.9	0.9	0.5
	Plain:									
473	From home recipe using enriched flour	1 pancake	27	50	60	2	2	0.5	0.8	0.5
474	From mix (with enriched flour), egg, milk, and oil added	1 pancake	27	54	60	2	2	0.5	0.9	0.5
	Piecrust, made with enriched flour and vegetable shortening, baked:									
475	From home recipe, 9-in diam.	1 pie shell	180	15	900	11	60	14.8	25.9	15.7
476	From mix, 9-in diam.	Piecrust for 2-crust pie	320	19	1,485	20	93	22.7	41.0	25.0
	Pies, piecrust made with enriched flour, vegetable shortening, 9-in diam.:									
	Apple:									
477	Whole	1 pie	945	48	2,420	21	105	27.4	44.4	26.5
478	Piece, 1/6 of pie	1 piece	158	48	405	3	18	4.6	7.4	4.4
	Blueberry:									
479	Whole	1 pie	945	51	2,285	23	102	25.5	44.4	27.4
480	Piece, 1/6 of pie	1 piece	158	51	380	4	17	4.3	7.4	4.6
	Cherry:									
481	Whole	1 pie	945	47	2,465	25	107	28.4	46.3	27.4
482	Piece, 1/6 of pie	1 piece	158	47	410	4	18	4.7	7.7	4.6
	Creme:									
483	Whole	1 pie	910	43	2,710	20	139	90.1	23.7	6.4
484	Piece, 1/6 of pie	1 piece	152	43	455	3	23	15.0	4.0	1.1
	Custard:									
485	Whole	1 pie	910	58	1,985	56	101	33.7	40.0	19.1
486	Piece, 1/6 of pie	1 piece	152	58	330	9	17	5.6	6.7	3.2
	Lemon meringue:									
487	Whole	1 pie	840	47	2,140	31	86	26.0	34.4	17.6
488	Piece, 1/6 of pie	1 piece	140	47	355	5	14	4.3	5.7	2.9
	Peach:									
489	Whole	1 pie	945	48	2,410	24	101	24.6	43.5	26.5
490	Piece, 1/6 of pie	1 piece	158	48	405	4	17	4.1	7.3	4.4

[25] Made with vegetable shortening.

Nutrients in Indicated Quantity													
Cholesterol	Carbohydrate	Calcium	Phosphorus	Iron	Potassium	Sodium	Vitamin A value (IU)	Vitamin A value (RE)	Thiamin	Riboflavin	Niacin	Ascorbic acid	Item No.
Milligrams	Grams	Milligrams	Milligrams	Milligrams	Milligrams	Milligrams	International units	Retinol equivalents	Milligrams	Milligrams	Milligrams	Milligrams	
112	17	72	85	1.3	86	257	110	32	0.12	0.16	1.0	Tr	460
0	39	14	85	2.1	103	1	0	0	0.23	0.13	1.8	0	461
0	24	8	53	1.3	64	1	0	0	0.15	0.08	1.2	0	462
0	32	11	70	1.7	85	1	0	0	0.20	0.11	1.5	0	463
19	20	54	46	0.9	47	198	40	9	0.10	0.11	0.9	1	464
24	19	60	125	1.4	99	189	230	30	0.11	0.13	1.3	3	465
23	21	66	59	0.9	57	169	80	15	0.11	0.11	0.9	Tr	466
45	22	15	90	0.9	54	225	50	11	0.10	0.17	1.1	Tr	467
28	24	27	182	1.7	50	385	100	14	0.08	0.12	1.9	0	468
42	22	30	128	1.3	31	291	90	16	0.09	0.09	0.8	Tr	469
50	37	16	94	2.6	70	3	110	34	0.22	0.13	1.9	0	470
5	26	14	41	0.4	33	450	0	0	0.05	0.03	0.6	0	471
20	6	59	91	0.4	66	125	60	17	0.04	0.05	0.2	Tr	472
16	9	27	38	0.5	33	115	30	10	0.06	0.07	0.5	Tr	473
16	8	36	71	0.7	43	160	30	7	0.09	0.12	0.8	Tr	474
0	79	25	90	4.5	90	1,100	0	0	0.54	0.40	5.0	0	475
0	141	131	272	9.3	179	2,602	0	0	1.06	0.80	9.9	0	476
0	360	76	208	9.5	756	2,844	280	28	1.04	0.76	9.5	9	477
0	60	13	35	1.6	126	476	50	5	0.17	0.13	1.6	2	478
0	330	104	217	12.3	945	2,533	850	85	1.04	0.85	10.4	38	479
0	55	17	36	2.1	158	423	140	14	0.17	0.14	1.7	6	480
0	363	132	236	9.5	992	2,873	4,160	416	1.13	0.85	9.5	0	481
0	61	22	40	1.6	166	480	700	70	0.19	0.14	1.6	0	482
46	351	273	919	6.8	796	2,207	1,250	391	0.36	0.89	6.4	0	483
8	59	46	154	1.1	133	369	210	65	0.06	0.15	1.1	0	484
1010	213	874	1,028	9.1	1,247	2,612	2,090	573	0.82	1.91	5.5	0	485
169	36	146	172	1.5	208	436	350	96	0.14	0.32	0.9	0	486
857	317	118	412	8.4	420	2,369	1,430	395	0.59	0.84	5.0	25	487
143	53	20	69	1.4	70	395	240	66	0.10	0.14	0.8	4	488
0	361	95	274	11.3	1,408	2,533	6,900	690	1.04	0.95	14.2	28	489
0	60	16	46	1.9	235	423	1,150	115	0.17	0.16	2.4	5	490

[36] Made with vegetable oil.

Table 2. Nutritive Value of the Edible Part of Food (Continued)

(Tr indicates nutrient present in trace amount.)

Item No.	Foods, approximate measures, units, and weight (weight of edible portion only)			Water	Food energy	Protein	Fat	Fatty acids: Saturated	Fatty acids: Monounsaturated	Fatty acids: Polyunsaturated
	Grain Products—Con.		Grams	Percent	Calories	Grams	Grams	Grams	Grams	Grams
	Pies, piecrust made with enriched flour, vegetable shortening, 9-inch diam.:									
	Pecan:									
491	Whole	1 pie	825	20	3,450	42	189	28.1	101.5	47.0
492	Piece, 1/6 of pie	1 piece	138	20	575	7	32	4.7	17.0	7.9
	Pumpkin:									
493	Whole	1 pie	910	59	1,920	36	102	38.2	40.0	18.2
494	Piece, 1/6 of pie	1 piece	152	59	320	6	17	6.4	6.7	3.0
	Pies, fried:									
495	Apple	1 pie	85	43	255	2	14	5.8	6.6	0.6
496	Cherry	1 pie	85	42	250	2	14	5.8	6.7	0.6
	Popcorn, popped:									
497	Air-popped, unsalted	1 cup	8	4	30	1	Tr	Tr	0.1	0.2
498	Popped in vegetable oil, salted	1 cup	11	3	55	1	3	0.5	1.4	1.2
499	Sugar syrup coated	1 cup	35	4	135	2	1	0.1	0.3	0.6
	Pretzels, made with enriched flour:									
500	Stick, 2-1/4 in long	10 pretzels	3	3	10	Tr	Tr	Tr	Tr	Tr
501	Twisted, dutch, 2-3/4 by 2-5/8 in	1 pretzel	16	3	65	2	1	0.1	0.2	0.2
502	Twisted, thin, 3-1/4 by 2-1/4 by 1/4 in	10 pretzels	60	3	240	6	2	0.4	0.8	0.6
	Rice:									
503	Brown, cooked, served hot	1 cup	195	70	230	5	1	0.3	0.3	0.4
	White, enriched:									
	Commercial varieties, all types:									
504	Raw	1 cup	185	12	670	12	1	0.2	0.2	0.3
505	Cooked, served hot	1 cup	205	73	225	4	Tr	0.1	0.1	0.1
506	Instant, ready-to-serve, hot	1 cup	165	73	180	4	0	0.1	0.1	0.1
	Parboiled:									
507	Raw	1 cup	185	10	685	14	1	0.1	0.1	0.2
508	Cooked, served hot	1 cup	175	73	185	4	Tr	Tr	Tr	0.1
	Rolls, enriched:									
	Commercial:									
509	Dinner, 2-1/2-in diam., 2 in high	1 roll	28	32	85	2	2	0.5	0.8	0.6
510	Frankfurter and hamburger (8 per 11-1/2-oz pkg.)	1 roll	40	34	115	3	2	0.5	0.8	0.6
511	Hard, 3-3/4-in diam., 2 in high	1 roll	50	25	155	5	2	0.4	0.5	0.6
512	Hoagie or submarine, 11-1/2 by 3 by 2-1/2 in	1 roll	135	31	400	11	8	1.8	3.0	2.2
	From home recipe:									
513	Dinner, 2-1/2-in diam., 2 in high	1 roll	35	26	120	3	3	0.8	1.2	0.9
	Spaghetti, enriched, cooked:									
514	Firm stage, "al dente," served hot	1 cup	130	64	190	7	1	0.1	0.1	0.3
515	Tender stage, served hot	1 cup	140	73	155	5	1	0.1	0.1	0.2
516	Toaster pastries	1 pastry	54	13	210	2	6	1.7	3.6	0.4
517	Tortillas, corn	1 tortilla	30	45	65	2	1	0.1	0.3	0.6
	Waffles, made with enriched flour, 7-in diam.:									
518	From home recipe	1 waffle	75	37	245	7	13	4.0	4.9	2.6
519	From mix, egg and milk added	1 waffle	75	42	205	7	8	2.7	2.9	1.5
	Wheat flours:									
	All-purpose or family flour, enriched:									
520	Sifted, spooned	1 cup	115	12	420	12	1	0.2	0.1	0.5
521	Unsifted, spooned	1 cup	125	12	455	13	1	0.2	0.1	0.5
522	Cake or pastry flour, enriched, sifted, spooned	1 cup	96	12	350	7	1	0.1	0.1	0.3
523	Self-rising, enriched, unsifted, spooned	1 cup	125	12	440	12	1	0.2	0.1	0.5
524	Whole-wheat, from hard wheats, stirred	1 cup	120	12	400	16	2	0.3	0.3	1.1

Nutrients in Indicated Quantity													
Cholesterol	Carbohydrate	Calcium	Phosphorus	Iron	Potassium	Sodium	Vitamin A value (IU)	Vitamin A value (RE)	Thiamin	Riboflavin	Niacin	Ascorbic acid	Item No.
Milligrams	Grams	Milligrams	Milligrams	Milligrams	Milligrams	Milligrams	International units	Retinol equivalents	Milligrams	Milligrams	Milligrams	Milligrams	
569	423	388	850	27.2	1,015	1,823	1,320	322	1.82	0.99	6.6	0	491
95	71	65	142	4.6	170	305	220	54	0.30	0.17	1.1	0	492
655	223	464	628	8.2	1,456	1,947	22,480	2,493	0.82	1.27	7.3	0	493
109	37	78	105	1.4	243	325	3,750	416	0.14	0.21	1.2	0	494
14	31	12	34	0.9	42	326	30	3	0.09	0.06	1.0	1	495
13	32	11	41	0.7	61	371	190	19	0.06	0.06	0.6	1	496
0	6	1	22	0.2	20	Tr	10	1	0.03	0.01	0.2	0	497
0	6	3	31	0.3	19	86	20	2	0.01	0.02	0.1	0	498
0	30	2	47	0.5	90	Tr	30	3	0.13	0.02	0.4	0	499
0	2	1	3	0.1	3	48	0	0	0.01	0.01	0.1	0	500
0	13	4	15	0.3	16	258	0	0	0.05	0.04	0.7	0	501
0	48	16	55	1.2	61	966	0	0	0.19	0.15	2.6	0	502
0	50	23	142	1.0	137	0	0	0	0.18	0.04	2.7	0	503
0	149	44	174	5.4	170	9	0	0	0.81	0.06	6.5	0	504
0	50	21	57	1.8	57	0	0	0	0.23	0.02	2.1	0	505
0	40	5	31	1.3	0	0	0	0	0.21	0.02	1.7	0	506
0	150	111	370	5.4	278	17	0	0	0.81	0.07	6.5	0	507
0	41	33	100	1.4	75	0	0	0	0.19	0.02	2.1	0	508
Tr	14	33	44	0.8	36	155	Tr	Tr	0.14	0.09	1.1	Tr	509
Tr	20	54	44	1.2	56	241	Tr	Tr	0.20	0.13	1.6	Tr	510
Tr	30	24	46	1.4	49	313	0	0	0.20	0.12	1.7	0	511
Tr	72	100	115	3.8	128	683	0	0	0.54	0.33	4.5	0	512
12	20	16	36	1.1	41	98	30	8	0.12	0.12	1.2	0	513
0	39	14	85	2.0	103	1	0	0	0.23	0.13	1.8	0	514
0	32	11	70	1.7	85	1	0	0	0.20	0.11	1.5	0	515
0	38	104	104	2.2	91	248	520	52	0.17	0.18	2.3	4	516
0	13	42	55	0.6	43	1	80	8	0.05	0.03	0.4	0	517
102	26	154	135	1.5	129	445	140	39	0.18	0.24	1.5	Tr	518
59	27	179	257	1.2	146	515	170	49	0.14	0.23	0.9	Tr	519
0	88	18	100	5.1	109	2	0	0	0.73	0.46	6.1	0	520
0	95	20	109	5.5	119	3	0	0	0.80	0.50	6.6	0	521
0	76	16	70	4.2	91	2	0	0	0.58	0.38	5.1	0	522
0	93	331	583	5.5	113	1,349	0	0	0.80	0.50	6.6	0	523
0	85	49	446	5.2	444	4	0	0	0.66	0.14	5.2	0	524

Table 2. Nutritive Value of the Edible Part of Food (Continued)

(Tr indicates nutrient present in trace amount.)

Item No.	Foods, approximate measures, units, and weight (weight of edible portion only)			Water	Food energy	Protein	Fat	Fatty acids: Saturated	Fatty acids: Monounsaturated	Fatty acids: Polyunsaturated
	Legumes, Nuts, and Seeds		Grams	Percent	Calories	Grams	Grams	Grams	Grams	Grams
	Almonds, shelled:									
525	Slivered, packed	1 cup	135	4	795	27	70	6.7	45.8	14.8
526	Whole	1 oz	28	4	165	6	15	1.4	9.6	3.1
	Beans, dry:									
	Cooked, drained:									
527	Black	1 cup	171	66	225	15	1	0.1	0.1	0.5
528	Great Northern	1 cup	180	69	210	14	1	0.1	0.1	0.6
529	Lima	1 cup	190	64	260	16	1	0.2	0.1	0.5
530	Pea (navy)	1 cup	190	69	225	15	1	0.1	0.1	0.7
531	Pinto	1 cup	180	65	265	15	1	0.1	0.1	0.5
	Canned, solids and liquid:									
	White with:									
532	Frankfurters (sliced)	1 cup	255	71	365	19	18	7.4	8.8	0.7
533	Pork and tomato sauce	1 cup	255	71	310	16	7	2.4	2.7	0.7
534	Pork and sweet sauce	1 cup	255	66	385	16	12	4.3	4.9	1.2
535	Red kidney	1 cup	255	76	230	15	1	0.1	0.1	0.6
536	Black-eyed peas, dry, cooked (with residual cooking liquid)	1 cup	250	80	190	13	1	0.2	Tr	0.3
537	Brazil nuts, shelled	1 oz	28	3	185	4	19	4.6	6.5	6.8
538	Carob flour	1 cup	140	3	255	6	Tr	Tr	0.1	0.1
	Cashew nuts, salted:									
539	Dry roasted	1 cup	137	2	785	21	63	12.5	37.4	10.7
540		1 oz	28	2	165	4	13	2.6	7.7	2.2
541	Roasted in oil	1 cup	130	4	750	21	63	12.4	36.9	10.6
542		1 oz	28	4	165	5	14	2.7	8.1	2.3
543	Chestnuts, European (Italian), roasted, shelled	1 cup	143	40	350	5	3	0.6	1.1	1.2
544	Chickpeas, cooked, drained	1 cup	163	60	270	15	4	0.4	0.9	1.9
	Coconut:									
	Raw:									
545	Piece, about 2 by 2 by 1/2 in	1 piece	45	47	160	1	15	13.4	0.6	0.2
546	Shredded or grated	1 cup	80	47	285	3	27	23.8	1.1	0.3
547	Dried, sweetened, shredded	1 cup	93	13	470	3	33	29.3	1.4	0.4
548	Filberts (hazelnuts), chopped	1 cup	115	5	725	15	72	5.3	56.5	6.9
549		1 oz	28	5	180	4	18	1.3	13.9	1.7
550	Lentils, dry, cooked	1 cup	200	72	215	16	1	0.1	0.2	0.5
551	Macadamia nuts, roasted in oil, salted	1 cup	134	2	960	10	103	15.4	80.9	1.8
552		1 oz	28	2	205	2	22	3.2	17.1	0.4
	Mixed nuts, with peanuts, salted:									
553	Dry roasted	1 oz	28	2	170	5	15	2.0	8.9	3.1
554	Roasted in oil	1 oz	28	2	175	5	16	2.5	9.0	3.8
555	Peanuts, roasted in oil, salted	1 cup	145	2	840	39	71	9.9	35.5	22.6
556		1 oz	28	2	165	8	14	1.9	6.9	4.4
557	Peanut butter	1 tbsp	16	1	95	5	8	1.4	4.0	2.5
558	Peas, split, dry, cooked	1 cup	200	70	230	16	1	0.1	0.1	0.3
559	Pecans, halves	1 cup	108	5	720	8	73	5.9	45.5	18.1
560		1 oz	28	5	190	2	19	1.5	12.0	4.7
561	Pine nuts (pinyons), shelled	1 oz	28	6	160	3	17	2.7	6.5	7.3
562	Pistachio nuts, dried, shelled	1 oz	28	4	165	6	14	1.7	9.3	2.1
563	Pumpkin and squash kernels, dry, hulled	1 oz	28	7	155	7	13	2.5	4.0	5.9
564	Refried beans, canned	1 cup	290	72	295	18	3	0.4	0.6	1.4
565	Sesame seeds, dry, hulled	1 tbsp	8	5	45	2	4	0.6	1.7	1.9
566	Soybeans, dry, cooked, drained	1 cup	180	71	235	20	10	1.3	1.9	5.3
	Soy products:									
567	Miso	1 cup	276	53	470	29	13	1.8	2.6	7.3
568	Tofu, piece 2-1/2 by 2-3/4 by 1 in	1 piece	120	85	85	9	5	0.7	1.0	2.9
569	Sunflower seeds, dry, hulled	1 oz	28	5	160	6	14	1.5	2.7	9.3
570	Tahini	1 tbsp	15	3	90	3	8	1.1	3.0	3.5

[41] Cashews without salt contain 21 mg sodium per cup or 4 mg per oz.
[42] Cashews without salt contain 22 mg sodium per cup or 5 mg per oz.
[43] Macadamia nuts without salt contain 9 mg sodium per cup or 2 mg per oz.

Nutrients in Indicated Quantity

Cholesterol	Carbohydrate	Calcium	Phosphorus	Iron	Potassium	Sodium	Vitamin A value (IU)	Vitamin A value (RE)	Thiamin	Riboflavin	Niacin	Ascorbic acid	Item No.
Milligrams	Grams	Milligrams	Milligrams	Milligrams	Milligrams	Milligrams	International units	Retinol equivalents	Milligrams	Milligrams	Milligrams	Milligrams	
0	28	359	702	4.9	988	15	0	0	0.28	1.05	4.5	1	525
0	6	75	147	1.0	208	3	0	0	0.06	0.22	1.0	Tr	526
0	41	47	239	2.9	608	1	Tr	Tr	0.43	0.05	0.9	0	527
0	38	90	266	4.9	749	13	0	0	0.25	0.13	1.3	0	528
0	49	55	293	5.9	1,163	4	0	0	0.25	0.11	1.3	0	529
0	40	95	281	5.1	790	13	0	0	0.27	0.13	1.3	0	530
0	49	86	296	5.4	882	3	Tr	Tr	0.33	0.16	0.7	0	531
30	32	94	303	4.8	668	1,374	330	33	0.18	0.15	3.3	Tr	532
10	48	138	235	4.6	536	1,181	330	33	0.20	0.08	1.5	5	533
10	54	161	291	5.9	536	969	330	33	0.15	0.10	1.3	5	534
0	42	74	278	4.6	673	968	10	1	0.13	0.10	1.5	0	535
0	35	43	238	3.3	573	20	30	3	0.40	0.10	1.0	0	536
0	4	50	170	1.0	170	1	Tr	Tr	0.28	0.03	0.5	Tr	537
0	126	390	102	5.7	1,275	24	Tr	Tr	0.07	0.07	2.2	Tr	538
0	45	62	671	8.2	774	[41]877	0	0	0.27	0.27	1.9	0	539
0	9	13	139	1.7	160	[41]181	0	0	0.06	0.06	0.4	0	540
0	37	53	554	5.3	689	[42]814	0	0	0.55	0.23	2.3	0	541
0	8	12	121	1.2	150	[42]177	0	0	0.12	0.05	0.5	0	542
0	76	41	153	1.3	847	3	30	3	0.35	0.25	1.9	37	543
0	45	80	273	4.9	475	11	Tr	Tr	0.18	0.09	0.9	0	544
0	7	6	51	1.1	160	9	0	0	0.03	0.01	0.2	1	545
0	12	11	90	1.9	285	16	0	0	0.05	0.02	0.4	3	546
0	44	14	99	1.8	313	244	0	0	0.03	0.02	0.4	1	547
0	18	216	359	3.8	512	3	80	8	0.58	0.13	1.3	1	548
0	4	53	88	0.9	126	1	20	2	0.14	0.03	0.3	Tr	549
0	38	50	238	4.2	498	26	40	4	0.14	0.12	1.2	0	550
0	17	60	268	2.4	441	[43]348	10	1	0.29	0.15	2.7	0	551
0	4	13	57	0.5	93	[43]74	Tr	Tr	0.06	0.03	0.6	0	552
0	7	20	123	1.0	169	[44]190	Tr	Tr	0.06	0.06	1.3	0	553
0	6	31	131	0.9	165	[44]185	10	1	0.14	0.06	1.4	Tr	554
0	27	125	734	2.8	1,019	[45]626	0	0	0.42	0.15	21.5	0	555
0	5	24	143	0.5	199	[45]122	0	0	0.08	0.03	4.2	0	556
0	3	5	60	0.3	110	75	0	0	0.02	0.02	2.2	0	557
0	42	22	178	3.4	592	26	80	8	0.30	0.18	1.8	0	558
0	20	39	314	2.3	423	1	140	14	0.92	0.14	1.0	2	559
0	5	10	83	0.6	111	Tr	40	4	0.24	0.04	0.3	1	560
0	5	2	10	0.9	178	20	10	1	0.35	0.06	1.2	1	561
0	7	38	143	1.9	310	2	70	7	0.23	0.05	0.3	Tr	562
0	5	12	333	4.2	229	5	110	11	0.06	0.09	0.5	Tr	563
0	51	141	245	5.1	1,141	1,228	0	0	0.14	0.16	1.4	17	564
0	1	11	62	0.6	33	3	10	1	0.06	0.01	0.4	0	565
0	19	131	322	4.9	972	4	50	5	0.38	0.16	1.1	0	566
0	65	188	853	4.7	922	8,142	110	11	0.17	0.28	0.8	0	567
0	3	108	151	2.3	50	8	0	0	0.07	0.04	0.1	0	568
0	5	33	200	1.9	195	1	10	1	0.65	0.07	1.3	Tr	569
0	3	21	119	0.7	69	5	10	1	0.24	0.02	0.8	1	570

[44]Mixed nuts without salt contain 3 mg sodium per oz.
[45]Peanuts without salt contain 22 mg sodium per cup or 4 mg per oz.

Table 2. Nutritive Value of the Edible Part of Food (Continued)

(Tr indicates nutrient present in trace amount.)

Item No.	Foods, approximate measures, units, and weight (weight of edible portion only)			Water	Food energy	Protein	Fat	Fatty acids: Saturated	Fatty acids: Monounsaturated	Fatty acids: Polyunsaturated
			Grams	Percent	Calories	Grams	Grams	Grams	Grams	Grams
	Legumes, Nuts, and Seeds—Con.									
	Walnuts:									
571	Black, chopped	1 cup	125	4	760	30	71	4.5	15.9	46.9
572		1 oz	28	4	170	7	16	1.0	3.6	10.6
573	English or Persian, pieces or chips	1 cup	120	4	770	17	74	6.7	17.0	47.0
574		1 oz	28	4	180	4	18	1.6	4.0	11.1
	Meat and Meat Products									
	Beef, cooked:[46]									
	Cuts braised, simmered, or pot roasted:									
	Relatively fat such as chuck blade:									
575	Lean and fat, piece, 2-1/2 by 2-1/2 by 3/4 in	3 oz	85	43	325	22	26	10.8	11.7	0.9
576	Lean only from item 575	2.2 oz	62	53	170	19	9	3.9	4.2	0.3
	Relatively lean, such as bottom round:									
577	Lean and fat, piece, 4-1/8 by 2-1/4 by 1/2 in	3 oz	85	54	220	25	13	4.8	5.7	0.5
578	Lean only from item 577	2.8 oz	78	57	175	25	8	2.7	3.4	0.3
	Ground beef, broiled, patty, 3 by 5/8 in:									
579	Lean	3 oz	85	56	230	21	16	6.2	6.9	0.6
580	Regular	3 oz	85	54	245	20	18	6.9	7.7	0.7
581	Heart, lean, braised	3 oz	85	65	150	24	5	1.2	0.8	1.6
582	Liver, fried, slice, 6-1/2 by 2-3/8 by 3/8 in[47]	3 oz	85	56	185	23	7	2.5	3.6	1.3
	Roast, oven cooked, no liquid added:									
	Relatively fat, such as rib:									
583	Lean and fat, 2 pieces, 4-1/8 by 2-1/4 by 1/4 in	3 oz	85	46	315	19	26	10.8	11.4	0.9
584	Lean only from item 583	2.2 oz	61	57	150	17	9	3.6	3.7	0.3
	Relatively lean, such as eye of round:									
585	Lean and fat, 2 pieces, 2-1/2 by 2-1/2 by 3/8 in	3 oz	85	57	205	23	12	4.9	5.4	0.5
586	Lean only from item 585	2.6 oz	75	63	135	22	5	1.9	2.1	0.2
	Steak:									
	Sirloin, broiled:									
587	Lean and fat, piece, 2-1/2 by 2-1/2 by 3/4 in	3 oz	85	53	240	23	15	6.4	6.9	0.6
588	Lean only from item 587	2.5 oz	72	59	150	22	6	2.6	2.8	0.3
589	Beef, canned, corned	3 oz	85	59	185	22	10	4.2	4.9	0.4
590	Beef, dried, chipped	2.5 oz	72	48	145	24	4	1.8	2.0	0.2
	Lamb, cooked:									
	Chops, (3 per lb with bone):									
	Arm, braised:									
591	Lean and fat	2.2 oz	63	44	220	20	15	6.9	6.0	0.9
592	Lean only from item 591	1.7 oz	48	49	135	17	7	2.9	2.6	0.4
	Loin, broiled:									
593	Lean and fat	2.8 oz	80	54	235	22	16	7.3	6.4	1.0
594	Lean only from item 593	2.3 oz	64	61	140	19	6	2.6	2.4	0.4
	Leg, roasted:									
595	Lean and fat, 2 pieces, 4-1/8 by 2-1/4 by 1/4 in	3 oz	85	59	205	22	13	5.6	4.9	0.8
596	Lean only from item 595	2.6 oz	73	64	140	20	6	2.4	2.2	0.4
	Rib, roasted:									
597	Lean and fat, 3 pieces, 2-1/2 by 2-1/2 by 1/4 in	3 oz	85	47	315	18	26	12.1	10.6	1.5
598	Lean only from item 597	2 oz	57	60	130	15	7	3.2	3.0	0.5

[46] Outer layer of fat was removed to within approximately 1/2 inch of the lean. Deposits of fat within the cut were not removed.

[47] Fried in vegetable shortening.

Nutrients in Indicated Quantity

Cholesterol	Carbohydrate	Calcium	Phosphorus	Iron	Potassium	Sodium	Vitamin A value (IU)	Vitamin A value (RE)	Thiamin	Riboflavin	Niacin	Ascorbic acid	Item No.
Milligrams	Grams	Milligrams	Milligrams	Milligrams	Milligrams	Milligrams	International units	Retinol equivalents	Milligrams	Milligrams	Milligrams	Milligrams	
0	15	73	580	3.8	655	1	370	37	0.27	0.14	0.9	Tr	571
0	3	16	132	0.9	149	Tr	80	8	0.06	0.03	0.2	Tr	572
0	22	113	380	2.9	602	12	150	15	0.46	0.18	1.3	4	573
0	5	27	90	0.7	142	3	40	4	0.11	0.04	0.3	1	574
87	0	11	163	2.5	163	53	Tr	Tr	0.06	0.19	2.0	0	575
66	0	8	146	2.3	163	44	Tr	Tr	0.05	0.17	1.7	0	576
81	0	5	217	2.8	248	43	Tr	Tr	0.06	0.21	3.3	0	577
75	0	4	212	2.7	240	40	Tr	Tr	0.06	0.20	3.0	0	578
74	0	9	134	1.8	256	65	Tr	Tr	0.04	0.18	4.4	0	579
76	0	9	144	2.1	248	70	Tr	Tr	0.03	0.16	4.9	0	580
164	0	5	213	6.4	198	54	Tr	Tr	0.12	1.31	3.4	5	581
410	7	9	392	5.3	309	90	[48]30,690	[48]9,120	0.18	3.52	12.3	23	582
72	0	8	145	2.0	246	54	Tr	Tr	0.06	0.16	3.1	0	583
49	0	5	127	1.7	218	45	Tr	Tr	0.05	0.13	2.7	0	584
62	0	5	177	1.6	308	50	Tr	Tr	0.07	0.14	3.0	0	585
52	0	3	170	1.5	297	46	Tr	Tr	0.07	0.13	2.8	0	586
77	0	9	186	2.6	306	53	Tr	Tr	0.10	0.23	3.3	0	587
64	0	8	176	2.4	290	48	Tr	Tr	0.09	0.22	3.1	0	588
80	0	17	90	3.7	51	802	Tr	Tr	0.02	0.20	2.9	0	589
46	0	14	287	2.3	142	3,053	Tr	Tr	0.05	0.23	2.7	0	590
77	0	16	132	1.5	195	46	Tr	Tr	0.04	0.16	4.4	0	591
59	0	12	111	1.3	162	36	Tr	Tr	0.03	0.13	3.0	0	592
78	0	16	162	1.4	272	62	Tr	Tr	0.09	0.21	5.5	0	593
60	0	12	145	1.3	241	54	Tr	Tr	0.08	0.18	4.4	0	594
78	0	8	162	1.7	273	57	Tr	Tr	0.09	0.24	5.5	0	595
65	0	6	150	1.5	247	50	Tr	Tr	0.08	0.20	4.6	0	596
77	0	19	139	1.4	224	60	Tr	Tr	0.08	0.18	5.5	0	597
50	0	12	111	1.0	179	46	Tr	Tr	0.05	0.13	3.5	0	598

[48] Value varies widely.

Table 2. Nutritive Value of the Edible Part of Food (Continued)

(Tr indicates nutrient present in trace amount.)

Item No.	Foods, approximate measures, units, and weight (weight of edible portion only)			Water	Food energy	Protein	Fat	Fatty acids: Saturated	Fatty acids: Monounsaturated	Fatty acids: Polyunsaturated
	Meat and Meat Products—Con.		Grams	Percent	Calories	Grams	Grams	Grams	Grams	Grams
	Pork, cured, cooked:									
	Bacon:									
599	Regular----------------------	3 medium slices	19	13	110	6	9	3.3	4.5	1.1
600	Canadian-style----------------	2 slices--------	46	62	85	11	4	1.3	1.9	0.4
	Ham, light cure, roasted:									
601	Lean and fat, 2 pieces, 4-1/8 by 2-1/4 by 1/4 in---------	3 oz------------	85	58	205	18	14	5.1	6.7	1.5
602	Lean only from item 601------	2.4 oz----------	68	66	105	17	4	1.3	1.7	0.4
603	Ham, canned, roasted, 2 pieces, 4-1/8 by 2-1/4 by 1/4 in-----	3 oz------------	85	67	140	18	7	2.4	3.5	0.8
	Luncheon meat:									
604	Canned, spiced or unspiced, slice, 3 by 2 by 1/2 in----	2 slices--------	42	52	140	5	13	4.5	6.0	1.5
605	Chopped ham (8 slices per 6 oz pkg)--------------------	2 slices--------	42	64	95	7	7	2.4	3.4	0.9
	Cooked ham (8 slices per 8-oz pkg):									
606	Regular------------------	2 slices--------	57	65	105	10	6	1.9	2.8	0.7
607	Extra lean---------------	2 slices--------	57	71	75	11	3	0.9	1.3	0.3
	Pork, fresh, cooked:									
	Chop, loin (cut 3 per lb with bone):									
	Broiled:									
608	Lean and fat---------------	3.1 oz----------	87	50	275	24	19	7.0	8.8	2.2
609	Lean only from item 608----	2.5 oz----------	72	57	165	23	8	2.6	3.4	0.9
	Pan fried:									
610	Lean and fat---------------	3.1 oz----------	89	45	335	21	27	9.8	12.5	3.1
611	Lean only from item 610----	2.4 oz----------	67	54	180	19	11	3.7	4.8	1.3
	Ham (leg), roasted:									
612	Lean and fat, piece, 2-1/2 by 2-1/2 by 3/4 in------------	3 oz------------	85	53	250	21	18	6.4	8.1	2.0
613	Lean only from item 612------	2.5 oz----------	72	60	160	20	8	2.7	3.6	1.0
	Rib, roasted:									
614	Lean and fat, piece, 2-1/2 by 3/4 in---------------------	3 oz------------	85	51	270	21	20	7.2	9.2	2.3
615	Lean only from item 614------	2.5 oz----------	71	57	175	20	10	3.4	4.4	1.2
	Shoulder cut, braised:									
616	Lean and fat, 3 pieces, 2-1/2 by 2-1/2 by 1/4 in---------	3 oz------------	85	47	295	23	22	7.9	10.0	2.4
617	Lean only from item 616------	2.4 oz----------	67	54	165	22	8	2.8	3.7	1.0
	Sausages (See also Luncheon meats, items 604-607):									
618	Bologna, slice (8 per 8-oz pkg)	2 slices--------	57	54	180	7	16	6.1	7.6	1.4
619	Braunschweiger, slice (6 per 6-oz pkg)--------------------	2 slices--------	57	48	205	8	18	6.2	8.5	2.1
620	Brown and serve (10-11 per 8-oz pkg), browned-----------	1 link----------	13	45	50	2	5	1.7	2.2	0.5
621	Frankfurter (10 per 1-lb pkg), cooked (reheated)------------	1 frankfurter---	45	54	145	5	13	4.8	6.2	1.2
622	Pork link (16 per 1-lb pkg), cooked[50] ---------------------	1 link----------	13	45	50	3	4	1.4	1.8	0.5
	Salami:									
623	Cooked type, slice (8 per 8-oz pkg)------------------	2 slices--------	57	60	145	8	11	4.6	5.2	1.2
624	Dry type, slice (12 per 4-oz pkg)----------------------	2 slices--------	20	35	85	5	7	2.4	3.4	0.6
625	Sandwich spread (pork, beef)---	1 tbsp----------	15	60	35	1	3	0.9	1.1	0.4
626	Vienna sausage (7 per 4-oz can)	1 sausage-------	16	60	45	2	4	1.5	2.0	0.3
	Veal, medium fat, cooked, bone removed:									
627	Cutlet, 4-1/8 by 2-1/4 by 1/2 in, braised or broiled-------	3 oz------------	85	60	185	23	9	4.1	4.1	0.6
628	Rib, 2 pieces, 4-1/8 by 2-1/4 by 1/4 in, roasted-----------	3 oz------------	85	55	230	23	14	6.0	6.0	1.0

[49] Contains added sodium ascorbate. If sodium ascorbate is not added, ascorbic acid content is negligible.

Nutrients in Indicated Quantity													
Cholesterol	Carbohydrate	Calcium	Phosphorus	Iron	Potassium	Sodium	Vitamin A value (IU)	Vitamin A value (RE)	Thiamin	Riboflavin	Niacin	Ascorbic acid	Item No.
Milligrams	Grams	Milligrams	Milligrams	Milligrams	Milligrams	Milligrams	International units	Retinol equivalents	Milligrams	Milligrams	Milligrams	Milligrams	
16	Tr	2	64	0.3	92	303	0	0	0.13	0.05	1.4	6	599
27	1	5	136	0.4	179	711	0	0	0.38	0.09	3.2	10	600
53	0	6	182	0.7	243	1,009	0	0	0.51	0.19	3.8	0	601
37	0	5	154	0.6	215	902	0	0	0.46	0.17	3.4	0	602
35	Tr	6	188	0.9	298	908	0	0	0.82	0.21	4.3	[49]19	603
26	1	3	34	0.3	90	541	0	0	0.15	0.08	1.3	Tr	604
21	0	3	65	0.3	134	576	0	0	0.27	0.09	1.6	[49]8	605
32	2	4	141	0.6	189	751	0	0	0.49	0.14	3.0	[49]16	606
27	1	4	124	0.4	200	815	0	0	0.53	0.13	2.8	[49]15	607
84	0	3	184	0.7	312	61	10	3	0.87	0.24	4.3	Tr	608
71	0	4	176	0.7	302	56	10	1	0.83	0.22	4.0	Tr	609
92	0	4	190	0.7	323	64	10	3	0.91	0.24	4.6	Tr	610
72	0	3	178	0.7	305	57	10	1	0.84	0.22	4.0	Tr	611
79	0	5	210	0.9	280	50	10	2	0.54	0.27	3.9	Tr	612
68	0	5	202	0.8	269	46	10	1	0.50	0.25	3.6	Tr	613
69	0	9	190	0.8	313	37	10	3	0.50	0.24	4.2	Tr	614
56	0	8	182	0.7	300	33	10	2	0.45	0.22	3.8	Tr	615
93	0	6	162	1.4	286	75	10	3	0.46	0.26	4.4	Tr	616
76	0	5	151	1.3	271	68	10	1	0.40	0.24	4.0	Tr	617
31	2	7	52	0.9	103	581	0	0	0.10	0.08	1.5	[49]12	618
89	2	5	96	5.3	113	652	8,010	2,405	0.14	0.87	4.8	[49]6	619
9	Tr	1	14	0.1	25	105	0	0	0.05	0.02	0.4	0	620
23	1	5	39	0.5	75	504	0	0	0.09	0.05	1.2	[49]12	621
11	Tr	4	24	0.2	47	168	0	0	0.10	0.03	0.6	Tr	622
37	1	7	66	1.5	113	607	0	0	0.14	0.21	2.0	[49]7	623
16	1	2	28	0.3	76	372	0	0	0.12	0.06	1.0	[49]5	624
6	2	2	9	0.1	17	152	10	1	0.03	0.02	0.3	0	625
8	Tr	2	8	0.1	16	152	0	0	0.01	0.02	0.3	0	626
109	0	9	196	0.8	258	56	Tr	Tr	0.06	0.21	4.6	0	627
109	0	10	211	0.7	259	57	Tr	Tr	0.11	0.26	6.6	0	628

[50] One patty (8 per pound) of bulk sausage is equivalent to 2 links.

Table 2. Nutritive Value of the Edible Part of Food (Continued)
(Tr indicates nutrient present in trace amount.)

Item No.	Foods, approximate measures, units, and weight (weight of edible portion only)			Water	Food energy	Protein	Fat	Fatty acids: Saturated	Fatty acids: Monounsaturated	Fatty acids: Polyunsaturated
	Mixed Dishes and Fast Foods		Grams	Percent	Calories	Grams	Grams	Grams	Grams	Grams
	Mixed dishes:									
629	Beef and vegetable stew, from home recipe	1 cup	245	82	220	16	11	4.4	4.5	0.5
630	Beef potpie, from home recipe, baked, piece, 1/3 of 9-in diam. pie[51]	1 piece	210	55	515	21	30	7.9	12.9	7.4
631	Chicken a la king, cooked, from home recipe	1 cup	245	68	470	27	34	12.9	13.4	6.2
632	Chicken and noodles, cooked, from home recipe	1 cup	240	71	365	22	18	5.1	7.1	3.9
	Chicken chow mein:									
633	Canned	1 cup	250	89	95	7	Tr	0.1	0.1	0.8
634	From home recipe	1 cup	250	78	255	31	10	4.1	4.9	3.5
635	Chicken potpie, from home recipe, baked, piece, 1/3 of 9-in diam. pie[51]	1 piece	232	57	545	23	31	10.3	15.5	6.6
636	Chili con carne with beans, canned	1 cup	255	72	340	19	16	5.8	7.2	1.0
637	Chop suey with beef and pork, from home recipe	1 cup	250	75	300	26	17	4.3	7.4	4.2
	Macaroni (enriched) and cheese:									
638	Canned[52]	1 cup	240	80	230	9	10	4.7	2.9	1.3
639	From home recipe[38]	1 cup	200	58	430	17	22	9.8	7.4	3.6
640	Quiche Lorraine, 1/8 of 8-in diam. quiche[51]	1 slice	176	47	600	13	48	23.[illegible]	17.8	
	Spaghetti (enriched) in tomato sauce with cheese:									
641	Canned	1 cup	250	80	190	6	2	0.[illegible]	0.4	0.5
642	From home recipe	1 cup	250	77	260	9	9	3.0	3.6	1.2
	Spaghetti (enriched) with meatballs and tomato sauce:									
643	Canned	1 cup	250	78	260	12	10	2.4	3.9	3.1
644	From home recipe	1 cup	248	70	330	19	12	3.9	4.4	2.2
	Fast food entrees:									
	Cheeseburger:									
645	Regular	1 sandwich	112	46	300	15	15	7.3	5.6	1.0
646	4 oz patty	1 sandwich	194	46	525	30	31	15.1	12.2	1.4
	Chicken, fried. See Poultry and Poultry Products (items 656-659).									
647	Enchilada	1 enchilada	230	72	235	20	16	7.7	6.7	0.6
648	English muffin, egg, cheese, and bacon	1 sandwich	138	49	360	18	18	8.0	8.0	0.7
	Fish sandwich:									
649	Regular, with cheese	1 sandwich	140	43	420	16	23	6.3	6.9	7.7
650	Large, without cheese	1 sandwich	170	48	470	18	27	6.3	8.7	9.5
	Hamburger:									
651	Regular	1 sandwich	98	46	245	12	11	4.4	5.3	0.5
652	4 oz patty	1 sandwich	174	50	445	25	21	7.1	11.7	0.6
653	Pizza, cheese, 1/8 of 15-in diam. pizza[51]	1 slice	120	46	290	15	9	4.1	2.6	1.3
654	Roast beef sandwich	1 sandwich	150	52	345	22	13	3.5	6.9	1.8
655	Taco	1 taco	81	55	195	9	11	4.1	5.5	0.8

[38] Made with margarine.
[51] Crust made with vegetable shortening and enriched flour.

Nutrients in Indicated Quantity													
Cholesterol	Carbohydrate	Calcium	Phosphorus	Iron	Potassium	Sodium	Vitamin A value (IU)	Vitamin A value (RE)	Thiamin	Riboflavin	Niacin	Ascorbic acid	Item No.
Milligrams	Grams	Milligrams	Milligrams	Milligrams	Milligrams	Milligrams	International units	Retinol equivalents	Milligrams	Milligrams	Milligrams	Milligrams	
71	15	29	184	2.9	613	292	5,690	568	0.15	0.17	4.7	17	629
42	39	29	149	3.8	334	596	4,220	517	0.29	0.29	4.8	6	630
221	12	127	358	2.5	404	760	1,130	272	0.10	0.42	5.4	12	631
103	26	26	247	2.2	149	600	430	130	0.05	0.17	4.3	Tr	632
8	18	45	85	1.3	418	725	150	28	0.05	0.10	1.0	13	633
75	10	58	293	2.5	473	718	280	50	0.08	0.23	4.3	10	634
56	42	70	232	3.0	343	594	7,220	735	0.32	0.32	4.9	5	635
28	31	82	321	4.3	594	1,354	150	15	0.08	0.18	3.3	8	636
68	13	60	248	4.8	425	1,053	600	60	0.28	0.38	5.0	33	637
24	26	199	182	1.0	139	730	260	72	0.12	0.24	1.0	Tr	638
44	40	362	322	1.8	240	1,086	860	232	0.20	0.40	1.8	1	639
285	29	211	276	1.0	283	653	1,640	454	0.11	0.32	Tr	Tr	640
3	39	40	88	2.8	303	955	930	120	0.35	0.28	4.5	10	641
8	37	80	135	2.3	408	955	1,080	140	0.25	0.18	2.3	13	642
23	29	53	113	3.3	245	1,220	1,000	100	0.15	0.18	2.3	5	643
89	39	124	236	3.7	665	1,009	1,590	159	0.25	0.30	4.0	22	644
44	28	135	174	2.3	219	672	340	65	0.26	0.24	3.7	1	645
104	40	236	320	4.5	407	1,224	670	128	0.33	0.48	7.4	3	646
19	24	97	198	3.3	653	1,332	2,720	352	0.18	0.26	Tr	Tr	647
213	31	197	290	3.1	201	832	650	160	0.46	0.50	3.7	1	648
56	39	132	223	1.8	274	667	160	25	0.32	0.26	3.3	2	649
91	41	61	246	2.2	375	621	110	15	0.35	0.23	3.5	1	650
32	28	56	107	2.2	202	463	80	14	0.23	0.24	3.8	1	651
71	38	75	225	4.8	404	763	160	28	0.38	0.38	7.8	1	652
56	39	220	216	1.6	230	699	750	106	0.34	0.29	4.2	2	653
55	34	60	222	4.0	338	757	240	32	0.40	0.33	6.0	2	654
21	15	109	134	1.2	263	456	420	57	0.09	0.07	1.4	1	655

[52]Made with corn oil.

Table 2. Nutritive Value of the Edible Part of Food (Continued)
(Tr indicates nutrient present in trace amount.)

Item No.	Foods, approximate measures, units, and weight (weight of edible portion only)			Water	Food energy	Protein	Fat	Fatty acids: Saturated	Fatty acids: Monounsaturated	Fatty acids: Polyunsaturated
	Poultry and Poultry Products		Grams	Percent	Calories	Grams	Grams	Grams	Grams	Grams
	Chicken:									
	Fried, flesh, with skin:[53]									
	Batter dipped:									
656	Breast, 1/2 breast (5.6 oz with bones)	4.9 oz	140	52	365	35	18	4.9	7.6	4.3
657	Drumstick (3.4 oz with bones)	2.5 oz	72	53	195	16	11	3.0	4.6	2.7
	Flour coated:									
658	Breast, 1/2 breast (4.2 oz with bones)	3.5 oz	98	57	220	31	9	2.4	3.4	1.9
659	Drumstick (2.6 oz with bones)	1.7 oz	49	57	120	13	7	1.8	2.7	1.6
	Roasted, flesh only:									
660	Breast, 1/2 breast (4.2 oz with bones and skin)	3.0 oz	86	65	140	27	3	0.9	1.1	0.7
661	Drumstick, (2.9 oz with bones and skin)	1.6 oz	44	67	75	12	2	0.7	0.8	0.6
662	Stewed, flesh only, light and dark meat, chopped or diced	1 cup	140	67	250	38	9	2.6	3.3	2.2
663	Chicken liver, cooked	1 liver	20	68	30	5	1	0.4	0.3	0.2
664	Duck, roasted, flesh only	1/2 duck	221	64	445	52	25	9.2	8.2	3.2
	Turkey, roasted, flesh only:									
665	Dark meat, piece, 2-1/2 by 1-5/8 by 1/4 in	4 pieces	85	63	160	24	6	2.1	1.4	1.8
666	Light meat, piece, 4 by 2 by 1/4 in	2 pieces	85	66	135	25	3	0.9	0.5	0.7
	Light and dark meat:									
667	Chopped or diced	1 cup	140	65	240	41	7	2.3	1.4	2.0
668	Pieces (1 slice white meat, 4 by 2 by 1/4 in and 2 slices dark meat, 2-1/2 by 1-5/8 by 1/4 in)	3 pieces	85	65	145	25	4	1.4	0.9	1.2
	Poultry food products:									
	Chicken:									
669	Canned, boneless	5 oz	142	69	235	31	11	3.1	4.5	2.5
670	Frankfurter (10 per 1-lb pkg)	1 frankfurter	45	58	115	6	9	2.5	3.8	1.8
671	Roll, light (6 slices per 6 oz pkg)	2 slices	57	69	90	11	4	1.1	1.7	0.9
	Turkey:									
672	Gravy and turkey, frozen	5-oz package	142	85	95	8	4	1.2	1.4	0.7
673	Ham, cured turkey thigh meat (8 slices per 8-oz pkg)	2 slices	57	71	75	11	3	1.0	0.7	0.9
674	Loaf, breast meat (8 slices per 6-oz pkg)	2 slices	42	72	45	10	1	0.2	0.2	0.1
675	Patties, breaded, battered, fried (2.25 oz)	1 patty	64	50	180	9	12	3.0	4.8	3.0
676	Roast, boneless, frozen, seasoned, light and dark meat, cooked	3 oz	85	68	130	18	5	1.6	1.0	1.4
	Soups, Sauces, and Gravies									
	Soups:									
	Canned, condensed:									
	Prepared with equal volume of milk:									
677	Clam chowder, New England	1 cup	248	85	165	9	7	3.0	2.3	1.1
678	Cream of chicken	1 cup	248	85	190	7	11	4.6	4.5	1.6
679	Cream of mushroom	1 cup	248	85	205	6	14	5.1	3.0	4.6
680	Tomato	1 cup	248	85	160	6	6	2.9	1.6	1.1

[53] Fried in vegetable shortening.

Nutrients in Indicated Quantity													
Cho-les-terol	Carbo-hydrate	Calcium	Phos-phorus	Iron	Potas-sium	Sodium	Vitamin A value (IU)	Vitamin A value (RE)	Thiamin	Ribo-flavin	Niacin	Ascorbic acid	Item No.
Milli-grams	Grams	Milli-grams	Milli-grams	Milli-grams	Milli-grams	Milli-grams	Inter-national units	Retinol equiva-lents	Milli-grams	Milli-grams	Milli-grams	Milli-grams	
119	13	28	259	1.8	281	385	90	28	0.16	0.20	14.7	0	656
62	6	12	106	1.0	134	194	60	19	0.08	0.15	3.7	0	657
87	2	16	228	1.2	254	74	50	15	0.08	0.13	13.5	0	658
44	1	6	86	0.7	112	44	40	12	0.04	0.11	3.0	0	659
73	0	13	196	0.9	220	64	20	5	0.06	0.10	11.8	0	660
41	0	5	81	0.6	108	42	30	8	0.03	0.10	2.7	0	661
116	0	20	210	1.6	252	98	70	21	0.07	0.23	8.6	0	662
126	Tr	3	62	1.7	28	10	3,270	983	0.03	0.35	0.9	3	663
197	0	27	449	6.0	557	144	170	51	0.57	1.04	11.3	0	664
72	0	27	173	2.0	246	67	0	0	0.05	0.21	3.1	0	665
59	0	16	186	1.1	259	54	0	0	0.05	0.11	5.8	0	666
106	0	35	298	2.5	417	98	0	0	0.09	0.25	7.6	0	667
65	0	21	181	1.5	253	60	0	0	0.05	0.15	4.6	0	668
88	0	20	158	2.2	196	714	170	48	0.02	0.18	9.0	3	669
45	3	43	48	0.9	38	616	60	17	0.03	0.05	1.4	0	670
28	1	24	89	0.6	129	331	50	14	0.04	0.07	3.0	0	671
26	7	20	115	1.3	87	787	60	18	0.03	0.18	2.6	0	672
32	Tr	6	108	1.6	184	565	0	0	0.03	0.14	2.0	0	673
17	0	3	97	0.2	118	608	0	0	0.02	0.05	3.5	[54]0	674
40	10	9	173	1.4	176	512	20	7	0.06	0.12	1.5	0	675
45	3	4	207	1.4	253	578	0	0	0.04	0.14	5.3	0	676
22	17	186	156	1.5	300	992	160	40	0.07	0.24	1.0	3	677
27	15	181	151	0.7	273	1,047	710	94	0.07	0.26	0.9	1	678
20	15	179	156	0.6	270	1,076	150	37	0.08	0.28	0.9	2	679
17	22	159	149	1.8	449	932	850	109	0.13	0.25	1.5	68	680

[54]If sodium ascorbate is added, product contains 11 mg ascorbic acid.

Table 2. Nutritive Value of the Edible Part of Food (Continued)

(Tr indicates nutrient present in trace amount.)

Item No.	Foods, approximate measures, units, and weight (weight of edible portion only)			Water	Food energy	Protein	Fat	Fatty acids: Saturated	Fatty acids: Monounsaturated	Fatty acids: Polyunsaturated
	Soups, Sauces, and Gravies—Con.		Grams	Percent	Calories	Grams	Grams	Grams	Grams	Grams
	Soups:									
	Canned, condensed:									
	Prepared with equal volume of water:									
681	Bean with bacon	1 cup	253	84	170	8	6	1.5	2.2	1.8
682	Beef broth, bouillon, consomme	1 cup	240	98	15	3	1	0.3	0.2	Tr
683	Beef noodle	1 cup	244	92	85	5	3	1.1	1.2	0.5
684	Chicken noodle	1 cup	241	92	75	4	2	0.7	1.1	0.6
685	Chicken rice	1 cup	241	94	60	4	2	0.5	0.9	0.4
686	Clam chowder, Manhattan	1 cup	244	90	80	4	2	0.4	0.4	1.3
687	Cream of chicken	1 cup	244	91	115	3	7	2.1	3.3	1.5
688	Cream of mushroom	1 cup	244	90	130	2	9	2.4	1.7	4.2
689	Minestrone	1 cup	241	91	80	4	3	0.6	0.7	1.1
690	Pea, green	1 cup	250	83	165	9	3	1.4	1.0	0.4
691	Tomato	1 cup	244	90	85	2	2	0.4	0.4	1.0
692	Vegetable beef	1 cup	244	92	80	6	2	0.9	0.8	0.1
693	Vegetarian	1 cup	241	92	70	2	2	0.3	0.8	0.7
	Dehydrated:									
	Unprepared:									
694	Bouillon	1 pkt	6	3	15	1	1	0.3	0.2	Tr
695	Onion	1 pkt	7	4	20	1	Tr	0.1	0.2	Tr
	Prepared with water:									
696	Chicken noodle	1 pkt (6-fl-oz)	188	94	40	2	1	0.2	0.4	0.3
697	Onion	1 pkt (6-fl-oz)	184	96	20	1	Tr	0.1	0.2	0.1
698	Tomato vegetable	1 pkt (6-fl-oz)	189	94	40	1	1	0.3	0.2	0.1
	Sauces:									
	From dry mix:									
699	Cheese, prepared with milk	1 cup	279	77	305	16	17	9.3	5.3	1.6
700	Hollandaise, prepared with water	1 cup	259	84	240	5	20	11.6	5.9	0.9
701	White sauce, prepared with milk	1 cup	264	81	240	10	13	6.4	4.7	1.7
	From home recipe:									
702	White sauce, medium[55]	1 cup	250	73	395	10	30	9.1	11.9	7.2
	Ready to serve:									
703	Barbecue	1 tbsp	16	81	10	Tr	Tr	Tr	0.1	0.1
704	Soy	1 tbsp	18	68	10	2	0	0.0	0.0	0.0
	Gravies:									
	Canned:									
705	Beef	1 cup	233	87	125	9	5	2.7	2.3	0.2
706	Chicken	1 cup	238	85	190	5	14	3.4	6.1	3.6
707	Mushroom	1 cup	238	89	120	3	6	1.0	2.8	2.4
	From dry mix:									
708	Brown	1 cup	261	91	80	3	2	0.9	0.8	0.1
709	Chicken	1 cup	260	91	85	3	2	0.5	0.9	0.4
	Sugars and Sweets									
	Candy:									
710	Caramels, plain or chocolate	1 oz	28	8	115	1	3	2.2	0.3	0.1
	Chocolate:									
711	Milk, plain	1 oz	28	1	145	2	9	5.4	3.0	0.3
712	Milk, with almonds	1 oz	28	2	150	3	10	4.8	4.1	0.7
713	Milk, with peanuts	1 oz	28	1	155	4	11	4.2	3.5	1.5
714	Milk, with rice cereal	1 oz	28	2	140	2	7	4.4	2.5	0.2
715	Semisweet, small pieces (60 per oz)	1 cup or 6 oz	170	1	860	7	61	36.2	19.9	1.9
716	Sweet (dark)	1 oz	28	1	150	1	10	5.9	3.3	0.3
717	Fondant, uncoated (mints, candy corn, other)	1 oz	28	3	105	Tr	0	0.0	0.0	0.0
718	Fudge, chocolate, plain	1 oz	28	8	115	1	3	2.1	1.0	0.1
719	Gum drops	1 oz	28	12	100	Tr	Tr	Tr	Tr	0.1

[55] Made with enriched flour, margarine, and whole milk.

Nutrients in Indicated Quantity

Cholesterol	Carbohydrate	Calcium	Phosphorus	Iron	Potassium	Sodium	Vitamin A value (IU)	Vitamin A value (RE)	Thiamin	Riboflavin	Niacin	Ascorbic acid	Item No.
Milligrams	Grams	Milligrams	Milligrams	Milligrams	Milligrams	Milligrams	International units	Retinol equivalents	Milligrams	Milligrams	Milligrams	Milligrams	
3	23	81	132	2.0	402	951	890	89	0.09	0.03	0.6	2	681
Tr	Tr	14	31	0.4	130	782	0	0	Tr	0.05	1.9	0	682
5	9	15	46	1.1	100	952	630	63	0.07	0.06	1.1	Tr	683
7	9	17	36	0.8	55	1,106	710	71	0.05	0.06	1.4	Tr	684
7	7	17	22	0.7	101	815	660	66	0.02	0.02	1.1	Tr	685
2	12	34	59	1.9	261	1,808	920	92	0.06	0.05	1.3	3	686
10	9	34	37	0.6	88	986	560	56	0.03	0.06	0.8	Tr	687
2	9	46	49	0.5	100	1,032	0	0	0.05	0.09	0.7	1	688
2	11	34	55	0.9	313	911	2,340	234	0.05	0.04	0.9	1	689
0	27	28	125	2.0	190	988	200	20	0.11	0.07	1.2	2	690
0	17	12	34	1.8	264	871	690	69	0.09	0.05	1.4	66	691
5	10	17	41	1.1	173	956	1,890	189	0.04	0.05	1.0	2	692
0	12	22	34	1.1	210	822	3,010	301	0.05	0.05	0.9	1	693
1	1	4	19	0.1	27	1,019	Tr	Tr	Tr	0.01	0.3	0	694
Tr	4	10	23	0.1	47	627	Tr	Tr	0.02	0.04	0.4	Tr	695
2	6	24	24	0.4	23	957	50	5	0.05	0.04	0.7	Tr	696
0	4	9	22	0.1	48	635	Tr	Tr	0.02	0.04	0.4	Tr	697
0	8	6	23	0.5	78	856	140	14	0.04	0.03	0.6	5	698
53	23	569	438	0.3	552	1,565	390	117	0.15	0.56	0.3	2	699
52	14	124	127	0.9	124	1,564	730	220	0.05	0.18	0.1	Tr	700
34	21	425	256	0.3	444	797	310	92	0.08	0.45	0.5	3	701
32	24	292	238	0.9	381	888	1,190	340	0.15	0.43	0.8	2	702
0	2	3	3	0.1	28	130	140	14	Tr	Tr	0.1	1	703
0	2	3	38	0.5	64	1,029	0	0	0.01	0.02	0.6	0	704
7	11	14	70	1.6	189	1,305	0	0	0.07	0.08	1.5	0	705
5	13	48	69	1.1	259	1,373	880	264	0.04	0.10	1.1	0	706
0	13	17	36	1.6	252	1,357	0	0	0.08	0.15	1.6	0	707
2	14	66	47	0.2	61	1,147	0	0	0.04	0.09	0.9	0	708
3	14	39	47	0.3	62	1,134	0	0	0.05	0.15	0.8	3	709
1	22	42	35	0.4	54	64	Tr	Tr	0.01	0.05	0.1	Tr	710
6	16	50	61	0.4	96	23	30	10	0.02	0.10	0.1	Tr	711
5	15	65	77	0.5	125	23	30	8	0.02	0.12	0.2	Tr	712
5	13	49	83	0.4	138	19	30	8	0.07	0.07	1.4	Tr	713
6	18	48	57	0.2	100	46	30	8	0.01	0.08	0.1	Tr	714
0	97	51	178	5.8	593	24	30	3	0.10	0.14	0.9	Tr	715
0	16	7	41	0.6	86	5	10	1	0.01	0.04	0.1	Tr	716
0	27	2	Tr	0.1	1	57	0	0	Tr	Tr	Tr	0	717
1	21	22	24	0.3	42	54	Tr	Tr	0.01	0.03	0.1	Tr	718
0	25	2	Tr	0.1	1	10	0	0	0.00	Tr	Tr	0	719

Table 2. Nutritive Value of the Edible Part of Food (Continued)

(Tr indicates nutrient present in trace amount.)

Item No.	Foods, approximate measures, units, and weight (weight of edible portion only)			Water	Food energy	Protein	Fat	Fatty acids: Saturated	Fatty acids: Monounsaturated	Fatty acids: Polyunsaturated
	Sugars and Sweets—Con.		Grams	Percent	Calories	Grams	Grams	Grams	Grams	Grams
	Candy:									
720	Hard	1 oz	28	1	110	0	0	0.0	0.0	0.0
721	Jelly beans	1 oz	28	6	105	Tr	Tr	Tr	Tr	0.1
722	Marshmallows	1 oz	28	17	90	1	0	0.0	0.0	0.0
723	Custard, baked	1 cup	265	77	305	14	15	6.8	5.4	0.7
724	Gelatin dessert prepared with gelatin dessert powder and water	1/2 cup	120	84	70	2	0	0.0	0.0	0.0
725	Honey, strained or extracted	1 cup	339	17	1,030	1	0	0.0	0.0	0.0
726		1 tbsp	21	17	65	Tr	0	0.0	0.0	0.0
727	Jams and preserves	1 tbsp	20	29	55	Tr	Tr	0.0	Tr	Tr
728		1 packet	14	29	40	Tr	Tr	0.0	Tr	Tr
729	Jellies	1 tbsp	18	28	50	Tr	Tr	Tr	Tr	Tr
730		1 packet	14	28	40	Tr	Tr	Tr	Tr	Tr
731	Popsicle, 3-fl-oz size	1 popsicle	95	80	70	0	0	0.0	0.0	0.0
	Puddings:									
	Canned:									
732	Chocolate	5-oz can	142	68	205	3	11	9.5	0.5	0.1
733	Tapioca	5-oz can	142	74	160	3	5	4.8	Tr	Tr
734	Vanilla	5-oz can	142	69	220	2	10	9.5	0.2	0.1
	Dry mix, prepared with whole milk:									
	Chocolate:									
735	Instant	1/2 cup	130	71	155	4	4	2.3	1.1	0.2
736	Regular (cooked)	1/2 cup	130	73	150	4	4	2.4	1.1	0.1
737	Rice	1/2 cup	132	73	155	4	4	2.3	1.1	0.1
738	Tapioca	1/2 cup	130	75	145	4	4	2.3	1.1	0.1
	Vanilla:									
739	Instant	1/2 cup	130	73	150	4	4	2.2	1.1	0.2
740	Regular (cooked)	1/2 cup	130	74	145	4	4	2.3	1.0	0.1
	Sugars:									
741	Brown, pressed down	1 cup	220	2	820	0	0	0.0	0.0	0.0
	White:									
742	Granulated	1 cup	200	1	770	0	0	0.0	0.0	0.0
743		1 tbsp	12	1	45	0	0	0.0	0.0	0.0
744		1 packet	6	1	25	0	0	0.0	0.0	0.0
745	Powdered, sifted, spooned into cup	1 cup	100	1	385	0	0	0.0	0.0	0.0
	Syrups:									
	Chocolate-flavored syrup or topping:									
746	Thin type	2 tbsp	38	37	85	1	Tr	0.2	0.1	0.1
747	Fudge type	2 tbsp	38	25	125	2	5	3.1	1.7	0.2
748	Molasses, cane, blackstrap	2 tbsp	40	24	85	0	0	0.0	0.0	0.0
749	Table syrup (corn and maple)	2 tbsp	42	25	122	0	0	0.0	0.0	0.0
	Vegetables and Vegetable Products									
750	Alfalfa seeds, sprouted, raw	1 cup	33	91	10	1	Tr	Tr	Tr	0.1
751	Artichokes, globe or French, cooked, drained	1 artichoke	120	87	55	3	Tr	Tr	Tr	0.1
	Asparagus, green:									
	Cooked, drained:									
	From raw:									
752	Cuts and tips	1 cup	180	92	45	5	1	0.1	Tr	0.2
753	Spears, 1/2-in diam. at base	4 spears	60	92	15	2	Tr	Tr	Tr	0.1
	From frozen:									
754	Cuts and tips	1 cup	180	91	50	5	1	0.2	Tr	0.3
755	Spears, 1/2-in diam. at base	4 spears	60	91	15	2	Tr	0.1	Tr	0.1
756	Canned, spears, 1/2-in diam. at base	4 spears	80	95	10	1	Tr	Tr	Tr	0.1
757	Bamboo shoots, canned, drained	1 cup	131	94	25	2	1	0.1	Tr	0.2

[56] For regular pack; special dietary pack contains 3 mg sodium.

Nutrients in Indicated Quantity

Cholesterol	Carbohydrate	Calcium	Phosphorus	Iron	Potassium	Sodium	Vitamin A value (IU)	Vitamin A value (RE)	Thiamin	Riboflavin	Niacin	Ascorbic acid	Item No.
Milligrams	Grams	Milligrams	Milligrams	Milligrams	Milligrams	Milligrams	International units	Retinol equivalents	Milligrams	Milligrams	Milligrams	Milligrams	
0	28	Tr	2	0.1	1	7	0	0	0.10	0.00	0.0	0	720
0	26	1	1	0.3	11	7	0	0	0.00	Tr	Tr	0	721
0	23	1	2	0.5	2	25	0	0	0.00	Tr	Tr	0	722
278	29	297	310	1.1	387	209	530	146	0.11	0.50	0.3	1	723
0	17	2	23	Tr	Tr	55	0	0	0.00	0.00	0.0	0	724
0	279	17	20	1.7	173	17	0	0	0.02	0.14	1.0	3	725
0	17	1	1	0.1	11	1	0	0	Tr	0.01	0.1	Tr	726
0	14	4	2	0.2	18	2	Tr	Tr	Tr	0.01	Tr	Tr	727
0	10	3	1	0.1	12	2	Tr	Tr	Tr	Tr	Tr	Tr	728
0	13	2	Tr	0.1	16	5	Tr	Tr	Tr	0.01	Tr	1	729
0	10	1	Tr	Tr	13	4	Tr	Tr	Tr	Tr	Tr	1	730
0	18	0	0	Tr	4	11	0	0	0.00	0.00	0.0	0	731
1	30	74	117	1.2	254	285	100	31	0.04	0.17	0.6	Tr	732
Tr	28	119	113	0.3	212	252	Tr	Tr	0.03	0.14	0.4	Tr	733
1	33	79	94	0.2	155	305	Tr	Tr	0.03	0.12	0.6	Tr	734
14	27	130	329	0.3	176	440	130	33	0.04	0.18	0.1	1	735
15	25	146	120	0.2	190	167	140	34	0.05	0.20	0.1	1	736
15	27	133	110	0.5	165	140	140	33	0.10	0.18	0.6	1	737
15	25	131	103	0.1	167	152	140	34	0.04	0.18	0.1	1	738
15	27	129	273	0.1	164	375	140	33	0.04	0.17	0.1	1	739
15	25	132	102	0.1	166	178	140	34	0.04	0.18	0.1	1	740
0	212	187	56	4.8	757	97	0	0	0.02	0.07	0.2	0	741
0	199	3	Tr	0.1	7	5	0	0	0.00	0.00	0.0	0	742
0	12	Tr	Tr	Tr	Tr	Tr	0	0	0.00	0.00	0.0	0	743
0	6	Tr	Tr	Tr	Tr	Tr	0	0	0.00	0.00	0.0	0	744
0	100	1	Tr	Tr	4	2	0	0	0.00	0.00	0.0	0	745
0	22	6	49	0.8	85	36	Tr	Tr	Tr	0.02	0.1	0	746
0	21	38	60	0.5	82	42	40	13	0.02	0.08	0.1	0	747
0	22	274	34	10.1	1,171	38	0	0	0.04	0.08	0.8	0	748
0	32	1	4	Tr	7	19	0	0	0.00	0.00	0.0	0	749
0	1	11	23	0.3	26	2	50	5	0.03	0.04	0.2	3	750
0	12	47	72	1.6	316	79	170	17	0.07	0.06	0.7	9	751
0	8	43	110	1.2	558	7	1,490	149	0.18	0.22	1.9	49	752
0	3	14	37	0.4	186	2	500	50	0.06	0.07	0.6	16	753
0	9	41	99	1.2	392	7	1,470	147	0.12	0.19	1.9	44	754
0	3	14	33	0.4	131	2	490	49	0.04	0.06	0.6	15	755
0	2	11	30	0.5	122	[56]278	380	38	0.04	0.07	0.7	13	756
0	4	10	33	0.4	105	9	10	1	0.03	0.03	0.2	1	757

Table 2. Nutritive Value of the Edible Part of Food (Continued)

(Tr indicates nutrient present in trace amount.)

Item No.	Foods, approximate measures, units, and weight (weight of edible portion only)		Weight	Water	Food energy	Protein	Fat	Fatty acids: Saturated	Fatty acids: Monounsaturated	Fatty acids: Polyunsaturated
	Vegetables and Vegetable Products—Con.		Grams	Percent	Calories	Grams	Grams	Grams	Grams	Grams
	Beans:									
	Lima, immature seeds, frozen, cooked, drained:									
758	Thick-seeded types (Ford-hooks)	1 cup	170	74	170	10	1	0.1	Tr	0.3
759	Thin-seeded types (baby limas)	1 cup	180	72	190	12	1	0.1	Tr	0.3
	Snap:									
	Cooked, drained:									
760	From raw (cut and French style)	1 cup	125	89	45	2	Tr	0.1	Tr	0.2
761	From frozen (cut)	1 cup	135	92	35	2	Tr	Tr	Tr	0.1
762	Canned, drained solids (cut)	1 cup	135	93	25	2	Tr	Tr	Tr	0.1
	Beans, mature. See Beans, dry (items 527-535) and Black-eyed peas, dry (item 536).									
	Bean sprouts (mung):									
763	Raw	1 cup	104	90	30	3	Tr	Tr	Tr	0.1
764	Cooked, drained	1 cup	124	93	25	3	Tr	Tr	Tr	Tr
	Beets:									
	Cooked, drained:									
765	Diced or sliced	1 cup	170	91	55	2	Tr	Tr	Tr	Tr
766	Whole beets, 2-in diam.	2 beets	100	91	30	1	Tr	Tr	Tr	Tr
767	Canned, drained solids, diced or sliced	1 cup	170	91	55	2	Tr	Tr	Tr	0.1
768	Beet greens, leaves and stems, cooked, drained	1 cup	144	89	40	4	Tr	Tr	0.1	0.1
	Black-eyed peas, immature seeds, cooked and drained:									
769	From raw	1 cup	165	72	180	13	1	0.3	0.1	0.6
770	From frozen	1 cup	170	66	225	14	1	0.3	0.1	0.5
	Broccoli:									
771	Raw	1 spear	151	91	40	4	1	0.1	Tr	0.3
	Cooked, drained:									
	From raw:									
772	Spear, medium	1 spear	180	90	50	5	1	0.1	Tr	0.2
773	Spears, cut into 1/2-in pieces	1 cup	155	90	45	5	Tr	0.1	Tr	0.2
	From frozen:									
774	Piece, 4-1/2 to 5 in long	1 piece	30	91	10	1	Tr	Tr	Tr	Tr
775	Chopped	1 cup	185	91	50	6	Tr	Tr	Tr	0.1
	Brussels sprouts, cooked, drained:									
776	From raw, 7-8 sprouts, 1-1/4 to 1-1/2-in diam.	1 cup	155	87	60	4	1	0.2	0.1	0.4
777	From frozen	1 cup	155	87	65	6	1	0.1	Tr	0.3
	Cabbage, common varieties:									
778	Raw, coarsely shredded or sliced	1 cup	70	93	15	1	Tr	Tr	Tr	0.1
779	Cooked, drained	1 cup	150	94	30	1	Tr	Tr	Tr	0.2
	Cabbage, Chinese:									
780	Pak-choi, cooked, drained	1 cup	170	96	20	3	Tr	Tr	Tr	0.1
781	Pe-tsai, raw, 1-in pieces	1 cup	76	94	10	1	Tr	Tr	Tr	0.1
782	Cabbage, red, raw, coarsely shredded or sliced	1 cup	70	92	20	1	Tr	Tr	Tr	0.1
783	Cabbage, savoy, raw, coarsely shredded or sliced	1 cup	70	91	20	1	Tr	Tr	Tr	Tr

[57] For green varieties; yellow varieties contain 101 IU or 10 RE.
[58] For green varieties; yellow varieties contain 151 IU or 15 RE.
[59] For regular pack; special dietary pack contains 3 mg sodium.

Nutrients in Indicated Quantity													
Cholesterol	Carbohydrate	Calcium	Phosphorus	Iron	Potassium	Sodium	Vitamin A value (IU)	Vitamin A value (RE)	Thiamin	Riboflavin	Niacin	Ascorbic acid	Item No.
Milligrams	Grams	Milligrams	Milligrams	Milligrams	Milligrams	Milligrams	International units	Retinol equivalents	Milligrams	Milligrams	Milligrams	Milligrams	
0	32	37	107	2.3	694	90	320	32	0.13	0.10	1.8	22	758
0	35	50	202	3.5	740	52	300	30	0.13	0.10	1.4	10	759
0	10	58	49	1.6	374	4	[57]830	[57]83	0.09	0.12	0.8	12	760
0	8	61	32	1.1	151	18	[58]710	[58]71	0.06	0.10	0.6	11	761
0	6	35	26	1.2	147	[59]339	[60]470	[60]47	0.02	0.08	0.3	6	762
0	6	14	56	0.9	155	6	20	2	0.09	0.13	0.8	14	763
0	5	15	35	0.8	125	12	20	2	0.06	0.13	1.0	14	764
0	11	19	53	1.1	530	83	20	2	0.05	0.02	0.5	9	765
0	7	11	31	0.6	312	49	10	1	0.03	0.01	0.3	6	766
0	12	26	29	3.1	252	[61]466	20	2	0.02	0.07	0.3	7	767
0	8	164	59	2.7	1,309	347	7,340	734	0.17	0.42	0.7	36	768
0	30	46	196	2.4	693	7	1,050	105	0.11	0.18	1.8	3	769
0	40	39	207	3.6	638	9	130	13	0.44	0.11	1.2	4	770
0	8	72	100	1.3	491	41	2,330	233	0.10	0.18	1.0	141	771
0	10	82	86	2.1	293	20	2,540	254	0.15	0.37	1.4	113	772
0	9	71	74	1.8	253	17	2,180	218	0.13	0.32	1.2	97	773
0	2	15	17	0.2	54	7	570	57	0.02	0.02	0.1	12	774
0	10	94	102	1.1	333	44	3,500	350	0.10	0.15	0.8	74	775
0	13	56	87	1.9	491	33	1,110	111	0.17	0.12	0.9	96	776
0	13	37	84	1.1	504	36	910	91	0.16	0.18	0.8	71	777
0	4	33	16	0.4	172	13	90	9	0.04	0.02	0.2	33	778
0	7	50	38	0.6	308	29	130	13	0.09	0.08	0.3	36	779
0	3	158	49	1.8	631	58	4,370	437	0.05	0.11	0.7	44	780
0	2	59	22	0.2	181	7	910	91	0.03	0.04	0.3	21	781
0	4	36	29	0.3	144	8	30	3	0.04	0.02	0.2	40	782
0	4	25	29	0.3	161	20	700	70	0.05	0.02	0.2	22	783

[60] For green varieties; yellow varieties contain 142 IU or 14 RE.
[61] For regular pack; special dietary pack contains 78 mg sodium.

Table 2. Nutritive Value of the Edible Part of Food (Continued)

(Tr indicates nutrient present in trace amount.)

Item No.	Foods, approximate measures, units, and weight (weight of edible portion only)			Water	Food energy	Protein	Fat	Fatty acids: Saturated	Fatty acids: Monounsaturated	Fatty acids: Polyunsaturated
	Vegetables and Vegetable Products—Con.		Grams	Percent	Calories	Grams	Grams	Grams	Grams	Grams
	Carrots:									
	Raw, without crowns and tips, scraped:									
784	Whole, 7-1/2 by 1-1/8 in, or strips, 2-1/2 to 3 in long	1 carrot or 18 strips	72	88	30	1	Tr	Tr	Tr	0.1
785	Grated	1 cup	110	88	45	1	Tr	Tr	Tr	0.1
	Cooked, sliced, drained:									
786	From raw	1 cup	156	87	70	2	Tr	0.1	Tr	0.1
787	From frozen	1 cup	146	90	55	2	Tr	Tr	Tr	0.1
788	Canned, sliced, drained solids	1 cup	146	93	35	1	Tr	0.1	Tr	0.1
	Cauliflower:									
789	Raw, (flowerets)	1 cup	100	92	25	2	Tr	Tr	Tr	0.1
	Cooked, drained:									
790	From raw (flowerets)	1 cup	125	93	30	2	Tr	Tr	Tr	0.1
791	From frozen (flowerets)	1 cup	180	94	35	3	Tr	0.1	Tr	0.2
	Celery, pascal type, raw:									
792	Stalk, large outer, 8 by 1-1/2 in (at root end)	1 stalk	40	95	5	Tr	Tr	Tr	Tr	Tr
793	Pieces, diced	1 cup	120	95	20	1	Tr	Tr	Tr	0.1
	Collards, cooked, drained:									
794	From raw (leaves without stems)	1 cup	190	96	25	2	Tr	0.1	Tr	0.2
795	From frozen (chopped)	1 cup	170	88	60	5	1	0.1	0.1	0.4
	Corn, sweet:									
	Cooked, drained:									
796	From raw, ear 5 by 1-3/4 in	1 ear	77	70	85	3	1	0.2	0.3	0.5
	From frozen:									
797	Ear, trimmed to about 3-1/2 in long	1 ear	63	73	60	2	Tr	0.1	0.1	0.2
798	Kernels	1 cup	165	76	135	5	Tr	Tr	Tr	0.1
	Canned:									
799	Cream style	1 cup	256	79	185	4	1	0.2	0.3	0.5
800	Whole kernel, vacuum pack	1 cup	210	77	165	5	1	0.2	0.3	0.5
	Cowpeas. See Black-eyed peas, immature (items 769,770), mature (item 536).									
801	Cucumber, with peel, slices, 1/8 in thick (large, 2-1/8-in diam.; small, 1-3/4-in diam.)	6 large or 8 small slices	28	96	5	Tr	Tr	Tr	Tr	Tr
802	Dandelion greens, cooked, drained	1 cup	105	90	35	2	1	0.1	Tr	0.3
803	Eggplant, cooked, steamed	1 cup	96	92	25	1	Tr	Tr	Tr	0.1
804	Endive, curly (including escarole), raw, small pieces	1 cup	50	94	10	1	Tr	Tr	Tr	Tr
805	Jerusalem-artichoke, raw, sliced	1 cup	150	78	115	3	Tr	0.0	Tr	Tr
	Kale, cooked, drained:									
806	From raw, chopped	1 cup	130	91	40	2	1	0.1	Tr	0.3
807	From frozen, chopped	1 cup	130	91	40	4	1	0.1	Tr	0.3
808	Kohlrabi, thickened bulb-like stems, cooked, drained, diced	1 cup	165	90	50	3	Tr	Tr	Tr	0.1
	Lettuce, raw:									
	Butterhead, as Boston types:									
809	Head, 5-in diam	1 head	163	96	20	2	Tr	Tr	Tr	0.2
810	Leaves	1 outer or 2 inner leaves	15	96	Tr	Tr	Tr	Tr	Tr	Tr
	Crisphead, as iceberg:									
811	Head, 6-in diam	1 head	539	96	70	5	1	0.1	Tr	0.5
812	Wedge, 1/4 of head	1 wedge	135	96	20	1	Tr	Tr	Tr	0.1
813	Pieces, chopped or shredded	1 cup	55	96	5	1	Tr	Tr	Tr	0.1
814	Looseleaf (bunching varieties including romaine or cos), chopped or shredded pieces	1 cup	56	94	10	1	Tr	Tr	Tr	0.1

[62] For regular pack; special dietary pack contains 61 mg sodium.
[63] For yellow varieties; white varieties contain only a trace of vitamin A.

Nutrients in Indicated Quantity

Cholesterol	Carbohydrate	Calcium	Phosphorus	Iron	Potassium	Sodium	Vitamin A value (IU)	Vitamin A value (RE)	Thiamin	Riboflavin	Niacin	Ascorbic acid	Item No.
Milligrams	Grams	Milligrams	Milligrams	Milligrams	Milligrams	Milligrams	International units	Retinol equivalents	Milligrams	Milligrams	Milligrams	Milligrams	
0	7	19	32	0.4	233	25	20,250	2,025	0.07	0.04	0.7	7	784
0	11	30	48	0.6	355	39	30,940	3,094	0.11	0.06	1.0	10	785
0	16	48	47	1.0	354	103	38,300	3,830	0.05	0.09	0.8	4	786
0	12	41	38	0.7	231	86	25,850	2,585	0.04	0.05	0.6	4	787
0	8	37	35	0.9	261	[62]352	20,110	2,011	0.03	0.04	0.8	4	788
0	5	29	46	0.6	355	15	20	2	0.08	0.06	0.6	72	789
0	6	34	44	0.5	404	8	20	2	0.08	0.07	0.7	69	790
0	7	31	43	0.7	250	32	40	4	0.07	0.10	0.6	56	791
0	1	14	10	0.2	114	35	50	5	0.01	0.01	0.1	3	792
0	4	43	31	0.6	341	106	150	15	0.04	0.04	0.4	8	793
0	5	148	19	0.8	177	36	4,220	422	0.03	0.08	0.4	19	794
0	12	357	46	1.9	427	85	10,170	1,017	0.08	0.20	1.1	45	795
0	19	2	79	0.5	192	13	[63]170	[63]17	0.17	0.06	1.2	5	796
0	14	2	47	0.4	158	3	[63]130	[63]13	0.11	0.04	1.0	3	797
0	34	3	78	0.5	229	8	[63]410	[63]41	0.11	0.12	2.1	4	798
0	46	8	131	1.0	343	[64]730	[63]250	[63]25	0.06	0.14	2.5	12	799
0	41	11	134	0.9	391	[65]571	[63]510	[63]51	0.09	0.15	2.5	17	800
0	1	4	5	0.1	42	1	10	1	0.01	0.01	0.1	1	801
0	7	147	44	1.9	244	46	12,290	1,229	0.14	0.18	0.5	19	802
0	6	6	21	0.3	238	3	60	6	0.07	0.02	0.6	1	803
0	2	26	14	0.4	157	11	1,030	103	0.04	0.04	0.2	3	804
0	26	21	117	5.1	644	6	30	3	0.30	0.09	2.0	6	805
0	7	94	36	1.2	296	30	9,620	962	0.07	0.09	0.7	53	806
0	7	179	36	1.2	417	20	8,260	826	0.06	0.15	0.9	33	807
0	11	41	74	0.7	561	35	60	6	0.07	0.03	0.6	89	808
0	4	52	38	0.5	419	8	1,580	158	0.10	0.10	0.5	13	809
0	Tr	5	3	Tr	39	1	150	15	0.01	0.01	Tr	1	810
0	11	102	108	2.7	852	49	1,780	178	0.25	0.16	1.0	21	811
0	3	26	27	0.7	213	12	450	45	0.06	0.04	0.3	5	812
0	1	10	11	0.3	87	5	180	18	0.03	0.02	0.1	2	813
0	2	38	14	0.8	148	5	1,060	106	0.03	0.04	0.2	10	814

[64]For regular pack; special dietary pack contains 8 mg sodium.
[65]For regular pack; special dietary pack contains 6 mg sodium.

Table 2. Nutritive Value of the Edible Part of Food (Continued)

(Tr indicates nutrient present in trace amount.)

Item No.	Foods, approximate measures, units, and weight (weight of edible portion only)			Water	Food energy	Protein	Fat	Fatty acids: Saturated	Fatty acids: Monounsaturated	Fatty acids: Polyunsaturated
	Vegetables and Vegetable Products—Con.		Grams	Percent	Calories	Grams	Grams	Grams	Grams	Grams
	Mushrooms:									
815	Raw, sliced or chopped	1 cup	70	92	20	1	Tr	Tr	Tr	0.1
816	Cooked, drained	1 cup	156	91	40	3	1	0.1	Tr	0.3
817	Canned, drained solids	1 cup	156	91	35	3	Tr	0.1	Tr	0.2
818	Mustard greens, without stems and midribs, cooked, drained	1 cup	140	94	20	3	Tr	Tr	0.2	0.1
819	Okra pods, 3 by 5/8 in, cooked	8 pods	85	90	25	2	Tr	Tr	Tr	Tr
	Onions:									
	Raw:									
820	Chopped	1 cup	160	91	55	2	Tr	0.1	0.1	0.2
821	Sliced	1 cup	115	91	40	1	Tr	0.1	Tr	0.1
822	Cooked (whole or sliced), drained	1 cup	210	92	60	2	Tr	0.1	Tr	0.1
823	Onions, spring, raw, bulb (3/8-in diam.) and white portion of top	6 onions	30	92	10	1	Tr	Tr	Tr	Tr
824	Onion rings, breaded, par-fried, frozen, prepared	2 rings	20	29	80	1	5	1.7	2.2	1.0
	Parsley:									
825	Raw	10 sprigs	10	88	5	Tr	Tr	Tr	Tr	Tr
826	Freeze-dried	1 tbsp	0.4	2	Tr	Tr	Tr	Tr	Tr	Tr
827	Parsnips, cooked (diced or 2 in lengths), drained	1 cup	156	78	125	2	Tr	0.1	0.2	0.1
828	Peas, edible pod, cooked, drained	1 cup	160	89	65	5	Tr	0.1	Tr	0.2
	Peas, green:									
829	Canned, drained solids	1 cup	170	82	115	8	1	0.1	0.1	0.3
830	Frozen, cooked, drained	1 cup	160	80	125	8	Tr	0.1	Tr	0.2
	Peppers:									
831	Hot chili, raw	1 pepper	45	88	20	1	Tr	Tr	Tr	Tr
	Sweet (about 5 per lb, whole), stem and seeds removed:									
832	Raw	1 pepper	74	93	20	1	Tr	Tr	Tr	0.2
833	Cooked, drained	1 pepper	73	95	15	Tr	Tr	Tr	Tr	0.1
	Potatoes, cooked:									
	Baked (about 2 per lb, raw):									
834	With skin	1 potato	202	71	220	5	Tr	0.1	Tr	0.1
835	Flesh only	1 potato	156	75	145	3	Tr	Tr	Tr	0.1
	Boiled (about 3 per lb, raw):									
836	Peeled after boiling	1 potato	136	77	120	3	Tr	Tr	Tr	0.1
837	Peeled before boiling	1 potato	135	77	115	2	Tr	Tr	Tr	0.1
	French fried, strip, 2 to 3-1/2 in long, frozen:									
838	Oven heated	10 strips	50	53	110	2	4	2.1	1.8	0.3
839	Fried in vegetable oil	10 strips	50	38	160	2	8	2.5	1.6	3.8
	Potato products, prepared:									
	Au gratin:									
840	From dry mix	1 cup	245	79	230	6	10	6.3	2.9	0.3
841	From home recipe	1 cup	245	74	325	12	19	11.6	5.3	0.7
842	Hashed brown, from frozen	1 cup	156	56	340	5	18	7.0	8.0	2.1
	Mashed:									
	From home recipe:									
843	Milk added	1 cup	210	78	160	4	1	0.7	0.3	0.1
844	Milk and margarine added	1 cup	210	76	225	4	9	2.2	3.7	2.5
845	From dehydrated flakes (without milk), water, milk, butter, and salt added	1 cup	210	76	235	4	12	7.2	3.3	0.5
846	Potato salad, made with mayonnaise	1 cup	250	76	360	7	21	3.6	6.2	9.3
	Scalloped:									
847	From dry mix	1 cup	245	79	230	5	11	6.5	3.0	0.5
848	From home recipe	1 cup	245	81	210	7	9	5.5	2.5	0.4

[66] For regular pack; special dietary pack contains 3 mg sodium.
[67] For red peppers; green peppers contain 350 IU or 35 RE.
[68] For green peppers; red peppers contain 4,220 IU or 422 RE.

Nutrients in Indicated Quantity

Cholesterol	Carbohydrate	Calcium	Phosphorus	Iron	Potassium	Sodium	Vitamin A value (IU)	Vitamin A value (RE)	Thiamin	Riboflavin	Niacin	Ascorbic acid	Item No.
Milligrams	Grams	Milligrams	Milligrams	Milligrams	Milligrams	Milligrams	International units	Retinol equivalents	Milligrams	Milligrams	Milligrams	Milligrams	
0	3	4	73	0.9	259	3	0	0	0.07	0.31	2.9	2	815
0	8	9	136	2.7	555	3	0	0	0.11	0.47	7.0	6	816
0	8	17	103	1.2	201	663	0	0	0.13	0.03	2.5	0	817
0	3	104	57	1.0	283	22	4,240	424	0.06	0.09	0.6	35	818
0	6	54	48	0.4	274	4	490	49	0.11	0.05	0.7	14	819
0	12	40	46	0.6	248	3	0	0	0.10	0.02	0.2	13	820
0	8	29	33	0.4	178	2	0	0	0.07	0.01	0.1	10	821
0	13	57	48	0.4	319	17	0	0	0.09	0.02	0.2	12	822
0	2	18	10	0.6	77	1	1,500	150	0.02	0.04	0.1	14	823
0	8	6	16	0.3	26	75	50	5	0.06	0.03	0.7	Tr	824
0	1	13	4	0.6	54	4	520	52	0.01	0.01	0.1	9	825
0	Tr	1	2	0.2	25	2	250	25	Tr	0.01	Tr	1	826
0	30	58	108	0.9	573	16	0	0	0.13	0.08	1.1	20	827
0	11	67	88	3.2	384	6	210	21	0.20	0.12	0.9	77	828
0	21	34	114	1.6	294	[66]372	1,310	131	0.21	0.13	1.2	16	829
0	23	38	144	2.5	269	139	1,070	107	0.45	0.16	2.4	16	830
0	4	8	21	0.5	153	3	[67]4,840	[67]484	0.04	0.04	0.4	109	831
0	4	4	16	0.9	144	2	[68]390	[68]39	0.06	0.04	0.4	[69]95	832
0	3	3	11	0.6	94	1	[70]280	[70]28	0.04	0.03	0.3	[71]81	833
0	51	20	115	2.7	844	16	0	0	0.22	0.07	3.3	26	834
0	34	8	78	0.5	610	8	0	0	0.16	0.03	2.2	20	835
0	27	7	60	0.4	515	5	0	0	0.14	0.03	2.0	18	836
0	27	11	54	0.4	443	7	0	0	0.13	0.03	1.8	10	837
0	17	5	43	0.7	229	16	0	0	0.06	0.02	1.2	5	838
0	20	10	47	0.4	366	108	0	0	0.09	0.01	1.6	5	839
12	31	203	233	0.8	537	1,076	520	76	0.05	0.20	2.3	8	840
56	28	292	277	1.6	970	1,061	650	93	0.16	0.28	2.4	24	841
0	44	23	112	2.4	680	53	0	0	0.17	0.03	3.8	10	842
4	37	55	101	0.6	628	636	40	12	0.18	0.08	2.3	14	843
4	35	55	97	0.5	607	620	360	42	0.18	0.08	2.3	13	844
29	32	103	118	0.5	489	697	380	44	0.23	0.11	1.4	20	845
170	28	48	130	1.6	635	1,323	520	83	0.19	0.15	2.2	25	846
27	31	88	137	0.9	497	835	360	51	0.05	0.14	2.5	8	847
29	26	140	154	1.4	926	821	330	47	0.17	0.23	2.6	26	848

[69]For green peppers; red peppers contain 141 mg ascorbic acid.
[70]For green peppers; red peppers contain 2,740 IU or 274 RE.
[71]For green peppers; red peppers contain 121 mg ascorbic acid.

Table 2. Nutritive Value of the Edible Part of Food (Continued)
(Tr indicates nutrient present in trace amount.)

Item No.	Foods, approximate measures, units, and weight (weight of edible portion only)			Water	Food energy	Protein	Fat	Fatty acids: Saturated	Fatty acids: Monounsaturated	Fatty acids: Polyunsaturated
	Vegetables and Vegetable Products—Con.		Grams	Percent	Calories	Grams	Grams	Grams	Grams	Grams
849	Potato chips	10 chips	20	3	105	1	7	1.8	1.2	3.6
	Pumpkin:									
850	Cooked from raw, mashed	1 cup	245	94	50	2	Tr	0.1	Tr	Tr
851	Canned	1 cup	245	90	85	3	1	0.4	0.1	Tr
852	Radishes, raw, stem ends, rootlets cut off	4 radishes	18	95	5	Tr	Tr	Tr	Tr	Tr
853	Sauerkraut, canned, solids and liquid	1 cup	236	93	45	2	Tr	0.1	Tr	0.1
	Seaweed:									
854	Kelp, raw	1 oz	28	82	10	Tr	Tr	0.1	Tr	Tr
855	Spirulina, dried	1 oz	28	5	80	16	2	0.8	0.2	0.6
	Southern peas. See Black-eyed peas, immature (items 769,770), mature (item 536).									
	Spinach:									
856	Raw, chopped	1 cup	55	92	10	2	Tr	Tr	Tr	0.1
	Cooked, drained:									
857	From raw	1 cup	180	91	40	5	Tr	0.1	Tr	0.2
858	From frozen (leaf)	1 cup	190	90	55	6	Tr	0.1	Tr	0.2
859	Canned, drained solids	1 cup	214	92	50	6	1	0.2	Tr	0.4
860	Spinach souffle	1 cup	136	74	220	11	18	7.1	6.8	3.1
	Squash, cooked:									
861	Summer (all varieties), sliced, drained	1 cup	180	94	35	2	1	0.1	Tr	0.2
862	Winter (all varieties), baked, cubes	1 cup	205	89	80	2	1	0.3	0.1	0.5
	Sunchoke. See Jerusalem-artichoke (item 805).									
	Sweetpotatoes:									
	Cooked (raw, 5 by 2 in; about 2-1/2 per lb):									
863	Baked in skin, peeled	1 potato	114	73	115	2	Tr	Tr	Tr	0.1
864	Boiled, without skin	1 potato	151	73	160	2	Tr	0.1	Tr	0.2
865	Candied, 2-1/2 by 2-in piece	1 piece	105	67	145	1	3	1.4	0.7	0.2
	Canned:									
866	Solid pack (mashed)	1 cup	255	74	260	5	1	0.1	Tr	0.2
867	Vacuum pack, piece 2-3/4 by 1 in	1 piece	40	76	35	1	Tr	Tr	Tr	Tr
	Tomatoes:									
868	Raw, 2-3/5-in diam. (3 per 12 oz pkg.)	1 tomato	123	94	25	1	Tr	Tr	Tr	0.1
869	Canned, solids and liquid	1 cup	240	94	50	2	1	0.1	0.1	0.2
870	Tomato juice, canned	1 cup	244	94	40	2	Tr	Tr	Tr	0.1
	Tomato products, canned:									
871	Paste	1 cup	262	74	220	10	2	0.3	0.4	0.9
872	Puree	1 cup	250	87	105	4	Tr	Tr	Tr	0.1
873	Sauce	1 cup	245	89	75	3	Tr	0.1	0.1	0.2
874	Turnips, cooked, diced	1 cup	156	94	30	1	Tr	Tr	Tr	0.1
	Turnip greens, cooked, drained:									
875	From raw (leaves and stems)	1 cup	144	93	30	2	Tr	0.1	Tr	0.1
876	From frozen (chopped)	1 cup	164	90	50	5	1	0.2	Tr	0.3
877	Vegetable juice cocktail, canned	1 cup	242	94	45	2	Tr	Tr	Tr	0.1
	Vegetables, mixed:									
878	Canned, drained solids	1 cup	163	87	75	4	Tr	0.1	Tr	0.2
879	Frozen, cooked, drained	1 cup	182	83	105	5	Tr	0.1	Tr	0.1
880	Waterchestnuts, canned	1 cup	140	86	70	1	Tr	Tr	Tr	Tr

[1] Value not determined.
[72] With added salt; if none is added, sodium content is 58 mg.
[73] For regular pack; special dietary pack contains 31 mg sodium.
[74] With added salt; if none is added, sodium content is 24 mg.

Nutrients in Indicated Quantity

Cholesterol	Carbohydrate	Calcium	Phosphorus	Iron	Potassium	Sodium	Vitamin A value (IU)	Vitamin A value (RE)	Thiamin	Riboflavin	Niacin	Ascorbic acid	Item No.
Milligrams	Grams	Milligrams	Milligrams	Milligrams	Milligrams	Milligrams	International units	Retinol equivalents	Milligrams	Milligrams	Milligrams	Milligrams	
0	10	5	31	0.2	260	94	0	0	0.03	Tr	0.8	8	849
0	12	37	74	1.4	564	2	2,650	265	0.08	0.19	1.0	12	850
0	20	64	86	3.4	505	12	54,040	5,404	0.06	0.13	0.9	10	851
0	1	4	3	0.1	42	4	Tr	Tr	Tr	0.01	0.1	4	852
0	10	71	47	3.5	401	1,560	40	4	0.05	0.05	0.3	35	853
0	3	48	12	0.8	25	66	30	3	0.01	0.04	0.1	([1])	854
0	7	34	33	8.1	386	297	160	16	0.67	1.04	3.6	3	855
0	2	54	27	1.5	307	43	3,690	369	0.04	0.10	0.4	15	856
0	7	245	101	6.4	839	126	14,740	1,474	0.17	0.42	0.9	18	857
0	10	277	91	2.9	566	163	14,790	1,479	0.11	0.32	0.8	23	858
0	7	272	94	4.9	740	[72]683	18,780	1,878	0.03	0.30	0.8	31	859
184	3	230	231	1.3	201	763	3,460	675	0.09	0.30	0.5	3	860
0	8	49	70	0.6	346	2	520	52	0.08	0.07	0.9	10	861
0	18	29	41	0.7	896	2	7,290	729	0.17	0.05	1.4	20	862
0	28	32	63	0.5	397	11	24,880	2,488	0.08	0.14	0.7	28	863
0	37	32	41	0.8	278	20	25,750	2,575	0.08	0.21	1.0	26	864
8	29	27	27	1.2	198	74	4,400	440	0.02	0.04	0.4	7	865
0	59	77	133	3.4	536	191	38,570	3,857	0.07	0.23	2.4	13	866
0	8	9	20	0.4	125	21	3,190	319	0.01	0.02	0.3	11	867
0	5	9	28	0.6	255	10	1,390	139	0.07	0.06	0.7	22	868
0	10	62	46	1.5	530	[73]391	1,450	145	0.11	0.07	1.8	36	869
0	10	22	46	1.4	537	[74]881	1,360	136	0.11	0.08	1.6	45	870
0	49	92	207	7.8	2,442	[75]170	6,470	647	0.41	0.50	8.4	111	871
0	25	38	100	2.3	1,050	[76]50	3,400	340	0.18	0.14	4.3	88	872
0	18	34	78	1.9	909	[77]1,482	2,400	240	0.16	0.14	2.8	32	873
0	8	34	30	0.3	211	78	0	0	0.04	0.04	0.5	18	874
0	6	197	42	1.2	292	42	7,920	792	0.06	0.10	0.6	39	875
0	8	249	56	3.2	367	25	13,080	1,308	0.09	0.12	0.8	36	876
0	11	27	41	1.0	467	883	2,830	283	0.10	0.07	1.8	67	877
0	15	44	68	1.7	474	243	18,990	1,899	0.08	0.08	0.9	8	878
0	24	46	93	1.5	308	64	7,780	778	0.13	0.22	1.5	6	879
0	17	6	27	1.2	165	11	10	1	0.02	0.03	0.5	2	880

[75] With no added salt; if salt is added, sodium content is 2,070 mg.
[76] With no added salt; if salt is added, sodium content is 998 mg.
[77] With salt added.

Table 2. Nutritive Value of the Edible Part of Food (Continued)

(Tr indicates nutrient present in trace amount.)

Item No.	Foods, approximate measures, units, and weight (weight of edible portion only)			Water	Food energy	Protein	Fat	Fatty acids: Saturated	Fatty acids: Monounsaturated	Fatty acids: Polyunsaturated
	Miscellaneous Items		Grams	Percent	Calories	Grams	Grams	Grams	Grams	Grams
	Baking powders for home use:									
	Sodium aluminum sulfate:									
881	With monocalcium phosphate monohydrate	1 tsp	3	2	5	Tr	0	0.0	0.0	0.0
882	With monocalcium phosphate monohydrate, calcium sulfate	1 tsp	2.9	1	5	Tr	0	0.0	0.0	0.0
883	Straight phosphate	1 tsp	3.8	2	5	Tr	0	0.0	0.0	0.0
884	Low sodium	1 tsp	4.3	1	5	Tr	0	0.0	0.0	0.0
885	Catsup	1 cup	273	69	290	5	1	0.2	0.2	0.4
886		1 tbsp	15	69	15	Tr	Tr	Tr	Tr	Tr
887	Celery seed	1 tsp	2	6	10	Tr	1	Tr	0.3	0.1
888	Chili powder	1 tsp	2.6	8	10	Tr	Tr	0.1	0.1	0.2
	Chocolate:									
889	Bitter or baking	1 oz	28	2	145	3	15	9.0	4.9	0.5
	Semisweet, see Candy, (item 715).									
890	Cinnamon	1 tsp	2.3	10	5	Tr	Tr	Tr	Tr	Tr
891	Curry powder	1 tsp	2	10	5	Tr	Tr	([1])	([1])	([1])
892	Garlic powder	1 tsp	2.8	6	10	Tr	Tr	Tr	Tr	Tr
893	Gelatin, dry	1 envelope	7	13	25	6	Tr	Tr	Tr	Tr
894	Mustard, prepared, yellow	1 tsp or individual packet	5	80	5	Tr	Tr	Tr	0.2	Tr
	Olives, canned:									
895	Green	4 medium or 3 extra large	13	78	15	Tr	2	0.2	1.2	0.1
896	Ripe, Mission, pitted	3 small or 2 large	9	73	15	Tr	2	0.3	1.3	0.2
897	Onion powder	1 tsp	2.1	5	5	Tr	Tr	Tr	Tr	Tr
898	Oregano	1 tsp	1.5	7	5	Tr	Tr	Tr	Tr	0.1
899	Paprika	1 tsp	2.1	10	5	Tr	Tr	Tr	Tr	0.2
900	Pepper, black	1 tsp	2.1	11	5	Tr	Tr	Tr	Tr	Tr
	Pickles, cucumber:									
901	Dill, medium, whole, 3-3/4 in long, 1-1/4-in diam.	1 pickle	65	93	5	Tr	Tr	Tr	Tr	0.1
902	Fresh-pack, slices 1-1/2-in diam., 1/4 in thick	2 slices	15	79	10	Tr	Tr	Tr	Tr	Tr
903	Sweet, gherkin, small, whole, about 2-1/2 in long, 3/4-in diam.	1 pickle	15	61	20	Tr	Tr	Tr	Tr	Tr
	Popcorn. See Grain Products, (items 497-499).									
904	Relish, finely chopped, sweet	1 tbsp	15	63	20	Tr	Tr	Tr	Tr	Tr
905	Salt	1 tsp	5.5	0	0	0	0	0.0	0.0	0.0
906	Vinegar, cider	1 tbsp	15	94	Tr	Tr	0	0.0	0.0	0.0
	Yeast:									
907	Baker's, dry, active	1 pkg	7	5	20	3	Tr	Tr	0.1	Tr
908	Brewer's, dry	1 tbsp	8	5	25	3	Tr	Tr	Tr	0.0

[1]Value not determined.

Nutrients in Indicated Quantity													
Cholesterol	Carbohydrate	Calcium	Phosphorus	Iron	Potassium	Sodium	Vitamin A value (IU)	Vitamin A value (RE)	Thiamin	Riboflavin	Niacin	Ascorbic acid	Item No.
Milligrams	Grams	Milligrams	Milligrams	Milligrams	Milligrams	Milligrams	International units	Retinol equivalents	Milligrams	Milligrams	Milligrams	Milligrams	
0	1	58	87	0.0	5	329	0	0	0.00	0.00	0.0	0	881
0	1	183	45	0.0	4	290	0	0	0.00	0.00	0.0	0	882
0	1	239	359	0.0	6	312	0	0	0.00	0.00	0.0	0	883
0	1	207	314	0.0	891	Tr	0	0	0.00	0.00	0.0	0	884
0	69	60	137	2.2	991	2,845	3,820	382	0.25	0.19	4.4	41	885
0	4	3	8	0.1	54	156	210	21	0.01	0.01	0.2	2	886
0	1	35	11	0.9	28	3	Tr	Tr	0.01	0.01	0.1	Tr	887
0	1	7	8	0.4	50	26	910	91	0.01	0.02	0.2	2	888
0	8	22	109	1.9	235	1	10	1	0.01	0.07	0.4	0	889
0	2	28	1	0.9	12	1	10	1	Tr	Tr	Tr	1	890
0	1	10	7	0.6	31	1	20	2	0.01	0.01	0.1	Tr	891
0	2	2	12	0.1	31	1	0	0	0.01	Tr	Tr	Tr	892
0	0	1	0	0.0	2	6	0	0	0.00	0.00	0.0	0	893
0	Tr	4	4	0.1	7	63	0	0	Tr	0.01	Tr	Tr	894
0	Tr	8	2	0.2	7	312	40	4	Tr	Tr	Tr	0	895
0	Tr	10	2	0.2	2	68	10	1	Tr	Tr	Tr	0	896
0	2	8	7	0.1	20	1	Tr	Tr	0.01	Tr	Tr	Tr	897
0	1	24	3	0.7	25	Tr	100	10	0.01	Tr	0.1	1	898
0	1	4	7	0.5	49	1	1,270	127	0.01	0.04	0.3	1	899
0	1	9	4	0.6	26	1	Tr	Tr	Tr	0.01	Tr	0	900
0	1	17	14	0.7	130	928	70	7	Tr	0.01	Tr	4	901
0	3	5	4	0.3	30	101	20	2	Tr	Tr	Tr	1	902
0	5	2	2	0.2	30	107	10	1	Tr	Tr	Tr	1	903
0	5	3	2	0.1	30	107	20	2	Tr	Tr	0.0	1	904
0	0	14	3	Tr	Tr	2,132	0	0	0.00	0.00	0.0	0	905
0	1	1	1	0.1	15	Tr	0	0	0.00	0.00	0.0	0	906
0	3	3	90	1.1	140	4	Tr	Tr	0.16	0.38	2.6	Tr	907
0	3	[78]17	140	1.4	152	10	Tr	Tr	1.25	0.34	3.0	Tr	908

[78]Value may vary from 6 to 60 mg.

Table 3.—Yield of Cooked Meat per Pound of Raw Meat as Purchased

Retail cut and method of cooking	Yield after cooking (less drippings): Parts weighed	Weight
		Ounces
Chops or steaks for broiling or frying:		
With bone and relatively large amount of fat, such as pork or lamb chops; beef rib, sirloin, or porterhouse steaks.	Lean, bone, and fat	10-12
	Lean and fat	7-10
	Lean only	5-7
Without bone and with very little fat, such as round of beef, veal steaks.	Lean and fat	12-13
	Lean only	9-12
Ground meat for broiling or frying, such as beef, lamb, or pork patties.	Patties	9-13
Roast for oven cooking (no liquid added):		
With bone and relatively large amount of fat, such as beef rib, loin, chuck; lamb shoulder, leg; pork, fresh or cured.	Lean, bone, and fat	10-12
	Lean and fat	8-10
	Lean only	6-9
Without bone.	Lean and fat	10-12
	Lean only	7-10
Cuts for pot roasting, simmering, braising, stewing:		
With bone and relatively large amount of fat, such as beef chuck, pork shoulder.	Lean, bone, and fat	10-11
	Lean and fat	8-9
	Lean only	6-8
Without bone and with relatively small amount of fat, such as trimmed beef, veal.	Lean with adhering fat	9-11

Table 4.—Recommended Daily Dietary Allowances (RDA)[1]

(Designed for the maintenance of good nutrition of practically all healthy persons in the United States.)

Sex-age category	Age (Persons)		Weight (Persons)		Height (Persons)		Food energy	Protein	Minerals: Calcium	Minerals: Phosphorus	Minerals: Iron	Vitamin A		Thiamin	Riboflavin	Niacin	Ascorbic acid
	Years From	*To*	*Kilograms*	*Pounds*	*Centimeters*	*Inches*	*Calories*	*Grams*	*Milligrams*	*Milligrams*	*Milligrams*	*Retinol equivalents*[2]	*International units*[3]	*Milligrams*	*Milligrams*	*Milligrams*	*Milligrams*
Infants	0	0.5	6	13	60	24	kg × 115 lb × 52.3	kg × 2.2 lb × 1.0	360	240	10	420	1,400	0.3	0.4	6	35
	0.5	1	9	20	71	28	kg × 105 lb × 47.7	kg × 2.0 lb × 0.9	540	360	15	400	2,000	.5	6	8	35
Children	1	3	13	29	90	35	1,300	23	800	800	15	400	2,000	.7	.8	9	45
	4	6	20	44	112	44	1,700	30	800	800	10	500	2,500	.9	1.0	11	45
	7	10	28	62	132	52	2,400	34	800	800	10	700	3,300	1.2	1.4	16	45
Males	11	14	45	99	157	62	2,700	45	1,200	1,200	18	1,000	5,000	1.4	1.6	18	50
	15	18	66	145	176	69	2,800	56	1,200	1,200	18	1,000	5,000	1.4	1.7	18	60
	19	22	70	154	177	70	2,900	56	800	800	10	1,000	5,000	1.5	1.7	19	60
	23	50	70	154	178	70	2,700	56	800	800	10	1,000	5,000	1.4	1.6	18	60
	51+		70	154	178	70	2,400	56	800	800	10	1,000	5,000	1.2	1.4	16	60
Females	11	14	46	101	157	62	2,200	46	1,200	1,200	18	800	4,000	1.1	1.3	15	50
	15	18	55	120	163	64	2,100	46	1,200	1,200	18	800	4,000	1.1	1.3	14	60
	19	22	55	120	163	64	2,100	44	800	800	18	800	4,000	1.1	1.3	14	60
	23	50	55	120	163	64	2,000	44	800	800	18	800	4,000	1.0	1.2	13	60
	51+		55	120	163	64	[4]1,800	44	800	800	10	800	4,000	1.0	1.2	13	60
Pregnant							+300	+30	+400	+400	[5]18+	+200	+1,000	+.4	+.3	+2	+20
Lactating							+500	+20	+400	+400	18	+400	+2,000	+.5	+.5	+5	+40

1. Source: Adapted from Recommended Dietary Allowances, 9th ed., 1980, 185 pp. Washington DC: National Academy of Sciences, National Research Council. Also available in libraries. This publication tabulates the RDA for selected nutrients, discusses the basis for all RDA, and reviews current knowledge of the dietary needs for other nutrients.

2. 1 retinol equivalent = 1 μg retinol or 6 μg beta-carotene.

3. 1 international unit = 0.3 μg retinol or 0.6 μg beta-carotene.

4. After age 75 years, energy requirement is 2,050 calories for males and 1,600 calories for females.

5. The increased requirement cannot be met by ordinary diets; therefore the use of supplemental iron is recommended.

NOTE—The Recommended Daily Dietary Allowances (RDA) should not be confused with the U.S. Recommended Daily Allowances (U.S. RDA). The RDA are amounts of nutrients recommended by the Food and Nutrition Board of the National Research Council and are considered adequate for maintenance of good nutrition in healthy persons in the United States. The allowances are revised from time to time in accordance with newer knowledge of nutritional needs.

The U.S. RDA are the amounts of protein, vitamins, and minerals established by the Food and Drug Administration as standards for nutrition labeling. These allowances were derived from the RDA set by the Food and Nutrition Board. The U.S. RDA for most nutrients approximates the highest RDA of the sex-age categories in this table, excluding the allowances for pregnant and lactating females. Therefore, a diet that furnishes the U.S. RDA for a nutrient will furnish the RDA for most people and more than the RDA for many. U.S. RDA are protein, 45 grams (eggs, fish, meat, milk, poultry), 65 grams (other foods); vitamin A, 5,000 International Units; thiamin, 1.5 milligrams; riboflavin, 1.7 milligrams; niacin, 20 milligrams; ascorbic acid, 60 milligrams; calcium, 1 gram; phosphorus, 1 gram; iron, 18 milligrams. For additional information on U.S. RDA, see the "Federal Register," vol. 38, no. 49 (March 14, 1973), pp. 6959-6960, and Agriculture Information Bulletin 382, "Nutrition Labeling—Tools for Its Use."

Table 5—Food Sources of Additional Nutrients

Vitamins

Vitamin B_6	Vitamin B_{12} (present in foods of animal origin only)	Vitamin D
Bananas	Cheese	Egg yolk
Fish (most)	Fish	Liver
Liver and kidney	Liver and kidney	Saltwater fish
Meat	Meat	Vitamin D milk
Poultry	Milk	
Potatoes and sweetpotatoes	Shellfish	
Whole-grain cereals	Whole egg and egg yolk	
Yeast		

Vitamin E	Folacin
Margarine	Dark-green vegetables
Nuts	Dry beans and peas
Peanuts and peanut butter	Liver
Vegetable oils	Wheat germ
Whole-grain cereals	Yeast

Minerals

Iodine	Magnesium	Zinc
Iodized salt	Bananas	Cocoa
Seafood	Cocoa	Dry beans and peas
	Dark-green vegetables (most)	Meat
	Dry beans and peas	Poultry
	Milk	Shellfish
	Nuts	Whole-grain cereals
	Whole-grain cereals	

Table 6—Amount of Fat That Provides 30 and 35 Percent of Calories at Specified Calorie Levels

Calories per day in diet	Amount of fat that provides— 30% of calories	35% of calories
	Grams	*Grams*
1,500	50	58
2,000	67	78
2,500	83	97
3,000	100	117

GLOSSARY

A

Achilles tendinitis: an inflammation of the Achilles tendon.

acute injury: a single event injury.

acute stress: life event which requires immediate response to a threat; Type I stress.

adenosine triphosphate (ATP): the sole immediate source of energy for muscular contraction.

adherence: maintaining a program; i.e., staying with an exercise program and not "dropping out."

adrenal glands: a small, triangular shaped pair of glands located on top of the kidneys that secrete hormones including adrenaline (epinephrine) directly into the bloodstream.

aerobic exercise: a form of exercise that increases respiration, intake of oxygen, heart rate, and cardiovascular fitness.

aerobic training: conditioning that involves repeated prolonged exercise bouts in which a large amount of aerobic energy is used (also called endurance training).

aerobics: prolonged exercise in which the muscles rely heavily on oxidative (aerobic) metabolism for energy.

alarm phase: stage of General Adaptation Syndrome characterized by increased arousal.

aldosterone: a hormone secreted by the adrenal gland (cortex) and is associated with chronic stress and the elevation of blood pressure.

amenorrhea: complete cessation of menstrual cycle for 90 days or more.

amino acids: the building blocks that compose protein.

anaerobics: high intensity activity in which the muscles must rely on the production of energy without adequate oxygen.

angina pectoris: pain in the chest.

anorexia nervosa: an eating disorder characterized by low caloric intake and reverse weight loss.

anterior knee pain: also known as chondromalacia patella.

anxiety: an emotional state characterized by uneasiness, apprehension, or fear.

atherosclerosis: a form of hardening of the arteries in which a substance known as plaque gradually accumulates on artery walls, causing the blood vessels to lose elasticity and the arterial openings to narrow.

atherosclerotic plaque: a buildup of fat, smooth muscle, and cell components which can constrict the size of an arterial vessel and reduce blood flow.

athletic amenorrhea: cessation of the menstrual cycle associated with heavy sustained exercise training.

autogenic training: self generated relaxation training associated with interal feelings of heaviness, warmth, etc.

autonomic nervous system: a portion of the peripheral nervous system associated with neural control of body organ function. Consists of the sympathetic and parasympathetic systems.

B

B-cells: specialized lymphocytes which are the site of antibody production.

ballistic stretching: exercises characterized by bouncing movements.

belief systems: opinions people use to guide behavior. Beliefs may be correct or incorrect. Their use in guiding behavior is the important aspect.

bioelectric impedance: method of measuring body composition through the ability of the fat-free mass to conduct a small electrical current.

biofeedback training: relaxation training characterized by equipment display of physiological function to the person.

blister: a collection of fluid under the outer layer of the skin produced by repeated friction or pressure against the skin.

blood glucose: carbohydrate found in blood derived from liver glycogen or digested meal.

body composition: the major components that make up the body's weight - fat-free mass (FFM) and the fat mass (FM).

breathholding: not allowing air to be exchanged during exercise; a dangerous practice when straining against a load.

bulimia: an eating disorder characterized by excessive eating followed by vomiting or laxative use.

bursitis: an inflammation of the bursa sac.

C

caffeine: a naturally occurring stimulant found in coffee and tea; often added to soft drinks and over-the-counter medicines.

calcific bursitis: calcium deposits from an overused tendon producing an inflammation of the bursa sac.

calcium: a silvery, metallic element that is the most abundant mineral in the body; an adequate supply of the calcium is essential for the growth and maintenance of the skeletal system and to a broad range of bodily functions; the main dietary sources of calcium are dairy products, eggs, green vegetables, fruit, and fish.

calcium carbonate: a source of calcium obtained from oyster shell which contains 40% calcium and 60% carbonate.

carbohydrates (CHO): the foods that provide the primary fuel for the body. Carbohydrate stores in the body include muscle and liver glycogen and blood glucose.

carbon monoxide (CO): A colorless, odorless, and highly toxic gas formed as a byproduct during the incomplete combustion of fossil fuels; it is also found in coal gas, the exhaust of internal combustion engines, and cigarette smoke.

cardiac output: the amount of blood pumped by the heart each minute (heart rate x stroke volume).

cardiovascular disease: any of several diseases of the heart and its blood vessels.

cardiovascular fitness: status of the heart, lungs, and blood vessels usually assessed in terms of maximal oxygen consumption or lactate threshold.

catecholamines: hormones adrenalin and noradrenalin released from the adrenal medulla and noradrenalin released from sympathetic nerves as part of the "fight or flight" response of the sympathetic nervous system.

cerebrovascular disease: injury to the brain through a thrombosis or clot in a blood vessel of the brain; also called a stroke.

cholesterol: a fat-like substance found in animal foods and also manufactured by the body. Cholesterol is essential to nerve and brain cell function and to the synthesis of sex hormones and is also a component of bile acids used to aid fat digestion. It is also a part of atherosclerotic plaques that accumulate on artery walls (see "Coronary artery disease").

chondromalacia patella: a grinding sound and pain when the knee is bent caused by a wearing away of the underlying bone, also known as anterior pain.

chronic injury: also known as overuse injury.

chronic stress: in which the body responds over a long period of time because immediate resolution is not possible.

circuit resistance training (CRT): a method of weight lifting characterized by lighter weights (~60% 1 RM), greater repetitions (~12-15), and shorter rest periods (15-30 sec) than strength resistance training.

cirrhosis (of the liver): a disease that causes scarring and decreased functioning of the liver. It can be caused by chronic liver inflammation, hepatitis B, or chronic alcoholism.

climacteric: the gradual changes from reproductive to nonreproductive years in women.

cognitive dissonance: mental state of confusion when beliefs are not matched in reality or when expectancies are not matched by results. May decrease exercise motivation.

commitment: a strong sense of involvement in personal events.

compartment syndrome: swollen muscles cutting off the blood supply, also called shin splints.

complete proteins: proteins that contain all the essential amino acids required by the body.

complex carbohydrates: foods rich in starches such as pasta, breads, rice, and potatoes.

concentric contraction: dynamic movement in which muscular tension is greater than external resistance and the muscle shortens.

constant resistance: load which does not change throughout the range of motion; also known as isotonic resistance.

contractility: the state of the muscle's ability to contract, i.e., a change in tension for a given period of time.

cool-down: a period following an exercise session in which the intensity of the exercise is gradually decreased allowing muscle temperature and blood flow to gradually be reduced.

coronary artery disease: disease of the blood vessels near the heart in which the arteries become narrowed and clogged with raised patches known as atherosclerotic plaque. Atherosclerotic plaque consists of decaying muscle cells, fibrous tissue, clumps of blood platelets, cholesterol, lipoproteins, and sometimes calcium.

cortical bone: more solid, outer layer of bone.

cortisol: a hormone secreted by the adrenal gland (cortex) associated with the metabolic effects of chronic stress.

creatine phosphate (CP): an indirect energy source which can quickly replenish ATP.

creeping obesity: the slow, almost unnoticed process.

cues: stimuli to behave a certain way.

D

decibels: a measure of the loudness or intensity of sound.

dehydration: reduction of tissue fluids to levels which may affect exercise performance.

density: ratio of the mass of a body to its volume.

determinents of health: elements which dictate the wellness status of an individual.

detraining: loss of conditioning due to a cessation of exercise training.

diet: the sum total of the foods eaten.

dimensions of health: the many aspects of living which produce total well-being.

dimensions of physical fitness: components of life-style which determine the overall fitness of an individual.

dislocation: a complete disjoining of two bones at a joint site.

E

eating disorders: problems associated with abnormal food intake and large changes in body weight.

eccentric contraction: dynamic movement in which muscular tension is less than external resistance and the muscle lengthens.

elastic: the property of a muscle which allows it to return to its original shape after it has been subjected to a stretch.

elevated post-exercise oxygen consumption (EPOC): the increased oxygen consumption above the resting level following an activity.

enabling: skills and resources which help a person move toward a healthy life-style.

endorphin: a hormone secreted by the brain associated with euphoria and pain reduction.

environmental barriers: external or environmental impediments to exercise. Examples include: conveniences of exercise facility, time to exercise, and family interruptions.

epinephrine: a hormone produced by the adrenal gland (medulla) associated with acute cardiovascular and metabolic stress reactions.

esophagus: the tubular structure located immediately behind the windpipe (trachea) that connects the mouth and the stomach.

essential fat: fat that is required for normal body functions.

estrogen: a female sex steroid which is involved in menstrual cycle regulation and in the female secondary sec characteristics.

exercise addiction: compulsion to exercise. May result from realistic or unrealistic factors.

exercise motivation: motivational factors specific to exercise. The desire/need to, importance of, and factors which influence exercising.

exercise training: repeating exercise bouts over several months or years.

exhaustion phase: the final stage of the General Adaptation Syndrome which is characterized by fatigue and disability or death.

expectancies: results which are expected. May be realistic or unrealistic. Expectancies may drive behavior.

F

fast-twitch fibers: muscle fibers which are high in anaerobic capacity, fast contracting, and quick to fatigue.

fat mass (FM): the non-active, storage tissue of the body.

fat-free mass (FFM): the functional, active tissues of the body, including skeletal muscle, bones, organs, and glands.

fat-soluble vitamins: vitamins that dissolve in the fats of the body.

fatigue fracture: also known as a stress fracture.

ferritin: the storage form of iron. Ferritin levels in the blood provide a good indication of iron stored in bone marrow.

fight or flight: a term coined by Dr. Walter Cannon to describe the bodily changes associated with an acute stress reaction.

flexibility: the range of motion about a joint.

follicular phase: stage of the reproductive cycle which follows menstruation.

fracture: a break or breaks in a bone.

free fatty acids (FFA): components of triglycerides which are used as an energy source during prolonged exercise.

frictional bursitis: an inflammation of the bursa sac due to repeated movements over the sac.

frostbite: a chilled condition of the body when fluids around the skin turn to ice crystals.

G

General Adaptation Syndrome (GAS): a term coined by Dr. Hans Selye to describe the changes in body function and structure associated with chronic stress.

genital irritation: friction producing irritation around the genital area.

gingivitis: an inflammation of the gums especially around the margins of the teeth.

glycogen: The stored form of carbohydrate found in muscle and liver and a primary source of energy during exercise.

H

hardiness: a term coined by Dr. Suzanne Kobasa to describe the social and personality characteristics of persons who remain healthy despite experiencing high levels of stressful life events.

HDL cholesterol: a lipid compound containing cholesterol removed from the arteries; also termed the "good" form of cholesterol because high levels are desirable and reduce the risk of heart disease.

health behavior: actions, habits, and components of life-style which affect health, either positively or negatively.

health behavior change: alterations in behavior to produce better health.

health status: general overall well-being, including physical and mental health.

healthful living: performing life-style behavior which contribute to total well-being.

heart attack: the sudden death of part of the heart muscle. Also known as myocardial infarction.

heart rate reserve (HRR): The difference between maximal heart rate minus resting heart rate.

heat exhaustion: a condition caused by dehydration and a drop of blood volume.

heat stroke: a potentially life-threatening condition caused by extremely high body temperatures.

high impact: weight bearing exercises in which the center of gravity is raised and lowered significantly.

hostility: ill feelings toward people.

human wholeness: achieving one's individual potential.

hydrostatic weighing: also known as densitometry, this is the method of determining body fat content by the volume of water displaced during submersion.

hypertension: a chronic condition of high blood pressure, leading to increased risk for cardiovascular disease, stroke, and kidney disease.

hyperventilation: increased rate and depth of breathing in which excess carbon dioxide is exhaled.

hypoglycemia: low blood sugar.

hypothermia: a dramatic lowering of body temperature due to cold air, cold wind and wet conditions.

hypoxia: reduced oxygen in a tissue.

I

iliotibial band friction syndrome: friction between the iliotibial band and the knee causing irritation.

incomplete proteins: proteins method of measuring body composition using the speed with which infrared waves pass through body tissues of different densities.

infrared reactance: body composition techniques which relies on differences in absorption of infared rays by fat and lean tissue.

iron deficiency anemia: severe loss of iron characterized by depletion of iron reserves and hemoglobin levels below 11g/dl.

iron depletion: loss of iron from iron stores characterized by decreased serum ferritin levels.

insulin: a hormone that assists in transporting sugar across the cell membranes in the body.

insulin overshoot: excess insulin production caused by high intake of simple sugars.

isokinetic contraction: a dynamic movement in which the speed of muscle shortening is maintained constant by the machine resistance mechanism.

J

journaling: a relaxation technique in which daily activities and feelings are recorded.

L

lactate threshold: the workload at which significant amounts of lactic acid accumulate in blood.

LDL cholesterol: A form of cholesterol that is deposited in the walls of arteries, contributing to the process of atherosclerosis. It is increased by overconsumption of saturated fat and cholesterol and contributes to the risk of heart disease.

lean body mass (LBM): weight of the body excluding body fat.

life-style diseases: illnesses which are a result of improper life-style behavior, rather than of genetic or organic causes.

lipids: fats; substances characterized by insolubility in blood.

load-deformation curve: a graphic display of the strength of a material based on how much "give" that material can withstand before failure as a load is placed upon it.

locus of control: feelings of being in charge and control versus others being in control, or versus feelings of not being able to affect/influence and outcome.

long-haul concept: a method of weight loss or weight control which is base on small reductions of daily caloric intake or brief exercise bouts over a prolonged period.

low back pain: pain usually occurring in the lumbar region of the back, most often a muscle strain.

low impact: weight bearing exercise characterized by lower knee action and reduced center of gravity movement.

luteal phase: the female reproductive cycle from ovulation (release of egg from ovary) to the onset of the next menses.

M

maintenance training: a reduced, temporary training program used to prevent detraining.

major minerals: minerals such as calcium, phosphorous, sodium, potassium, and magnesium which are required in larger amounts for normal bodily function.

malnourished: when an individual's diet is lacking in the essential elements to maintain a normal, healthy existence.

maximal oxygen uptake or consumption (VO_2 max): The greatest amount of oxygen taken up and utilized by the body during heavy exercise ($L \bullet min^{-1}$ or $ml \bullet kg^{-1} \bullet min^{-1}$).

melanoma: a skin cancer originating in the pigment-secreting cells of the skin that is highly malignant and may cause death.

menopause: the cessation of menstruation in the female, typically between the ages of 45 and 50.

menstrual cycle: reproductive cycle with phases of follicular, ovulation, luteal and menstration.

metabolic equivalent (MET): metabolic equivalent; unit of exercise intensity in which 1 MET is equal to resting metabolism.

minerals: inorganic substances which serve a wide variety of uses in the body.
motivation: anything that moves a person to action. Why people behave as they do.
muscular balance: appropriate strength relationship between opposing muscles or the same muscle on both sides of the body.
muscle cramp: painful involuntary contractions of a muscle.
muscle hypertrophy: An increase in muscle girth in response to weight training resulting from an increase in muscle fiber size, an increase in connective tissue, and an increase in blood supply to the muscle.
muscle soreness: painful condition usually brought on by eccentric muscle contractions or negative work.
myocardial oxygen consumption: amount of oxygen (energy) used by the heart.

N

neural adaptations: Improvements in neuromuscular function, i.e., motor unit recruitment, which can contribute to strength gains during a resistance training program.
nicotine: a poisonous alkaloid that is the chief psychoactive ingredient of tobacco.
norepinephrine: a hormone produced by the adrenal gland (medulla) associated with acute stress reactions; chemically related to epinephrine.

O

obese: the excess storage of body fat.
obesity: the excessive accumulation of fat in the body to a level that, depending on the age, frame size, and height of the affected person, is considered undesirable.
oligomenorrhea: irregular menstrual cycle; infrequent cycle.
oral contraceptives (OC): synthetic estrogen and/or progestine used to prevent ovulation.
osteoarthritis: a degenerative wearing away of the cartilage between bones.
osteoporosis: increased porosity of the bones, leading to weakness and a greater likelihood of fractures.
overload: exposing a system, such as skeletal muscle, to a greater workload than it is accustomed.
overuse injury: a repetitive event injury, one which takes a long time to develop, see chronic injury.
oxygen consumption or uptake (VO_2): the amount of oxygen used to produce energy during rest, exercise, or recovery.

P

pancreas: a long, tapered irregularly shaped gland behind the stomach that secretes a variety of digestive enzymes and hormones including insulin, which regulates the level of glucose (sugar) in the blood.
passive stretching: a stretching technique where one person actively moves another person's limbs through a range of motion.
patellar tendinitis: an inflammation of the patellar tendon.
patellofemoral pain: also known as runner's knee.
pathologist: a person who studies disease, particularly its causes, processes, and effects on the body.
perceived need: why people believe they must exercise. Knowledge or belief that exercise is necessary for certain reasons, e.g., lose weight, live longer, have more energy.
perceptual barriers: internal impediments to exercise based upon interpretations and perceptions of a situation.
periodization: phases of a long-term resistance training program ranging from rest to peak effort.
periostitis: an inflammation of the bone covering.
personal health responsibility (PHR): being accountable for one's own health status.
personal wellness assessment: self evaluation of life-style behavior.
plantar fasciitis: an inflammation of the plantar fascia in the foot.
pleasure principle: motivation due to enjoyment. The more enjoyable an activity/behavior the more likely participation in the activity.
podiatrist: a medical professional who specializes in treating disorders of the feet.

power training: conditioning for power (strength x speed) usually with high speed movements.

predisposing: values and attitudes which help one move toward a healthier life-style.

pregnancy: carrying the fetus by a female for approximately nine months.

progesterone: a female sex steroid produced by the ovaries after ovulation (luteal phase) which is important for preparing the uterine lining for the implantation of a fertilized ovum.

progressive relaxation: a technique used to relieve stress in which muscle

s are voluntarily tensed and relaxed to gain the sensation of muscular signals.

proprioceptive neuromuscular facilitation (PNF): a stretching technique characterized by a stretch, isometric contraction of the muscle being stretched, and then further stretch of the same muscle.

R

rating of perceived exertion (RPE): the personal evaluation of the difficulty of an exercise.

Raynaud's Syndrome: a condition characterized by constriction or spasm of blood vessels in the hands and feet resulting in coldness of tissue, pain, and in severe cases loss of tissue.

recovery energy: also known as EPOC; calories burned after an exercise bout.

reinforcing: social norms which help one move toward a healthier life-style.

relative outcome: perceived value of exercise results when weighed against other alternatives which vie for exercise time/effort.

relaxation: a reduction in tension in a muscle group to very low levels.

resolution: a return to the normal unstimulated state.

resistance phase: the second stage of the General Adaptation Syndrome in which the body attempts to resist or adopt to the stressor.

resistance training: exercise in which the muscles are overloaded with the use of weights, bands, hydraulics, etc.

resting heart rate: the heart rate (beats per minute) while an individual is completely at rest, most accurately determined while still lying down following a night's sleep.

resolution: a return to the normal unstimulated state.

R.I.C.E.: an injury treatment composed of rest, ice, compression, and elevation.

runner's knee.: soreness and discomfort around the kneecap and the retinaculum.

S

saturated fat: organic acids containing carbon, oxygen, and the maximum quantity of hydrogen possible, combined with an oily alcohol called glycerol. Palm oil, coconut oil, and most animal fats are highly saturated.

sciatica: a compression of the sciatic nerve causing pain in the

lower back and leg.

self-efficacy: how each person regards him/herself ability to perform or accomplish a task. Closely related to self-esteem, but can be situation specific.

sel-image: the concept that a person has toward oneself and one's perception of how others view him/her.

self-esteem: how each person regards him/herself. One's own internal value assessment.

set-point: the hypothesized regulatory mechanism located in the brain that controls body weight.

shin splints: unspecific pain along the tibia.

simple sugars: smallest molecules of carbohydrates.

significant emotional event (SEE): a happening which carries a powerful impact on an individual.

skinfold: the layer of skin and fat covering the surface of the body.

skinfold caliper: an instrument to measure the thickness of a double fold of fat and skin on the surface of the body.

slow-twitch fibers: muscle fibers which are high in aerobic capacity, slow contracting, and fatigue resistant.

social facilitation: the effect of the presence of others upon behavior. Usually viewed as improvements in performance due to the presence of others. However, decrements may also result.

social readjustment rating scale (SRRS): a point system used to quantify the stress caused by recent life events.

social support: the support provided by family, friends, co-workers, neighbors, and organizations.

sodium: a mineral that helps regulates the body's water balance, maintain normal heart rhythm, and is vital to the transmission of impulses by the nervous system; the best known source of dietary sodium is sodium chloride (NaCl), table salt.

spot reduction: the process of decreasing the amount of fat in a specific area such as the waist.

sprain: a stretch or tear of the ligamentous fibers that connect bones to bones.

static resistance: immovable resistance.

static stretching: a stretching technique characterized by a long, slow stretch through a range of motion with a hold at the end of the stretch.

stitch-in-the-side: undefined pain under the ribs, usually occurs near the diaphragm and is caused by deficient muscle blood flow.

storage fat: the fat that is placed in reserve to serve as an energy source, a cushion, and insulation.

strain: a stretch or tear of a muscle or its tendon attachment.

strength training: exercising the muscle with resistance to improve the ability to move a load.

stress: any external stimulus, whether physical or psychological, that necessitates resistance, change, or adaptation by the individual.

stress fracture: a slight crack or microfracture in the bone caused by repeated stresses, also called fatigue fracture.

stress relaxation: a reduced tension in the tendon or muscle allowing for a longer stretch.

stretch reflex: an involuntary muscular resonse stimulated by rapid elongation of the muscle.

stretching: motion which extends the connective tissue in and around the muscle.

stroke volume: the amount of blood pressure by the heart with each beat.

subluxation: a partial separation of two bones at a joint.

supercompensation: the cellular rebuilding process which occurs after the muscle has been exercised.

sympathetic nervous system (SNS): a branch of the autonomic nervous system whose activity prepares the body for activity.

T

T-cells: specialized lymphocytes which perform numerous immune functions including the destruction of pathogenic microbes.

talk test: the ability to carry on a conversation during an exercise bout.

target heart rate (THR): estimated exercise heart rate to achieve cardiovascular fitness gains.

tendinitis: an inflammation of the tendon or tendon sheath.

tension: the electrical activity in a muscle group.

tension signal: the sensations or feelings associated with a muscle group that is tensed or braced.

testosterone: A male sex hormone (androgen) responsible for muscle enlargement, reproductive function, and male secondary sex characteristics.

thrombosis: coagulation of the blood into a clot that impedes circulation.

tibial stress fracture: another name for shin splints, see also stress fracture.

tibial stress syndrome: another name for shin splints, see also stress fracture.

tone: leanness and muscle firmness usually in a specific body area.

trabecular bone: ends the bone which is thinner and contains bone marrow.

trace minerals: minerals such as iron, zinc, copper, iodine, and chromium which are required in small amounts to maintain normal body function.

triglycerides (TG): storage form of fat found in adipose tissue and muscle.

Type-A behavior pattern: a behavior pattern characterized by polyphasic behavior, hurry sickness, inability to relax, hypercompetitive nature, hard driving behavior, and free floating hostility; associated with higher rates of coronary artery disease and sudden death.

Type I fibers: slow-twitch muscle fibers.

Type I stress: acute stress which requires an immediate response to a threat.

Type II stress: chronic stress characterized by a long term response because an immediate resolution is not possible.

Type IIa fibers: fast-twitch muscle fibers which have intermediate anaerobic and aerobic capacities.

Type IIb fibers: fast-twitch muscle fibers which are highest in anaerobic capacity.

U

ulnar neuropathy: an irritation of the ulnar nerve causing numbnes on the outside of the arm and hand.

undermuscled: when an individual has less muscle mass than considered adequate for normal daily function.

undernourished: when an individual's diet contains less than the required number of calories for a normal healthy existence.

underweight: when an individual is more than 20% below the recommended weight for a given height.

unsaturated fats: fats that do not have all their carbon bonds occupied.

V

variable resistance: load which is altered throughout the range of motion; linear (one direction) and compound (multidirection).

viscoelastic: containing both vicous and elastic properties.

viscous: the property of a muscle which allows a permanent deformation once a stretch has been applied.

visualization: a relaxation technique in which one thinks back and relives a pleasant experience or scene.

W

warming-up: the elevation of muscle temperature to allow for a greater range of motion or muscle extensibility.

water-soluble vitamins: vitamins that dissolve in the water of the body.

weight-bearing: exercise in which the legs support the body weight; walking is a weight-bearing activity but cycling is not.

wellness: quality of life involving the interaction of the physical, intellectual, emotional, social, spiritual, and vocational dimensions of the person.

wellness life-style behaviors: aspects of life-style which promote wellness or health.

Y

yo-yo diet: a pattern of losing weight and regaining it over relatively short periods of time.

INDEX

A

Achilles tendinitis, 204
acute injury, 197
acute stress, 161
addiction (exercise), 191
adenosine triphosphate (ATP), 47
adherence, 67
adrenal glands, 23
aerobic exercise, 20, 49
aerobic training, 53
alarm phase, 163
aldosterone, 165
amenorrhea, 149
amino acids, 134
anaerobics, 47
angina pectoris, 70
anorexia nervosa, 157
anterior knee pain, 204
anxiety, 26
atherosclerosis, 19
atherosclerotic plaque, 19
athletic amenorrhea, 147
autogenic training, 175
autonomic nervous system, 164

B

ballistic stretching, 91
barriers, 188
B-Calls, 164
belief systems,
bioelectric impedance, 127
biofeedback training, 176
blister, 207
blood glucose, 47
body composition, 125
breathholding, 63
bulimia, 157
bursitis, 200

C

caffeine, 173
calcific bursitis, 201
calcium, 23
calcium carbonate, 156
caloric expenditure, 43
calorie balance inventory, 261
carbohydrates (CHO), 47, 131
carbon monoxide (CO), 18
cardiac output, 52-54
cardiovascular disease, 17
cardiovascular fitness, 73
catecholamines, 62
cerebrovascular disease, 22
cholesterol, 18
chondromalacia patella, 204, 205
chronic injury, 199-201
chronic stress, 167
circuit resistance training (CRT), 84, 121
cirrhosis (of the liver), 17
climacteric, 153
cognitive dissonance, 188
commitment, 170
compartment syndrome, 206
complete proteins, 135
complex carbohydrates, 132
concentric contraction, 105
constant resistance, 108
contractility, 53
contraction, 105
cool-down, 62
coronary artery disease, 17
cortical bone, 153
cortisol, 163
creatine phosphate (CP), 47
creeping obesity, 126
cues, 42

D

decibels, 172
dehydration, 68
density, 127
determinents of health, 5
detraining, 57
diet, 130
dimensions of health, 4
dimensions of physical fitness, 3
dislocation, 197-198

E

eating disorders, 147
eccentric contraction, 105
elastic, 91
elevated post-exercise oxygen consumption (EPOC), 141
enabling, 34
endorphin, 164
environmental barriers, 188
epinephrine, 162
esophagus, 22
essential fat, 125
estrogen, 147
exercise addiction, 191-194
exercise motivation, 185-186
exercise training, 53
exhaustion phase, 163
expectancy, 187

F

fast-twitch fibers, 48
fat mass (FM), 125
fat-free mass (FFM), 125
fat-soluble vitamins, 137
fatigue fracture, 201
ferritin, 155
fight or flight 161,
fitness tests, 269, 273
flexibility, 89
flexibility tests, 215-229
follicular phase, 148
fracture, 197
free fatty acids (FFA), 49
frictional bursitis, 200
frostbite, 211

G

General Adaptation Syndrome (GAS), 162
gingivitis, 166
glycogen, 49

H

hardiness, 170
HDL cholesterol, 19
health behavior, 31
health behavior change, 31, 37
health status, 73
healthful living, 4-7
heart attack, 17
heart rate reserve (HRR), 63
heat exhaustion, 210
heat stroke, 210
high impact, 76
hostility, 168, 251
human wholeness, 7
hydrostatic weighing, 127
hypertension, 23, 165
hypertrophy (muscle),
hyperventilation, 66
hypoglycemia, 143
hypothermia, 211
hypoxia, 151

I

iliotibial band friction syndrome, 205
incomplete proteins, 135
infrared reactance, 128
injury, 197-208
insulin, 131
insulin overshoot, 131
iron deficiency anemia, 155
iron depletion, 155
isokinetic contraction, 105

J

journaling, 179

L

lactate threshold, 55
LDL cholesterol, 19
lean body mass (LBM), 125
life-style diseases, 12
lipids, 57
load-deformation curve, 202
locus of control, 186
long-haul concept, 139
low back pain, 205, 206
low impact, 76
luteal phase, 148

M

maintenance, 42
maintenance training, 57, 113
major minerals, 137
malnourished, 130
maximal oxygen consumption (VO_2 max), 50, 148
melanoma, 22
menopause, 17, 153
menstrual cycle, 149
metabolic equivalent (MET), 64
minerals, 137
motivation, 185
muscle cramp, 207
muscle hypertrophy, 147
muscle soreness, 207, 208
muscular balance, 117
myocardial oxygen consumption, 69

N

neural adaptations, 147
nicotine, 22
norepinephrine, 162

O

obese, 127
obesity, 26
oligomenorrhea, 149
oral contraceptives, 150
osteoarthritis, 201
osteoporosis, 24, 147
overload, 113
overuse injury, 199-201
oxygen consumption (VO_2), 52
oxygen uptake, 52

P

pancreas, 27
passive stretching, 93
patellar tendinitis, 204, 205
patellofemoral pain, 205
pathologist, 19
perceived need, 186

perceptual barriers, 188-189
periodization, 115
periostitis, 206
personal health responsibility (PHR), 6
personal wellness assessment, 41
plantar fasciitis, 206
pleasure principle, 192
podiatrist, 77
posture tests, 231
power training, 116
predisposing, 34
pregnancy, 150
progesterone, 148
progressive relaxation, 174
proprioceptive neuromuscular facilitation (PNF), 93

R

rating of perceived exertion (RPE), 65
Raynaud's Syndrome, 165
recovery energy, 51
reinforcing, 34
relative outcome, 188, 189
relaxation, 165
resistance phase, 163
resistance training, 112
resolution, 162
resting heart rate, 20
R.I.C.E., 198
runner's knee, 205

S

saturated fats, 19, 132
self efficacy, 186, 189
self image, 186, 189
self-esteem, 189
set-point, 139
shin splints, 131
simple sugars, 131
significant emotional event (SEE), 29
skinfold, 128
skinfold caliper, 128
slow-twitch fibers, 48
social facilitation, 190
social readjustment rating scale (SRRS), 171
social support, 171
sodium, 23
spot reduction, 118
sprain, 194
static resistance, 107
static stretching, 72
stitch-in-the-side, 28
storage fat, 125
strain, 199
strength testing, 273
strength training, 113
stress, 26
stress evaluation, 237, 245, 247
stress fracture, 149, 201
stress reflex, 91
stress relaxation, 92
stretching, 89
stroke volume, 52-54, 148
subluxation, 197
supercompensation, 113
sympathetic nervous system (SNS), 161

T

T-cells, 164
talk test, 66
target heart rate (THR), 63
tendinitis, 200
tension, 167
tension signal, 175
testosterone, 147
thrombosis, 27
tibial stress syndrome, 206
tibial stress fracture, 206
tone, 118
trabecular bone, 153
trace minerals, 137
triglycerides (TG), 49
Type-A behavior pattern, 168
Type I fibers, 48
Type I stress, 161
Type II stress, 162
Type IIa fibers, 48
Type IIb fibers, 48

U

ulnar neuropathy, 208
undermuscled, 141
undernourished, 130
underweight, 141
unsaturated fats, 132

V

variable resistance, 109
viscoelastic, 91
viscous, 91
visualization, 177

W

waist/hip ratio (WHR), 257
warming-up, 87
water-soluble vitamins, 135
weight-bearing, 73
wellness life-style behaviors, 8, 29
wellness, 3, 29
workout records, 279

Y

yo-yo diet, 138